Color Atlas of Endo-Otoscopy

Examination–Diagnosis–Treatment

Mario Sanna, MD
Professor of Otolaryngology
Department of Head and Neck Surgery
University of Chieti
Chieti, Italy
Director
Gruppo Otologico
Piacenza and Rome, Italy

Alessandra Russo, MD
Otologist and Skull Base Surgeon
Gruppo Otologico
Piacenza and Rome, Italy

Antonio Caruso, MD
Otologist and Skull Base Surgeon
Gruppo Otologico
Piacenza and Rome, Italy

Abdelkader Taibah, MD
Neurosurgeon, Otologist, and Skull Base Surgeon
Gruppo Otologico
Piacenza and Rome, Italy

Gianluca Piras, MD
Otologist and Skull Base Surgeon
Gruppo Otologico
Piacenza and Rome, Italy

With the collaboration of
Fernando Mancini, Hiroshi Sunose, Enrico Piccirillo, Lorenzo Lauda, Annalisa Giannuzzi, Sampath Chandra Prasad Rao

1007 illustrations

Thieme
Stuttgart • New York • Delhi • Rio de Janeiro

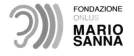

Library of Congress Cataloging-in-Publication Data is available from the publisher.

© 2017 by Georg Thieme Verlag KG

Thieme Publishers Stuttgart
Rüdigerstrasse 14, 70469 Stuttgart, Germany
+49 [0]711 8931 421, customerservice@thieme.de

Thieme Publishers New York
333 Seventh Avenue, New York, NY 10001 USA
+1 800 782 3488, customerservice@thieme.com

Thieme Publishers Delhi
A-12, Second Floor, Sector-2, Noida-201301
Uttar Pradesh, India
+91 120 45 566 00, customerservice@thieme.in

Thieme Publishers Rio de Janeiro, Thieme Publicações Ltda.
Edifício Rodolpho de Paoli, 25º andar
Av. Nilo Peçanha, 50 – Sala 2508
Rio de Janeiro 20020-906 Brasil
Tel: +55 21 3172-2297 / +55 21 3172-1896

Cover design: Thieme Publishing Group
Typesetting by DiTech Process Solutions, India

Printed in India by Replika Press Pvt. Ltd.   5 4 3 2 1

ISBN 978-3-13-241523-2

Also available as an e-book:
eISBN 978-3-13-241524-9

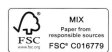

Contents

Preface

Despite advances in diagnostic techniques and imaging modalities, otoscopy remains the cornerstone in the diagnosis of otologic diseases. Every otolaryngologist, pediatrician, or even general practitioner dealing with ear diseases should have a good knowledge of otoscopy. This atlas is based on 30 years of experience in Gruppo Otologico in the treatment of otologic and neurotologic disorders, with more than 32,000 surgical operations and 300,000 consultations. It presents a vast collection of otoscopic views of a variety of lesions that can affect the ear and temporal bone. Many examples are given for each disease so that the reader becomes acquainted with the variable presentations each pathology can have.

While otoscopy alone can establish the diagnosis in some cases, parameters such as history or audiological and neuroradiological evaluation are required in others. An important aspect of this atlas is that it juxtaposes, when appropriate, the clinical picture, radiological diagnosis, and intraoperative findings with the otoscopic findings of the patient. Needless to say, every patient should be considered as a whole, and in some particular cases, the otoscopic findings might only be the "tip of the iceberg." Otalgia, otorrhea, and granulations in the external auditory canal are manifestations of otitis externa, but when they persist, particularly in the elderly, they should arouse suspicion of malignancy. Otitis media with effusion can be a simple disease when seen in children, whereas unilateral persistent otitis media with effusion in an adult may be the only sign of a nasopharyngeal carcinoma. A small attic perforation in the presence of facial nerve paralysis and sensorineural hearing loss may be all that is seen in a giant petrous bone cholesteatoma. The manifestation of an aural polyp can vary from a mucosal polyp associated with chronic suppurative otitis media to the much less common but more dangerous temporal bone paraganglioma. A small retrotympanic mass may represent an anomalous anatomy such as a high jugular bulb or an aberrant carotid artery. It may also represent frank pathology such as facial nerve neuroma, congenital cholesteatoma, or even en-plaque meningioma.

In each chapter, a surgical summary that lists the different approaches for the management of the pathology dealt with is provided. Throughout the book, emphasis is on how the otoscopic view and the clinical picture may affect the choice of treatment and the surgical technique.

At the end of this atlas, a chapter on postsurgical conditions is presented. The presence of previous surgery poses special difficulties because of the distorted anatomy. Moreover, the otologist should be able to distinguish between what is considered to be normal postsurgical healing and complications that need further intervention.

Our goal is to offer an easy-to-consult book for residents, specialists, and general practitioners. So, this first-step approach to patients with otologic diseases can open a wider view on complete knowledge of otology, neurotology, skull base pathology and surgery, and neuroradiology.

Drs. Russo, Taibah, Caruso, and Gianluca Piras, a new young colleague who has been working with us for the past year, helped to accomplish this work with their active and enthusiastic participation. A special thank goes to the other members of Gruppo Otologico, for their contribution in the realization of this book: Drs. Piccirillo, Lauda, Giannuzzi, and Prasad.

The authors would like to thank Mr. Stephan Konnry at Thieme Publishers for his excellent cooperation and help. Thanks also go to Paolo Piazza, neuroradiologist, for his continuous cooperation and to Fernando Mancini for the illustrations included in the book.

Mario Sanna, MD

Contributors

Antonio Caruso, MD
Otologist and Skull Base Surgeon
Gruppo Otologico
Piacenza and Rome, Italy

Annalisa Giannuzzi, MD, PhD
Otologist and Skull Base Surgeon
Gruppo Otologico
Piacenza and Rome, Italy

Lorenzo Lauda, MD
ENT and Skull Base Surgeon
Gruppo Otologico
Piacenza and Rome, Italy

Fernando Mancini, MD
ENT and Skull Base Surgeon
Gruppo Otologico
Piacenza and Rome, Italy

Enrico Piccirillo, MD
ENT and Skull Base Surgeon
Gruppo Otologico
Piacenza and Rome, Italy

Gianluca Piras, MD
Otologist and Skull Base Surgeon
Gruppo Otologico
Piacenza and Rome, Italy

Sampath Chandra Prasad Rao, MS, DNB, FEB-ORLHNS
ENT and Skull Base Surgeon
Gruppo Otologico
Piacenza and Rome, Italy

Alessandra Russo, MD
Otologist and Skull Base Surgeon
Gruppo Otologico
Piacenza and Rome, Italy

Mario Sanna, MD
Professor of Otolaryngology
Department of Head and Neck Surgery
University of Chieti
Chieti, Italy
Director
Gruppo Otologico
Piacenza and Rome, Italy

Hiroshi Sunose
Department of Otolaryngology
Medical Center East
Tokyo Women's Medical University
Tokyo, Japan

Abdelkader Taibah, MD
Neurosurgeon, Otologist, and Skull Base Surgeon
Gruppo Otologico
Piacenza and Rome, Italy

Chapter 1

Methods of Otoscopy

1 Methods of Otoscopy

Abstract
This chapter explains how we routinely perform otoscopy. With the help of a microscope and endoscope, each clinical condition can be easily studied, recorded, and printed for a deeper analysis. Performing a proper otoscopy is the first step for the correct management of the whole pathology of the temporal bone and skull base.

Keywords: otoscopy, microscope, endoscope, instant photography

A preliminary examination is performed using a head mirror or an otoscope.

For proper otoscopy, the external auditory canal should be cleaned. Few instruments are used for this step, namely, aural speculi of different sizes, a Billeau ear loop, Hartman auricular forceps, and suction tips (▶ Fig. 1.1). In cases with a history of recurrent otitis, we prefer to clean the ear with the aid of a microscope (▶ Fig. 1.2).

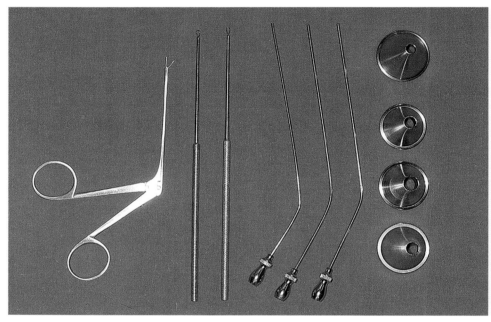

Fig. 1.1 Instruments used for cleaning the external auditory canal.

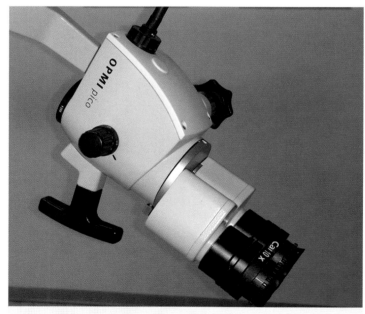

Fig. 1.2 Microscope used as an aid in cleaning the ear.

The use of a rigid 0-degree 6-cm endoscope (▶ Fig. 1.3) connected to a video system enables the patient to see the pthology involving his/her ear (▶ Fig. 1.4). The rigid 30-degree endoscope allows evaluation of attic retraction pockets, the extent of which cannot always be determined using the microscope or the 0-degree endoscope (▶ Fig. 1.5).

Instant photography has also been used in the operating room. A copy of the important steps of the operation is given to the patient while another copy is kept in the patient's chart. The patient is also photographed during the follow-up visit. Thus, for each patient pre-, intra-, and postoperative photographic documentation is obtained.

During the past years, a camera mounted to the endoscope was used for obtaining photos (▶ Fig. 1.6); nowadays a digital customized system is used for collecting pictures on a laptop storage, with the possibility of collect otoscopic images on a patient's chart. So, the advent of computerized systems (▶ Fig. 1.7) allows virtual storaging of all the photos or videos, with the advantage of reducing times of acquisition, modification, and deletion. Furthermore, a deeper clinical analysis could be assessed.

In all the cases, the examiner sits to the side of the patient whose head is slightly tilted toward the contralateral side. The examiner holds the camera attached to the endoscope with his right hand. With the ring and middle finger of the left hand, the

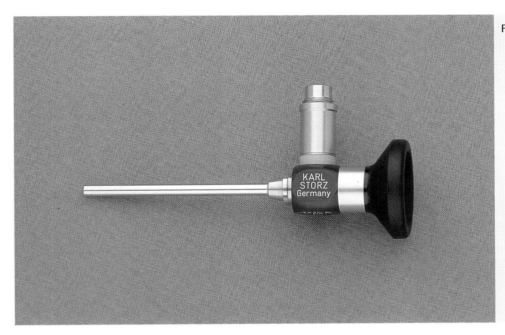

Fig. 1.3 A rigid 0-degree 6-cm endoscope.

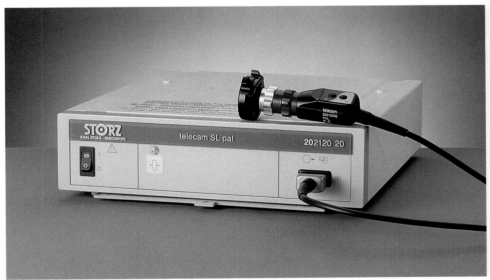

Fig. 1.4 The endoscope can be connected to a video system such as this.

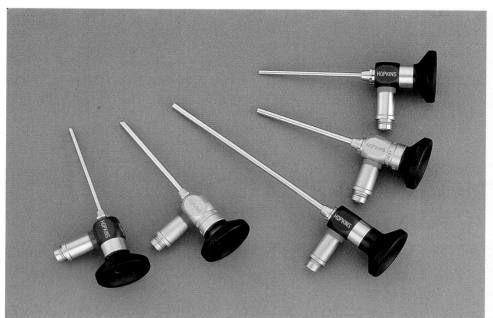

Fig. 1.5 A series of rigid endoscopes.

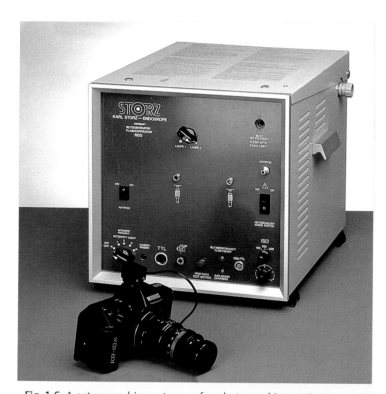

Fig. 1.6 A setup used in past years for photographing patients.

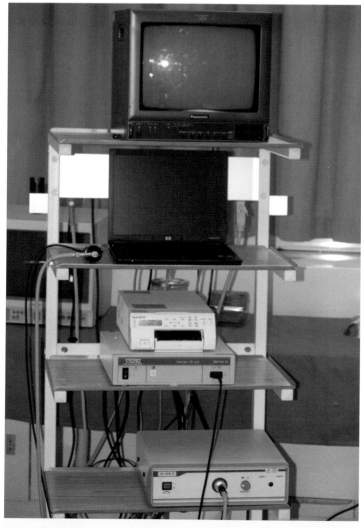

Fig. 1.7 A modern setup of computerized systems for digital collection of patients' photos.

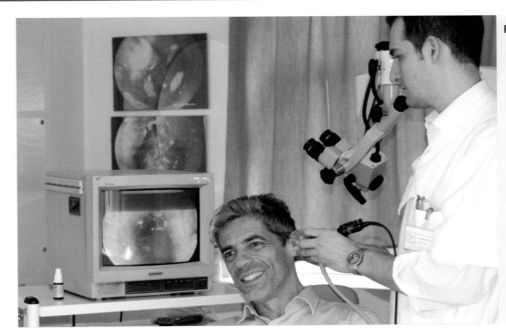

Fig. 1.8 Examination of a patient in progress.

examiner pulls the patient's auricle backward and outwards to straighten the external auditory canal. The endoscope is advanced over the index finger of the examiner's left hand into the patient's external auditory canal. In this manner, any undue injury to the external auditory canal is prevented (▶ Fig. 1.8).

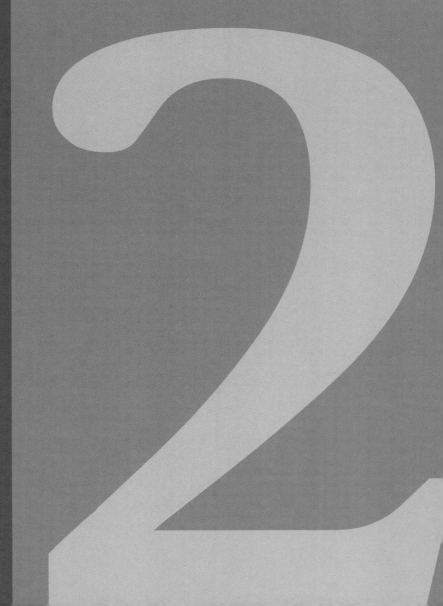

Chapter 2

The Normal Tympanic Membrane

2 The Normal Tympanic Membrane

Abstract

The normal tympanic membrane is thin, semi-transparent, pearly gray colored, and consists of three layers from the outside to the inside (epithelial, fibrous, and mucosal). The tympanic membrane not only acts as a sound wave transducer to the ossicular chain, but also has a protective function to the middle ear and serves as a sound amplifier. It is conventionally divided into four quadrants from two perpendicular lines passing through the umbo (anterosuperior, anteroinferior, posterosuperior, posteroinferior).

Keywords: tympanic membrane, tympanic layers, ossicular chain, tympanic quadrants

2.1 Anatomy

The tympanic membrane forms the major part of the lateral wall of the middle ear (see ▶ Fig. 2.1, ▶ Fig. 2.2, ▶ Fig. 2.3). It is thin, resistant, semi-transparent, has a pearly gray color, and is cone-like. The apex of the membrane lies at the umbo, which corresponds to the lowest part of the handle of the malleus. Most of the membrane circumference is thickened to form a fibrocartilaginous ring, the tympanic annulus, which sits in a groove in the tympanic bone called the tympanic sulcus. The fibrocartilaginous ring is deficient superiorly. This deficiency is known as the notch of Rivinus. The anterior and posterior malleolar folds extend from the short process of the malleus to the tympanic sulcus, thus forming the inferior limit of the pars flaccida of Shrapnell's membrane.

The membrane forms an obtuse angle with the posterior wall of the external auditory canal. It also forms an acute angle with the anterior wall of the canal. It is important to respect this acute angulation in the myringoplasty operation to maintain as much as possible the vibratory mechanism of the tympanic membrane and hence ensure maximum hearing improvement (see ▶ Fig. 2.4, ▶ Fig. 2.5, ▶ Fig. 2.6, ▶ Fig. 2.7, ▶ Fig. 2.8).

The external surface of the tympanic membrane is innervated by the auriculotemporal nerve and the auricular branch of the vagus nerve, whereas the inner surface is supplied by Jacobson's nerve, a branch of the glossopharyngeal nerve.

The blood supply is derived from the deep auricular and anterior tympanic arteries. Both are branches of the maxillary artery.

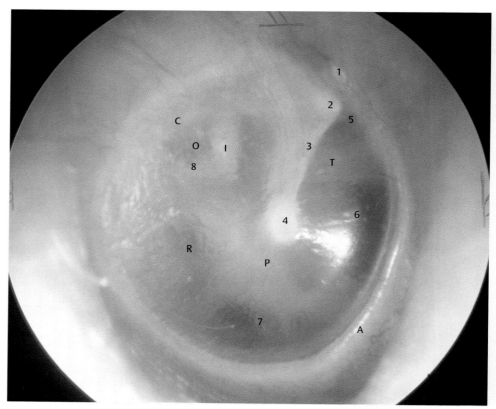

Fig. 2.1 Right ear. Normal tympanic membrane. 1, pars flaccida; 2, short process of the malleus; 3, handle of the malleus; 4, umbo; 5, supratubal recess; 6, tubal orifice; 7, hypotympanic air cells; 8, stapedius tendon; c, chorda tympani; I, incus; P, promontory; o, oval window; R, round window; T, tensor tympani; A, annulus.

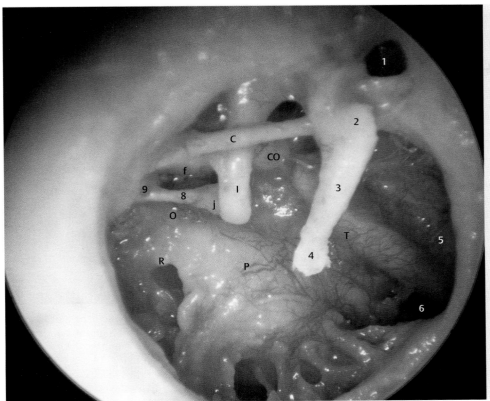

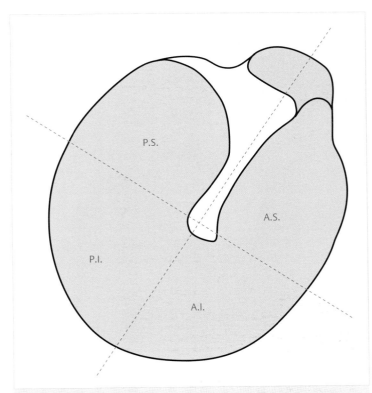

Fig. 2.3 Right ear. Division of the tympanic membrane into four quadrants: AS, anterosuperior; AI, anteroinferior; PS, posterosuperior; PI, posteroinferior. This division facilitates the description of different pathologic affections of the tympanic membrane.

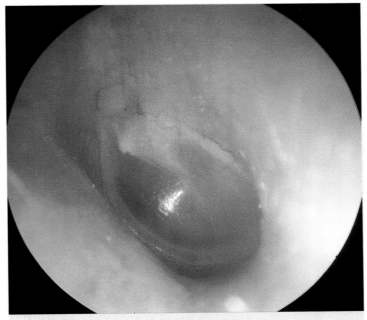

Fig. 2.4 Left ear. Normal tympanic membrane. Note the acute angle formed between the tympanic membrane and the anterior wall of the external auditory canal. The pars tensa with the short process of the handle of the malleus, the umbo, the cone of light, the annulus, and the pars flaccida are seen. Note also the presence of early exostosis in the superior wall of the external auditory canal.

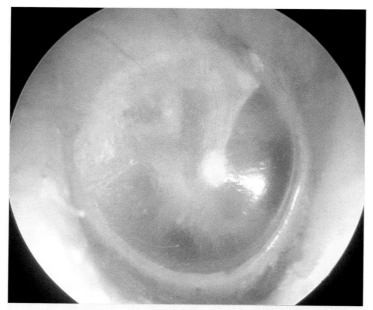

Fig. 2.5 Right ear. Normal tympanic membrane. In this case, the drum is very thin and transparent. The handle and short process of the malleus as well as the umbo and cone of light are well visualized. Through the transparent tympanic membrane, the region of the oval window, the long process of the incus, the posterior arc of the stapes, the incudostapedial joint, the round window, and the promontory can be distinguished. Anteriorly, at the region of the Eustachian tube, the tensor tympani canal and the supratubaric recess can be observed.

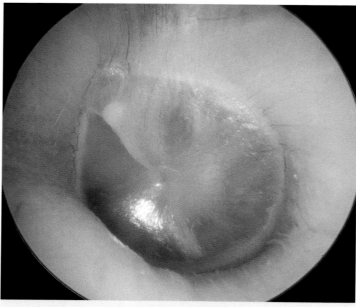

Fig. 2.6 Left ear. Normal tympanic membrane. The handle of the malleus and cone of light are well visualized through the tympanic membrane; the promontory, the area of the round window, and the air cells in the hypotympanum can be appreciated. The pars flaccida is visualized superior to the short process of the malleus.

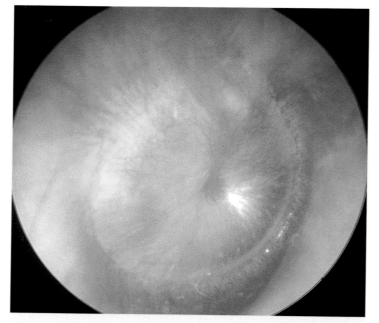

Fig. 2.7 Right ear. Normal tympanic membrane. The drum, however, is slightly thickened with an accentuated capillary network along the handle of the malleus. The increased thickness of the tympanic membrane obscures all the structures in the middle ear.

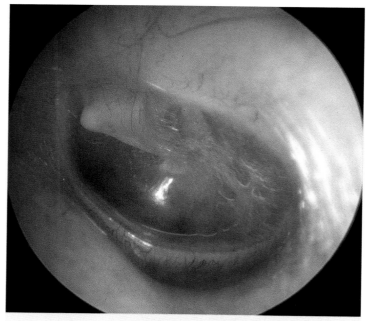

Fig. 2.8 Left ear. A normal tympanic membrane that is slightly thinned in the anterior quadrant and moderately thickened posteriorly.

2.2 Histology

The tympanic membrane consists of three layers: an outer epithelial layer continuous with the skin of the external auditory canal, a middle fibrous layer or lamina propria, and an inner mucosal layer continuous with the lining of the tympanic cavity.

The epidermis or outer layer is divided into the stratum corneum, the stratum granulosum, the stratum spinosum, and the stratum basale, which is the deepest layer that rests on the basement membrane.

The lamina propria is characterized by the presence of collagen fibers. In the pars tensa, these fibers are arranged in two basic layers: an outer radial layer that originates from the inferior part of the handle of the malleus and inserts in the annulus, and an inner circular layer that originates primarily from the short process of the malleus. Such a distinct arrangement, however, is absent in the pars flaccida.

The mucosal layer is formed mainly of a simple cuboidal or columnar epithelium. The free surface of the cells possesses numerous microvilli.

2.3 Physiology

The external ear has a protective function against the middle ear and serves as a sound amplifier. The external ear not only changes the perception of sound amplifying some frequencies, but also increases the directionality, due to the diffraction of the sound waves on the entire head and external ear, in particular the ear pavilion. The maximum amplification is ~20 dB for frequencies between 2 and 3 kHz. The tympanic membrane acts as a sound wave transducer to the ossicular chain.

Chapter 3

Diseases Affecting the External Auditory Canal

3

3 Diseases Affecting the External Auditory Canal

Abstract

Pathologies affecting the external auditory canal (EAC) are a wide spectrum of diseases that include: bony neoformations of the EAC (exostosis and osteomas), inflammatory diseases (external otitis, otomycosis, and inflammatory stenosis of the EAC), cholesteatoma of the EAC, benign tumors of the ear and skull base extending to the EAC (carcinoid tumor, meningiomas, facial nerve tumors, etc.), temporal bone fractures, and carcinoma of the EAC. Otoscopy is fundamental for the recognition of each clinical condition. Analysis of patient clinical history and symptoms are also of utmost importance to decide the proper therapeutic management, which is different depending on the pathology. For example, in case of exostosis and osteomas occluding the EAC a canalplasty is indicated, as well as a surgical treatment is the mainstay for most of the benign and malign tumors involving the EAC. Further radiological examinations (CT and MRI scans) are indicated in the suspect of a tumor.

Keywords: external auditory canal, exostosis, osteomas, otitis externa, otomycosis, cholesteatoma, meningioma, facial nerve tumor, temporal bone fractures, squamous cell carcinoma

3.1 Exostosis and Osteomas

Exostosis are defined as new bony growths in the osseous portion of the external auditory canal (EAC). They are usually multiple, bilateral, and are commonly sessile. They vary in shape, being either round, ovoid, or oblong. The condition is caused by periostitis secondary to exposure to cold water. This explains the high incidence of exostoses among divers and cold-water bathers. Histologically, they are formed from parallel layers of newly formed bone. It is postulated that the periosteum stimulates an osteogenic reaction with each exposure to cold water, causing this stratification. When exostoses are small, they are asymptomatic. Large lesions, however, can occlude the EAC and lead to conductive hearing loss or retention of wax and debris with subsequent otitis externa. In such cases, and in cases in which a hearing aid is to be fitted, surgical removal of exostoses is indicated. In some cases, surgery is technically difficult and special care is taken to preserve the skin of the EAC. Other structures at risk are the tympanic membrane and ossicular chain medially, the temporomandibular joint anteriorly, and the third segment of the facial nerve posteroinferiorly.

Osteoma is a true benign neoplasm of the bone of the EAC, usually unilateral and pedunculated. Histologically, it can be differentiated from exostosis by the absence of the laminated growth pattern.

According to the extent of both diseases, we developed a classification for EAC stenosis, which is based mainly on the amount of tympanic membrane otoscopically visible (▶ Table 3.1; ▶ Fig. 3.1, ▶ Fig. 3.2, ▶ Fig. 3.3, ▶ Fig. 3.4, ▶ Fig. 3.5, ▶ Fig. 3.6, ▶ Fig. 3.7, ▶ Fig. 3.8, ▶ Fig. 3.9, ▶ Fig. 3.10, ▶ Fig. 3.11, ▶ Fig. 3.12, ▶ Fig. 3.13, ▶ Fig. 3.14, ▶ Fig. 3.15, ▶ Fig. 3.16, ▶ Fig. 3.17, ▶ Fig. 3.18, ▶ Fig. 3.19, ▶ Fig. 3.20).

Table 3.1 Grading of external auditory canal stenosis

Grade	Severity	Otoendoscopic finding	Radiological finding*	Descriptive figures
0	No stenosis	All four quadrants of the pars tensa are perfectly visible. 100% of the pars tensa area is visible.	No narrowing of EAC	
I	Mild stenosis	One or more quadrants is/are partially visible. ≥75% of the pars tensa area is visible.	10–25% narrowing of EAC	

Table 3.1 Grading of external auditory canal stenosis (*continued*)

Grade	Severity	Otoendoscopic finding	Radiological finding*	Descriptive figures
II	Moderate stenosis	One of the quadrants is completely obscured. **50–75%** of the pars tensa area is visible.	25–50% narrowing of EAC	
III	Severe stenosis	Two of the quadrants are completely obscured. **25–50%** of the pars tensa area is visible.	50–75% narrowing of EAC	
IV	Near total stenosis	Three of the quadrants are completely obscured. **10–25%** of the pars tensa area is visible.	75–90% narrowing of EAC	
V	Total stenosis	None of the quadrants are visible. **0%** of the pars tensa area is visible.	90–100% narrowing of EAC	

*The degree of stenosis is calculated as a percentage of the maximum measurement available of the lesion against the maximum diameter of the EAC in axial and coronal cuts.

Abbreviation: EAC, external auditory canal.

15

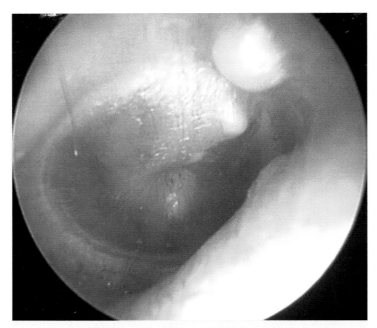

Fig. 3.1 Right ear. Small exostosis originating from the superior wall of the external auditory canal. A hump on the anterior wall precludes visualization of the anterior–inferior quadrant of the tympanic membrane.

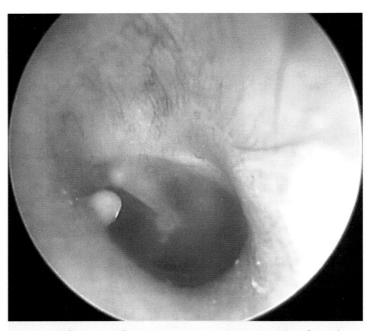

Fig. 3.2 Left ear. Small asymptomatic exostosis originating from the anterior wall of the external auditory canal.

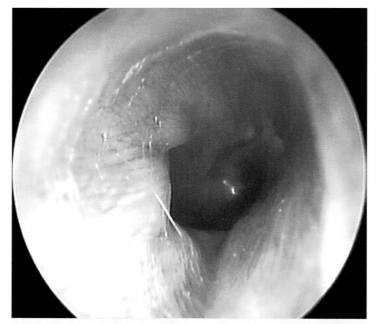

Fig. 3.3 Right ear. Exostosis originating from the inferior and posteriors wall of the external auditory canal. According to our classification, this is a Grade I stenosis. This case should be simply followed up.

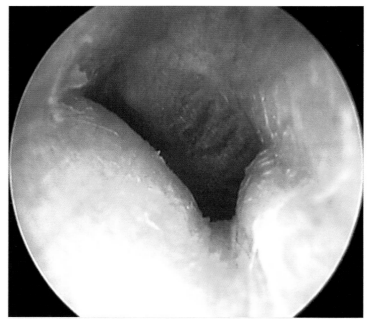

Fig. 3.4 Left ear. Bilateral Grade II stenosis of the external auditory canal for exostosis of the anterior wall. The tympanic membrane is viewable on its posterior quadrants. In this type of case, it is useful to photograph both ears for further follow-up within 1 to 2 years.

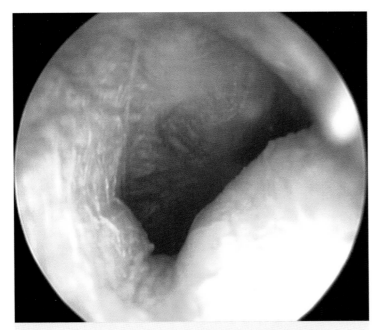

Fig. 3.5 Right ear. Same patient as in ▶ Fig. 3.4. Bilateral Grade II stenosis of the external auditory canal for exostosis of the anterior wall. The tympanic membrane is viewable on its posterior quadrants. In this type of case, it is useful to photograph both ears for further follow-up within 1 to 2 years.

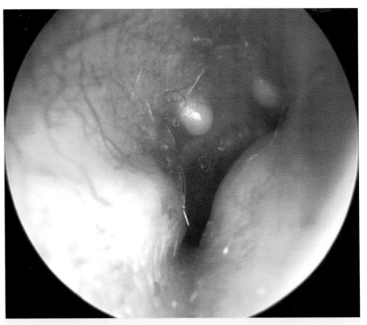

Fig. 3.6 Right ear. Grade III stenosis for exostosis originating from the anterior and posterior walls of the external auditory canal. Less than 50% of the tympanic membrane is viewable. The patient complains of hearing loss and frequent episodes of otitis externa secondary to retention of water and debris inside the canal. A canalplasty under local anesthesia is indicated to restore the size of the external auditory canal.

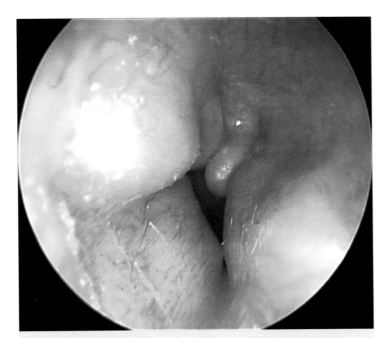

Fig. 3.7 Right ear. Grade IV stenosis. Less than 20% of the tympanic membrane is visible. The occurrence of conductive hearing loss is high in this type of stenosis, so surgery is recommended.

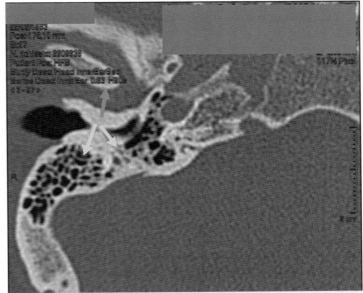

Fig. 3.8 This figure and ▶ Fig. 3.9 correspond to computed tomography (CT) scans (axial and coronal cuts), which show exostosis from each wall of the external auditory canal of the patient in ▶ Fig. 3.6 and ▶ Fig. 3.7. These bony lesions show radiopacity. A preoperative CT scan is not fundamental but could be useful to check the amount of bone removal anteriorly (avoiding the opening of the temporomandibular joint: *green arrow*), posteriorly (avoiding the opening of the mastoid air cells or an injury of the third portion of the facial nerve: *yellow arrows*), and medially (avoiding an injury of the tympanic membrane and of the ossicles).

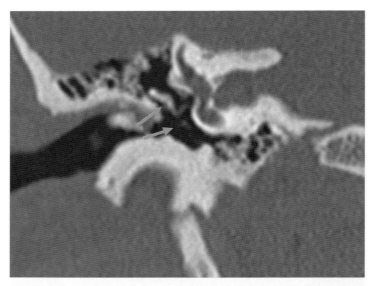

Fig. 3.9 Same patient as in ► Fig. 3.8. Computed tomography (CT) scans (axial and coronal cuts), which show exostosis from each wall of the external auditory canal. These bony lesions show radiopacity. A preoperative CT scan is not fundamental but could be useful to check the amount of bone removal anteriorly (avoiding the opening of the temporomandibular joint), posteriorly (avoiding the opening of the mastoid air cells or an injury of the third portion of the facial nerve), and medially (avoiding an injury of the tympanic membrane and of the ossicles: *blue arrows*).

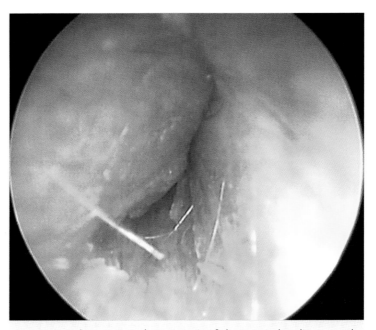

Fig. 3.10 Right ear. Complete stenosis of the external auditory canal. The tympanic membrane is not visible. As a first evaluation of complete stenosis is important to ensure the bony consistency of these lesions through a gentle pressure with a hook. The patient usually does not refer pain after the maneuver. A CT scan is indicated in this case to check the condition of the middle ear.

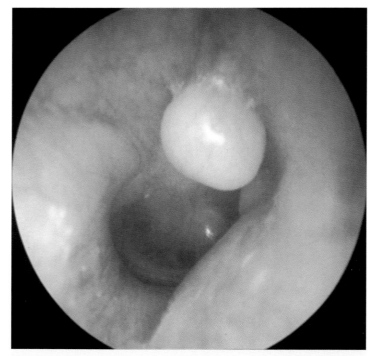

Fig. 3.11 Right ear. Osseous neoformation of the external auditory canal. In this case, given the pedunculated narrow base, an osteoma is a more probable diagnosis. This was confirmed by pathological examination of the removed specimen. Ample bone removal is performed in such cases to avoid recurrence.

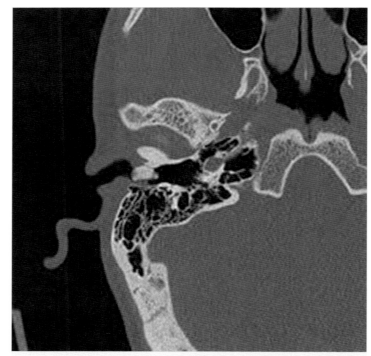

Fig. 3.12 Same patient. CT scan (axial cut) shows a pedunculated bony lesion of the anterosuperior wall of the external auditory canal.

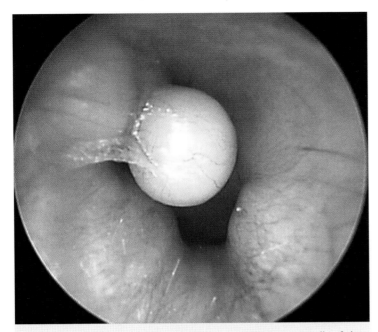

Fig. 3.13 Left ear. Exostoses of the posterior and anterior walls of the external auditory canal and osteoma of anterosuperior wall. The lesions allow only a limited view of the tympanic membrane (Grade III stenosis). In this case, regular follow-up is necessary because further growth of the lesions could lead to accumulation of debris and cerumen, necessitating surgical intervention.

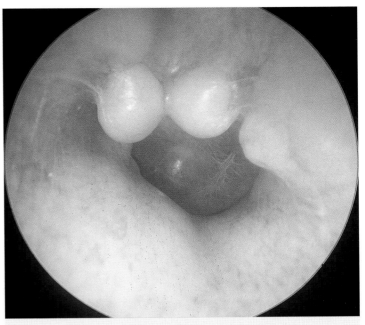

Fig. 3.14 Left ear. Osteomas of the superior wall of the external auditory canal. The pars flaccida of the tympanic membrane is not visible.

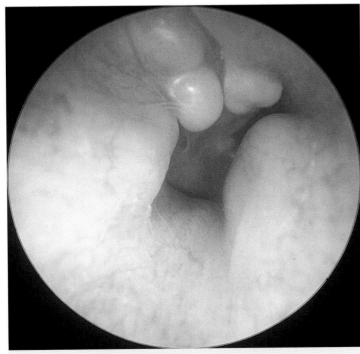

Fig. 3.15 Right ear. Same patient as in ▶ Fig. 3.14. Osteomas and exostoses allow visualization of the tympanic membrane only in the central part.

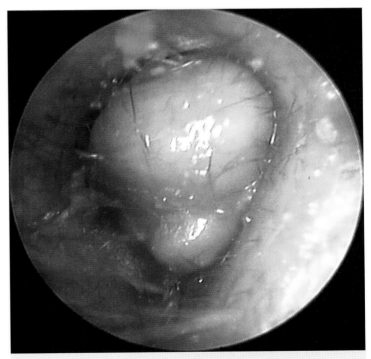

Fig. 3.16 Right ear. Osteoma occluding the external auditory canal with accumulation of wax and hearing loss. The pedicle of the lesion (anterior wall of the external auditory canal) is not well recognizable. Surgery is indicated in such case.

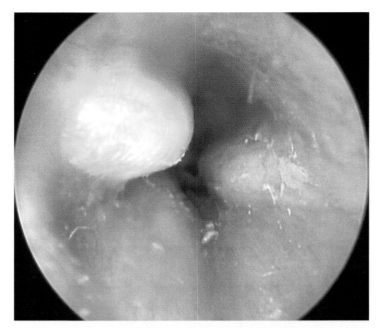

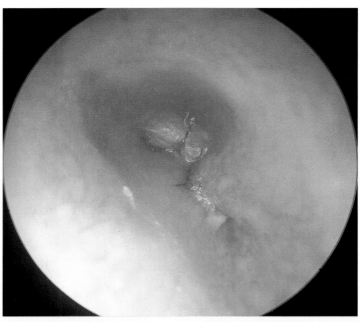

Fig. 3.17 Left ear. Exostoses with Grade III stenosis of the external auditory canal. A small perforation of the anteroinferior quadrant of the tympanic membrane is present. In this case, surgery includes a canalplasty combined with a myringoplasty.

Fig. 3.18 Left ear. Obstructing exostosis of the external auditory canal resulting in otitis externa due to accumulation of squamous debris inside the canal. Surgery is essential both to avoid the formation of cholesteatoma and to improve hearing.

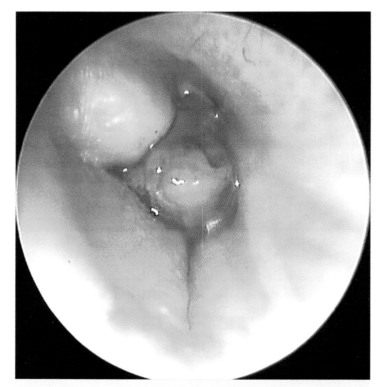

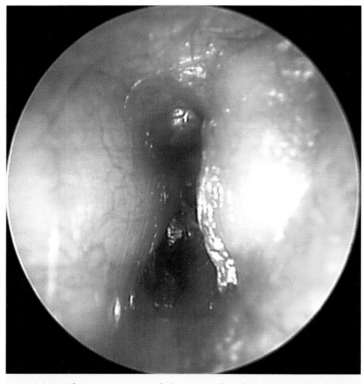

Fig. 3.19 Left ear. Exostosis of the external auditory canal with a polyp that occludes the meatus. Local therapy is indicated. In case of no response, a CT scan is mandatory to exclude pathology affecting the middle ear and/or the mastoid.

Fig. 3.20 Left ear. Exostoses of the external auditory canal with severe stenosis (Grade III). This condition facilitates retention of ear wax with the onset of conductive hearing loss.

3.1.1 Surgery for Exostosis and Osteoma: Canalplasty

Even if usually asymptomatic, exostosis and osteoma may grow occluding the EAC. Surgery is indicated in case of obstructing stenosis (with or without hearing loss), or in case of frequent otitis externa where it is necessary to fit a hearing aid. In cases where symptoms are minimal, it is useful to photograph the ear for further follow-up. In surgery, preservation and proper replacement of the meatal skin is important to prevent postoperative scarring and stenosis. Osteoma can be removed with a curette. However, if osteoma recurs, wide drilling of the bone around its base is indicated.

In limited cases in which wide exposure is not required (i.e., small osteoma), a transcanal approach could be used. The meatal skin is incised through an ear speculum and the skin over the osteoma is elevated. The osteoma is then removed with either a curette or a burr.

Surgical Steps

1. Retroauricular incision is used in most of the cases since this approach is wider and safer than the transcanal approach. The initial steps of surgery including skin incision, harvesting the temporalis fascia, and soft tissue incision.

2. In case of severe exostosis, there is no consistent landmark in the EAC since the tympanic membrane is obscured (▶ Fig. 3.21). If there is any space medially, the skin is detached from the bone and to push medially toward the tympanic membrane. The skin may be protected with an aluminum sheet with/without a small piece of cottonoid beneath the sheet.

3. If the space medial to bony protrusions is insufficient to contain the detached skin, the skin covering the bony overhang is detached and folded toward the contralateral wall. Protecting the skin with an aluminum sheet, a part of the protrusion is drilled medially (▶ Fig. 3.22).

4. The meatal skin covering another protrusion is detached, and the flap is then folded toward the space created by the drilling. The aluminum sheeting is repositioned between the bony wall and the meatal skin flap, and the bony protrusion is partially drilled medially.

5. After partly drilling the second bony protrusion, the meatal skin is repositioned, and the first protrusion is drilled further. In this way, the canal is gradually drilled from lateral to medial.

6. The mastoid segment of the facial nerve runs in the vicinity of the posterior meatal wall, 2 to 3 mm posterior to the annulus. The reported incidence of iatrogenic injury to the facial nerve during surgery for exostosis is very high. To avoid injury, it is important to restrict the area of drilling around the meatal

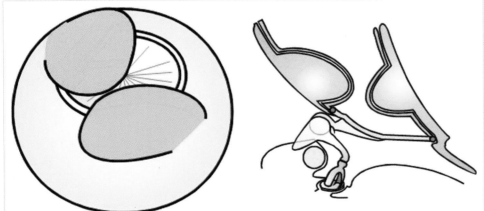

Fig. 3.21 The tympanic membrane is obscured in severe stenosis (no landmarks).

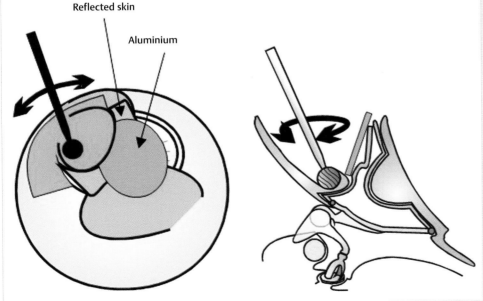

Reflected skin

Aluminium

Fig. 3.22 Skin flap folded on the opposite wall and protected with an aluminum sheet.

skin until the tympanic membrane is sufficiently visualized. Position of the tympanic membrane should be verified from time to time by replacing the meatal skin.

7. If protrusion still limits view of the tympanic membrane, the anterior canal wall may be drilled to help visualize the membrane, taking care not to damage the temporomandibular joint anteriorly (▶ Fig. 3.23). However, accidental exposure of the temporomandibular joint is better than damage of the facial nerve. Posterior canal should not be drilled too medially before verifying the area of drilling.

8. Using the meatal skin elevator (#2), quantity of bone to be drilled and distance from the annulus are estimated from time to time.

9. Removal of the final bony overhang may be conducted with a small curette (▶ Fig. 3.24). If the drill is used, care should be taken not to touch the short process of the malleus with a burr.

10. The exposed canal bone should be covered with the temporalis fascia. Longitudinal plastic cuts may be made in the meatal flap to assure intimate lining on the bone. Lateral meatal skin may also be cut longitudinally.

11. The external ear canal is packed with Gelfoam (see ▶ Fig. 3.25, ▶ Fig. 3.26, ▶ Fig. 3.27, ▶ Fig. 3.28, ▶ Fig. 3.29, ▶ Fig. 3.30).

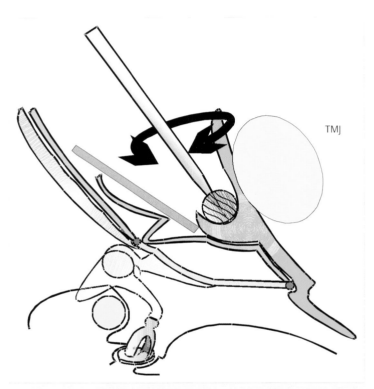

Fig. 3.23 Drilling of the anterior wall. TMJ, temporomandibular joint.

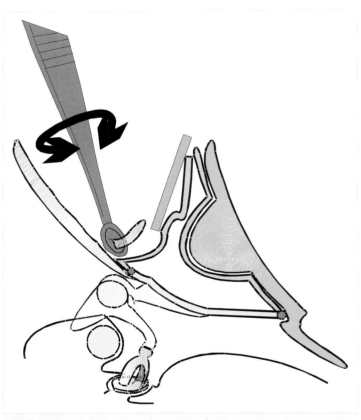

Fig. 3.24 Removal of the final bone overhang.

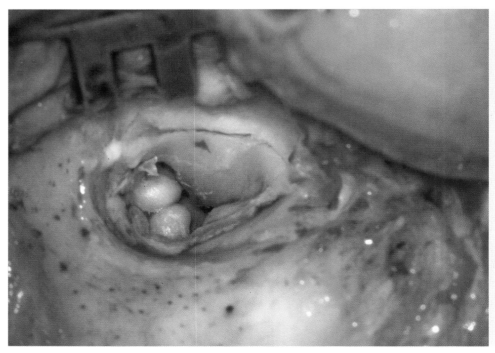

Fig. 3.25 Example of canalplasty. Right side. Exostoses of the anterior and posteroinferior walls of the external auditory canal and osteomas of the superior and posterior walls. A retroauricular approach has been performed and the meatal skin has been incised.

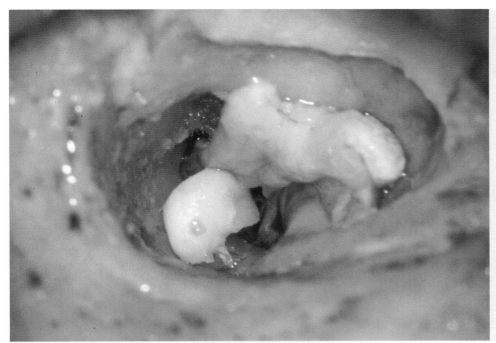

Fig. 3.26 The skin covering the exostoses has been detached and reflected anteriorly and medially. Osteomas are removed with a curette.

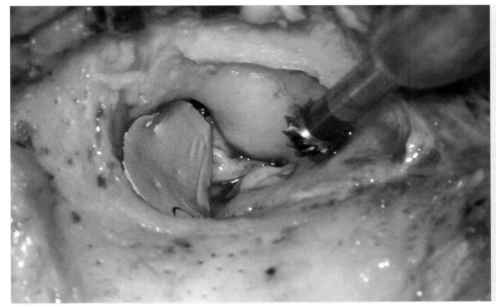

Fig. 3.27 The skin is pushed medially to the protrusions to make some room for drilling. To save time, most of the bone work is performed with cutting burrs.

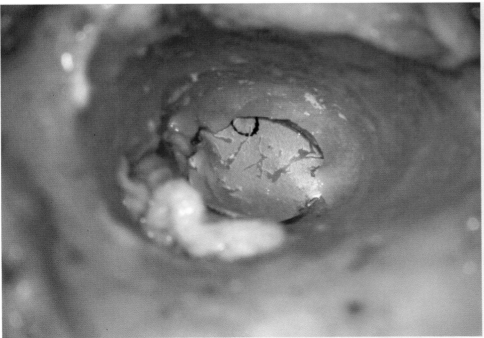

Fig. 3.28 The canalplasty has reached the area of the tympanic membrane. Some bone overhang remains near the tympanic membrane. The final bony overhang can be removed with a small diamond burr and a curette. Great care should be taken not to touch the lateral process of the malleus during drilling the anterosuperior wall.

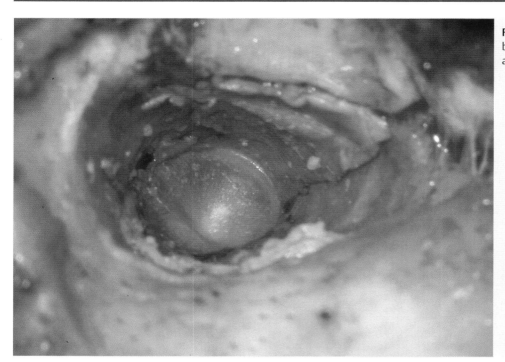

Fig. 3.29 The meatal skin is replaced over the bony wall. Note that the skin is well preserved, and the tympanic membrane remains intact.

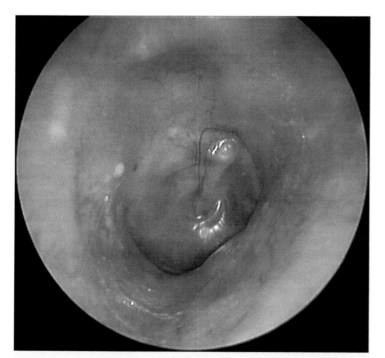

Fig. 3.30 Postoperative otoscopy (6 months). The external auditory canal has been perfectly calibrated. All the tympanic membrane is visible.

Summary

Surgery in cases of exostosis is indicated only in case with obstructing stenosis with or without hearing loss but with frequent otitis externa due to retention of debris. Surgery can be performed under local anesthesia, preferably using a postauricular incision. This approach allows excellent exposure of the whole meatus, thus minimizing the risk of injury to the tympanic membrane. In addition, it enables the surgeon to preserve the canal skin, thereby avoiding postoperative cicatricial stenosis. After dissecting the posterior limb, the flap is retained by the prongs of the self-retaining retractor. The skin of the anterior wall is incised medial to the tragus and is dissected in a lateral-to-medial direction. While drilling the exostosis, the skin of the canal is protected using an aluminum sheet (the cover of surgical sutures). Osteoma can be removed by using a curette. In case of recurrence, wide drilling of the bone around its base is also indicated.

3.2 External Auditory Canal Inflammatory Diseases

3.2.1 Eczema

Eczema is a dermo-epidermal process of reactive nature resulting from local or general factors. Local factors include allergy, topical medical preparations, or cosmetics, whereas general factors include hepatic or gastrointestinal dysfunction. It manifests by itching, a burning sensation, vesication, and sometimes serous otorrhea. Treatment consists of discontinuing the suspected causative irritant, correction of the systemic disturbances, as well as lavage with boric acid with alcohol and steroid lotion (see ▶ Fig. 3.31, ▶ Fig. 3.32).

3.2.2 Otitis Externa

Otitis externa is an inflammation of the skin of the EAC. The inflammation can be secondary to dermatitis (eczema) only, with no microbial infection, or it can be caused by active bacterial or fungal infection. In either case, but more often with infection, the ear canal skin swells and may become painful or tender to touch. Acute otitis externa is predominantly a microbial infection (i.e., *Pseudomonas aeruginosa*). Wax in the ear can combine with the swelling of the canal skin and any associated pus to block the canal and dampen hearing to varying degrees, creating a temporary conductive hearing loss. In more severe or untreated cases, the infection can spread to the soft tissues of the face that surround the adjacent parotid gland and the jaw joint, making chewing painful. The two factors that are required for external otitis to develop are: the presence of germs that can infect the skin and impairments in the integrity of the skin of the ear canal that allow infection to occur. However, if there are chronic skin conditions that affect the ear canal skin, such as atopic dermatitis, seborrheic dermatitis, psoriasis, or abnormalities of keratin production, or if there has been a break in the skin from trauma, even the normal bacteria found in the ear canal may cause infection and full-blown symptoms of external otitis. At the otoscopic examination, the canal appears red and swollen. Touching or moving the outer ear increases the pain, and this maneuver on physical exam is important in establishing the clinical diagnosis. Therapy consist of cleaning the ear with 2% alcohol boric, instillation of local antibiotic, oral antibiotic, and analgesic in advanced cases. *Necrotizing external otitis* (malignant otitis externa) is an uncommon form of external otitis that occurs mainly in elderly diabetics, being somewhat more likely and more severe when the diabetes is poorly controlled. Even less commonly, it can develop due to a severely compromised immune system. Beginning as infection of the external ear canal, there is extension of infection into the bony ear canal and the soft tissues deep to the bony canal with further extension to the skull base. Necrotizing external otitis requires oral or intravenous antibiotics for cure (fluoroquinolones plus cephalosporins), even for more than 2 weeks. Diabetes control is also an essential part of the treatment (see ▶ Fig. 3.33, ▶ Fig. 3.34, ▶ Fig. 3.35, ▶ Fig. 3.36, ▶ Fig. 3.37).

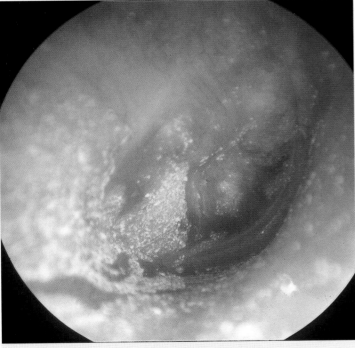

Fig. 3.31 Right ear. Chronic eczema of the external auditory canal. Squamous debris covering the skin of the external auditory canal can be observed. Successfully treated by the use of local steroid lotion.

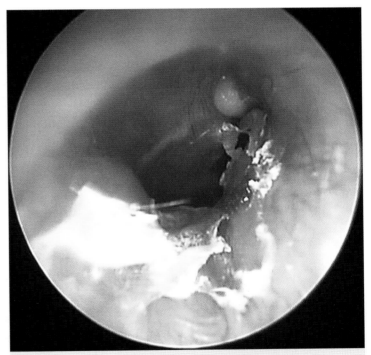

Fig. 3.32 Chronic eczema of the external auditory canal skin. Exostoses and osteoma are also evident. The accumulation of skin debris and wax could lead to external otitis.

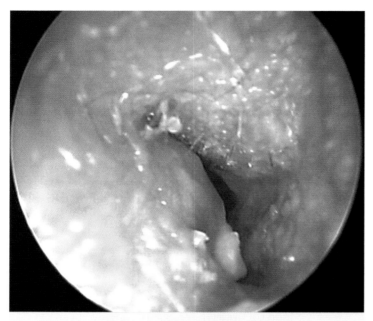

Fig. 3.33 Acute otitis externa. The external auditory canal appears swollen with skin debris and some otorrhea. The tympanic membrane is not visible. In case of no response after appropriate and prolonged therapy, it's important to exclude malignant disease that could get into differential diagnosis (i.e., carcinoma of the external auditory canal).

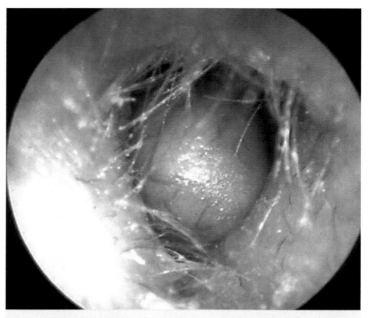

Fig. 3.34 A polyp-like mass is present in the external auditory canal. The patient, who had already undergone two tympanoplasties, complained of pain in the ear. He has suffered from diabetes for 15 years. A biopsy performed under local anesthesia excluded neoplastic disease. A scintigraphic examination confirmed the diagnosis of malignant external otitis. The patient was treated with a long course of antibiotic therapy, with final resolution of the pathology.

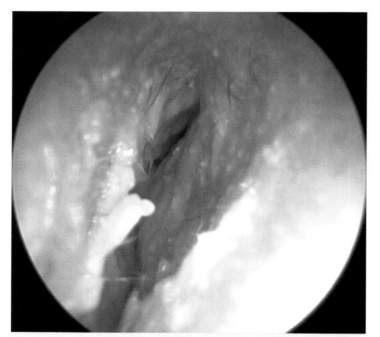

Fig. 3.35 Right ear. Malignant otitis externa in a 60-year-old patient affected by type I diabetes. The otoscopy is similar to that in ► Fig. 3.33. The patient had no remission with standard antibiotic therapies and developed skull base osteomyelitis (confirmed by CT scan, MRI, and scintigraphy). She further developed facial nerve and lower cranial nerves paralysis, which recovered after hospitalization and intravenous antibiotic therapy. The patient is still under antibiotic therapy (duration 4 months) with slight improvement of the clinical condition.

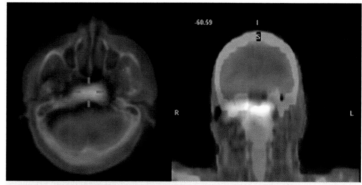

Fig. 3.36 Gallium[67] scintigraphy shows accumulation of the radio-nuclide at the level of the temporal bone, the temporomandibular joint, and the clivus. This technique is useful in diagnosis as well as for monitoring the response to treatment and detecting recurrence.

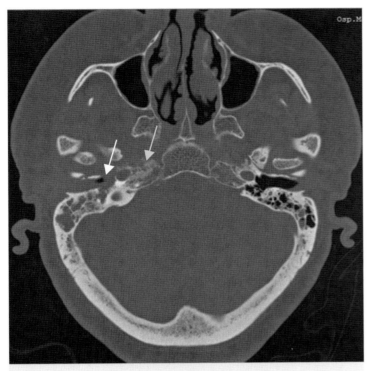

Fig. 3.37 CT scan. Axial view. Bone erosion is evident at the level of the anterior wall of the external auditory canal (*white arrow*) and the petrous apex (*yellow arrow*). The pathology completely involves the middle ear and the mastoid.

3.2.3 Foruncolosis

Foruncolosis is a pustular folliculitis by staphylococcal infection of a hair follicle. Infection occurs as a result of microabrasion or of decreased immunity, as in diabetics. It is characterized by severe pain. A tender swelling is seen in the cartilaginous part of the EAC, which may have a central necrotic part (see ▶ Fig. 3.38).

3.2.4 Otomycosis

Otomycosis is more common in tropical and subtropical countries. In the majority of cases, the isolated fungi are of the *Aspergillus* (*niger, fumigatus, flavescens, albus*) or the *Candida* species. Otomycosis is more common in immunocompromised patients and in diabetics. Local factors that favor fungal infections include chronic otorrhea and the presence of epithelial debris. Clinically, the patient complains of otorrhea, itching, and hearing loss. Therapy consists of cleaning the ear to remove all debris and the instillation of local antimycotic preparations as well as lavage with 2% alcohol boric acid drops (see ▶ Fig. 3.39, ▶ Fig. 3.40, ▶ Fig. 3.41, ▶ Fig. 3.42, ▶ Fig. 3.43).

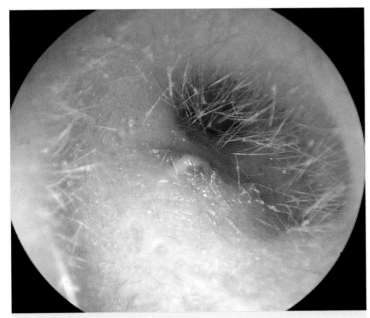

Fig. 3.38 A furuncle almost totally occluding the meatus. Pain is caused by distention of the richly innervated skin. A central necrotic part is seen.

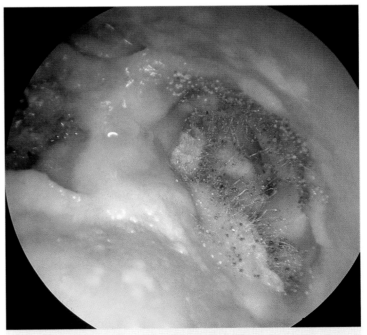

Fig. 3.39 Right ear. Radical mastoid cavity showing cholesteatoma with superimposed fungal infection.

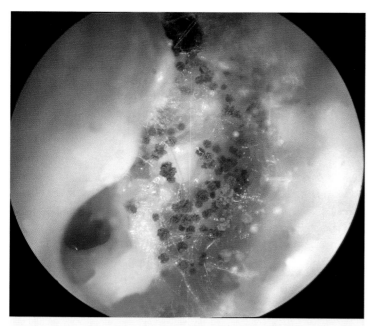

Fig. 3.40 An ear with chronic suppurative otitis media with choles- teatoma showing a superimposed fungal infection. The blackish fungal masses are early recognized. They should be removed before local antifungal solution is instilled.

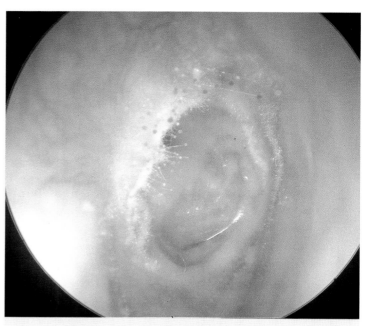

Fig. 3.41 Another example of otomycosis in a radical mastoid cavity.

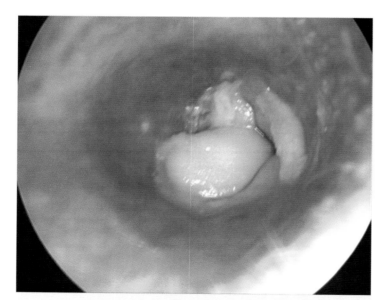

Fig. 3.42 Right ear. Otomycosis (*Candida* infection). The patient suffered from chronic otitis with occupational exposure to humid environments. The external auditory canal is filled with whitish lamellar material. Usually, it is not necessary to perform a culture of ear secretions and the diagnosis is clinical. The lack of response to a topical antibiotic therapy is a further confirmation of the fungal nature of the infection.

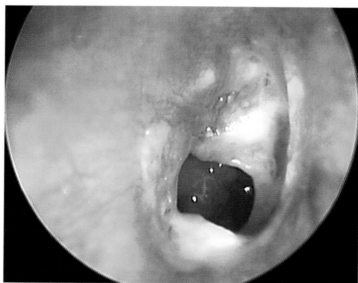

Fig. 3.43 Same ear after 10 days therapy with ear lavages and antimycotic drops. The external auditory canal is almost free from fungal secretions. A simple perforation of the inferior quadrants of the tympanic membrane is visible.

3.2.5 Myringitis and Meatal Stenosis

Myringitis is an inflammatory process that affects the tympanic membrane. Three forms are recognized: acute myringitis, bullous myringitis, and myringitis granulomatosa. Acute myringitis is usually seen in association with infection of the external ear (otitis externa) or middle ear (otitis media). It is characterized by hyperemia and the presence of purulent secretions. Therapy consist of administration of general and/or local antibiotics and local steroids. Bullous myringitis is commonly associated with viral upper respiratory tract infection. It is characterized by the presence of bullae filled with serosanguineous fluid. The bullae are located between the outer and the middle layers of the tympanic membrane. The patient complains of otalgia and hearing loss.

Therapy consist of antibiotics and steroids. In granulomatous myringitis, the outer epidermic layer of the tympanic membrane as well as the adjacent skin of the EAC are replaced by granulation tissue. It is generally seen in patients suffering from frequent episodes of otitis externa. In some cases, it may ultimately lead to stenosis of the most medial part of the EAC. It can usually be cured, however, by removing the granulation in the outpatient clinic using the microscope. This is followed by the administration of local steroid drops for nearly 1 month. In refractory cases, however, surgery in the form of canalplasty with free skin graft is necessary (see ▶ Fig. 3.44, ▶ Fig. 3.45, ▶ Fig. 3.46, ▶ Fig. 3.47, ▶ Fig. 3.48, ▶ Fig. 3.49, ▶ Fig. 3.50, ▶ Fig. 3.51, ▶ Fig. 3.52, ▶ Fig. 3.53, ▶ Fig. 3.54, ▶ Fig. 3.55, ▶ Fig. 3.56, ▶ Fig. 3.57, ▶ Fig. 3.58, ▶ Fig. 3.59).

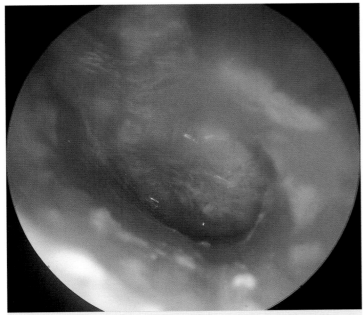

Fig. 3.44 Left ear. The tympanic membrane is characterized by thickening and hyperemia. In this case, the skin of the external auditory canal is also hyperemic. The tympanic membrane seems lateralized.

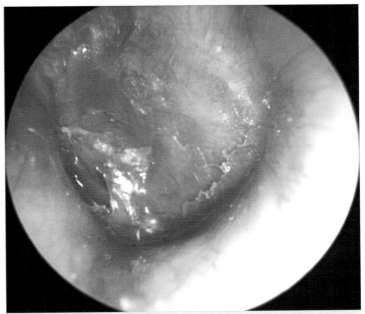

Fig. 3.45 Acute myringitis of a left tympanic membrane. The area of the malleus handle is hyperemic and the tympanic membrane seems lateralized. A small tympanic perforation is visible in the anterior–inferior quadrant.

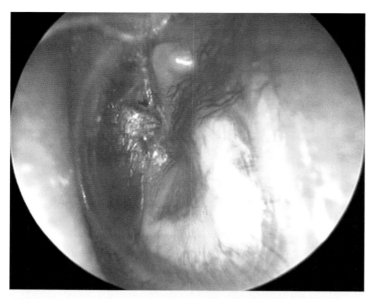

Fig. 3.46 Acute myringitis. The tympanic membrane over the malleus handle is hyperemic. A large tympanosclerosis plaque is visible on the posterior quadrants.

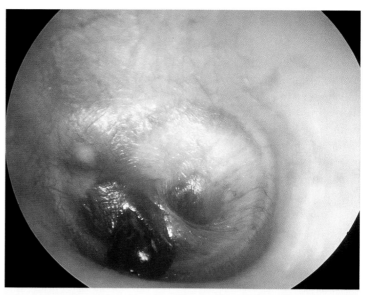

Fig. 3.47 Left tympanic membrane with a large bulla anterior to the malleus and a smaller one posterior to it.

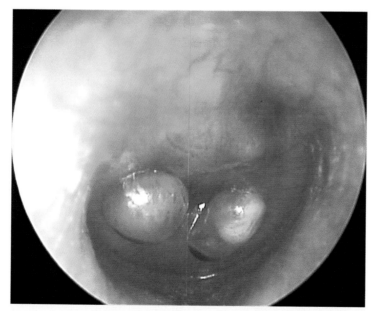

Fig. 3.48 Right bullous myringitis. The patient complained of a bad flu few days before the examination. Bleeding from the ear is quite common, due to the rupture of the bullae.

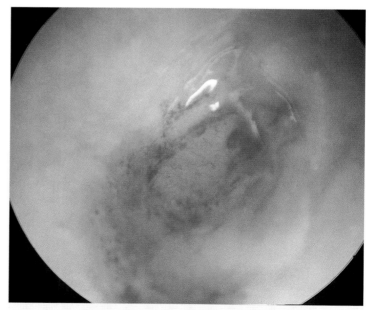

Fig. 3.49 Granulomatous myringitis. The granulomatous tissue has replaced the external skin layer of the tympanic membrane and part of the anterior wall of the external canal. This case was treated by removal of the granulation tissue under local anesthesia in the outpatient clinic. Local steroid drops were then administered for 1 month.

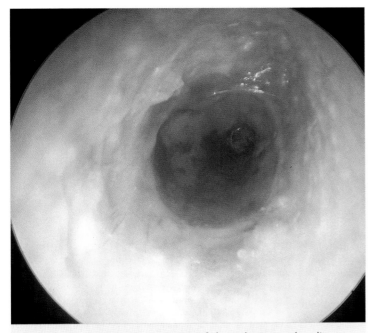

Fig. 3.50 Postinflammatory stenosis of the right external auditory canal of a 68-year-old woman. The patient complained of bilateral continuous otorrhea and hearing loss of 3 years' duration. The otorrhea in the left ear stopped 2 months before presentation. The granulations over the tympanic membrane were removed in the outpatient clinic. A cellophane sheet was inserted into the external auditory canal to avoid the reformation of stenosis. Local steroid drops were administered for 1 month. On follow-up, stenosis was already resolved and the granulation tissue in the external auditory canal was completely replaced by healthy skin.

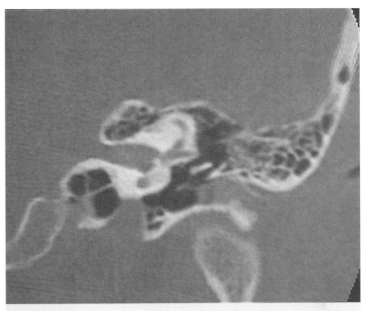

Fig. 3.51 CT of the same case. The bony walls of the external auditory canal are intact. The pathologic thick skin occupies the lumen of the external auditory canal.

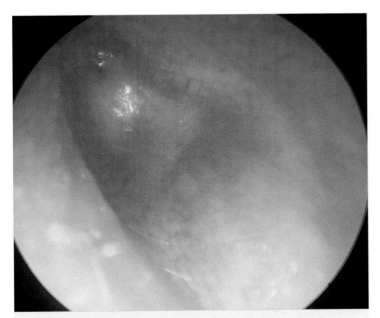

Fig. 3.52 Same patient, left ear (see also CT in ▶ Fig. 3.53). A canalplasty was performed on this side. After removal of the granulation tissue, myringoplasty and canalplasty were performed.

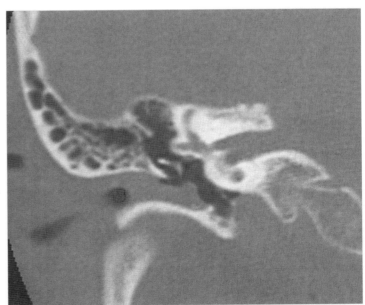

Fig. 3.53 The CT scan demonstrates a similar lesion on the contralateral side.

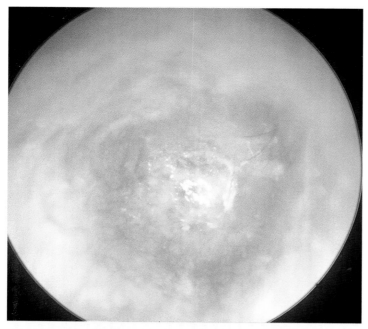

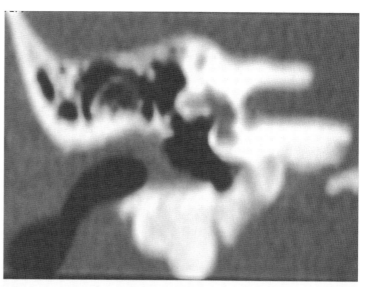

Fig. 3.55 The CT scan shows thickening of the tympanic membrane and normal bony canal.

Fig. 3.54 Right ear. Case similar to that seen in ▶ Fig. 3.44. The patient complained of intermittent otorrhea and hearing loss (see CT scan in ▶ Fig. 3.55).

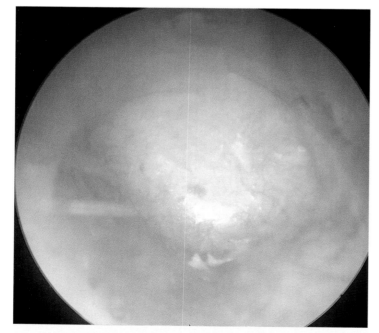

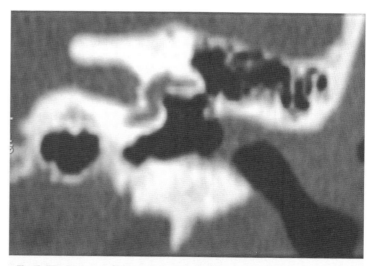

Fig. 3.57 CT scan of the previous case. The tympanic membrane is thickened and lateralized.

Fig. 3.56 Same patient, left ear. Two tympanoplasties were previously performed on this ear. Generally, revision surgery is better avoided in patients who have undergone multiple operations and present with canal stenosis associated with lateralization of the tympanic membrane (for postoperative stenosis of the external auditory canal, see Chapter 14).

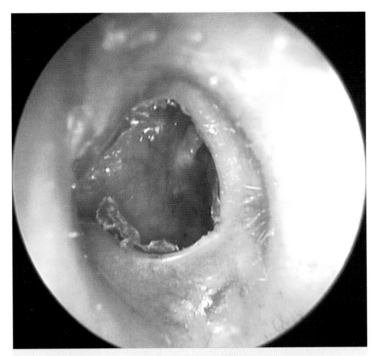

Fig. 3.58 Postinflammatory stenosis in a right canal wall down tympanoplasty. The patient complained of otorrhea and a recurrent cholesteatoma was found on the CT scan. A revision tympanoplasty was performed with removal of the external auditory canal scars. The risk of restenosis of the external auditory canal is very high in such cases.

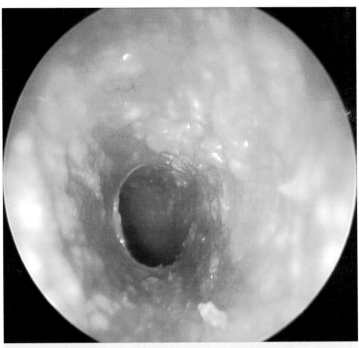

Fig. 3.59 Another case of postinflammatory stenosis on a left ear. The tympanic membrane is covered by scar tissue and only the anteroinferior quadrant is viewable.

3.2.6 Surgery for Postinflammatory Stenosis of the External Auditory Canal

Postinflammatory stenosis of the EAC is a difficult pathology to treat. In early cases, in which only granulation tissue is present, it is possible to remove the pathologic tissue (under local anesthesia in the outpatient clinic). Then, a plastic (polyethylene) sheet is inserted and left in place for ~20 days. Regular lavage is performed with 2% boric acid in 70% ethanol and local steroid lotions are applied during that period.

Surgery is doubtful in well-established cases, in which excessive scar tissue causes marked narrowing of the EAC and thickening of the tympanic membrane. In the majority of cases, restenosis occurs following surgical intervention. Therefore, it is preferable not to operate on the cases of unilateral postinflammatory stenosis.

Usually, for cases of bilateral involvement with marked hearing loss, hearing aids are prescribed. Bone-anchored hearing aids may be the choice if canal stenosis is severe. Surgery is nowadays indicated (in our group) only when the patient wants to try surgical correction for better hearing or there is difficulty in fitting hearing aids due to severe mixed hearing loss. If the surgery results in failure, canal wall down technique with preservation of the intact ossicular chain (modified Bondy's technique) is performed to prohibit recurrence of scar tissue proliferation in the canal.

In contrast, the results of treatment for postoperative stenosis are more encouraging. Surgery is indicated if the closure causes large air–bone gap. The scar tissue is usually formed lateral to the middle ear and fibrous layer of the tympanic membrane remains intact. Preservation of the fibrous layer of the tympanic membrane is a key for this surgery.

Surgical Steps

1. As in calibration of the EAC, retroauricular incision is performed and the posterior canal skin is incised. The depth of the meatus is then evaluated under direct vision. Then, another incision is made just medial to the bottom of the cul-de-sac skin leaving the scar tissue in the meatus. The lateral meatal skin is held anteriorly with a self-retaining retractor together with the auricle (see ▶ Fig. 3.60).

2. The scar tissue left over the tympanic membrane is then carefully elevated from the bony wall using a microraspatory (see ▶ Fig. 3.61).

3. The elevation of the scar tissue is carefully continued medially to reach the limbs. To avoid accidental damage to the inner and middle ear, the elevation should be started along the inferior wall where the ossicular chain is absent. Bulky scar tissue should be reduced with scissors. Care should be taken not to damage the limbs and not to get into the middle ear (see ▶ Fig. 3.62).

4. After reaching the limbs, direction of the dissection is changed parallel to the tympanic membrane. A correctly angled microraspatory should be used for the following dissection. Careful dissection of the annulus and its continuous structure from inferior to superior reveals the fibrous layer of the tympanic membrane. A clear plane of cleavage can usually be established between the fibrous layer and the scar tissue (see ▶ Fig. 3.63).

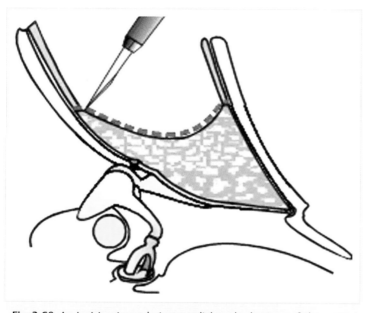

Fig. 3.60 An incision is made just medial to the bottom of the cul-de-sac.

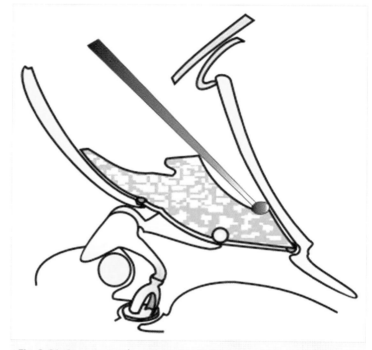

Fig. 3.61 Scar tissue elevation using a microraspatory.

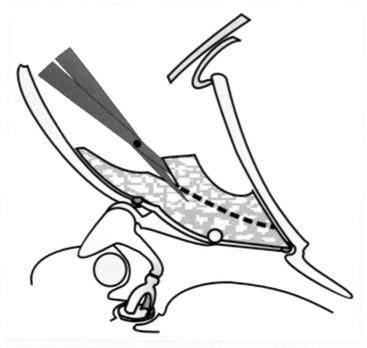

Fig. 3.62 Bulky scar tissue reduced with scissors.

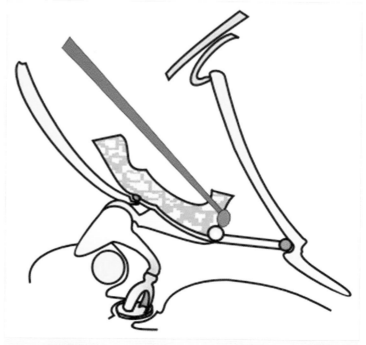

Fig. 3.63 Careful dissection from the annulus and fibrous layer of the tympanic membrane.

5. After removing the scar tissue, bony meatus is calibrated. Meticulous care should be taken not to touch the lateral process of the malleus with a burr. The tympanic membrane may be protected with a piece of aluminum sheet.

6. The cul-de-sac lateral meatal skin is opened and scar tissue around it, if any, is resected. The skin is mobilized by detaching it from the meatal cartilage for elongation. Longitudinal plastic cuts may be added to ensure intimate attachment of the skin to the bony meatus (see ▶ Fig. 3.64).

7. Split-thickness free skin graft is harvested from the posterior border of the retroauricular skin incision. The skin is grafted over the tympanic membrane and the bony meatus. The external meatus is partially packed with Gelfoam to secure the grafted skin. To prohibit postoperative scar formation, exposed bone should be covered with either the free skin graft or the lateral meatal skin flap as widely as possible (see ▶ Fig. 3.65).

8. The auricle is put back and the lateral meatal skin is replaced using a nasal speculum. Pieces of Silastic or plastic sheeting is placed over the skin and the tympanic membrane. The external meatus is further packed with Gelfoam (see ▶ Fig. 3.66, ▶ Fig. 3.67, ▶ Fig. 3.68, ▶ Fig. 3.69, ▶ Fig. 3.70).

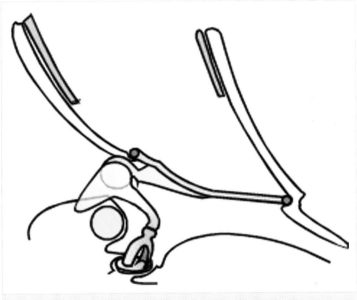

Fig. 3.64 Cul-de-sac opened and scar tissue removed.

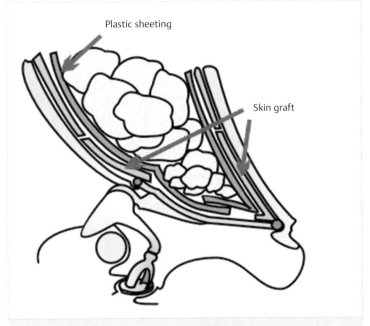

Fig. 3.65 External meatus packed with Gelfoam.

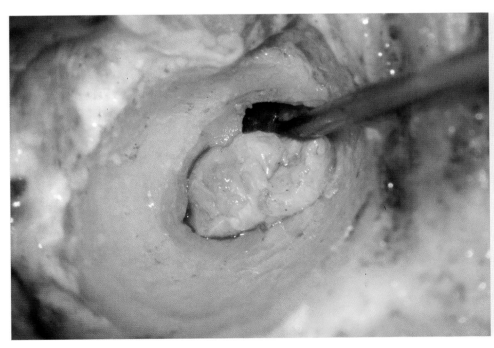

Fig. 3.66 A case of inflammatory stenosis. Left ear. The meatal skin is cut just medially to the scar tissue formed at the bottom of the external auditory canal and maintained with a self-retaining retractor. The lateral half of the bony meatus is already calibrated. Dissection of the scar tissue is carefully advanced medially with a microdissector.

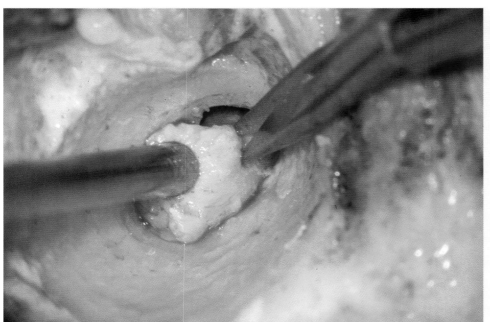

Fig. 3.67 The scar tissue is removed in piece-meal manner. The procedure makes some room for dissection and drilling, and reduces risk of adding excessive force to the ossicular chain.

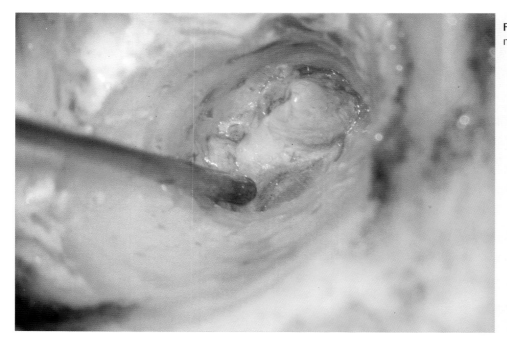

Fig. 3.68 The fibrous layer of the tympanic membrane is beginning to be seen.

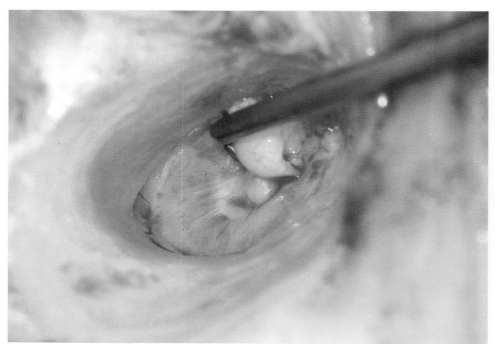

Fig. 3.69 The final part of the scar tissue is detached from the tympanic membrane.

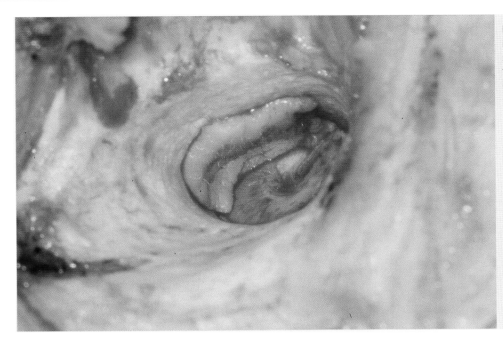

Fig. 3.70 The skin is grafted over the anterior meatal wall. The medial edge of the skin simultaneously covers the anterior edge of the tympanic membrane. The canal is packed with Gelfoam after replacing the vascular strip.

Summary

Postinflammatory stenosis of the external auditory canal is a difficult pathology to treat. In early cases, in which only granulation tissue is present, it is possible to remove the pathologic tissue (under local anesthesia in the outpatient clinic). This is followed by the insertion of a plastic (polyethylene) sheet to be left in place for ~20 days, during which regular lavage is performed with 2% boric acid in 70% alcohol and local steroid lotions are applied. Surgery is doubtful in well-established cases with excessive cicatricial tissue leading to marked narrowing of the external auditory canal and lateralization of the tympanic membrane (secondary to thickening of the latter). In the majority of cases, restenosis occurs following operative interference. Therefore, it is preferable not to operate in the case of unilateral postinflammatory stenosis. In bilateral cases with marked hearing loss, a hearing aid is prescribed. By contrast, postoperative stenosis has a better prognosis and the result of treatment are more encouraging.

3.3 Cholesteatoma of the External Auditory Canal

It is essential that the difference between cholesteatoma of the EAC and keratosis obturans should be clearly recognized. Keratosis obturans entails accumulation of desquamated squamous epithelium in the EAC forming an occluding cholesteatoma-like mass. This pathological condition generally involves both ears and occurs mainly in younger patients, whereas cholesteatoma of the EAC is usually unilateral and occurs in the elderly. In ~50% of patients, keratosis obturans is associated with bronchiectasis and chronic sinusitis. Removal of the mass is sufficient in keratosis obturans. However, cholesteatoma of the EAC requires some extent of surgical intervention. Small cholesteatoma of the EAC can be managed in the outpatient clinic by removing debris from the bone under local anesthesia. Larger cholesteatoma should be surgically removed using a retroauricular approach. Elevation of the meatal skin flap with or without the tympanic membrane, removal of the pathologic skin, and complete exposure of healthy bone by saucerizing sufficiently wide area with burrs are mandatory to avoid recurrence. A large bony defect should be obliterated with a piece of cartilage and bone paté. The temporalis fascia is laid over the area and the meatal skin flap is replaced over the fascia. Split-thickness free skin graft may be required to cover sufficiently both the fascia and the exposed bone.

Postoperative (iatrogenic) cholesteatoma of the EAC is generally located at the level of the anterior angle of the tympanic membrane. It usually originates from incorrect repositioning of the skin flaps at the end of the procedure. The cholesteatoma may look like exostosis in some case. Palpation of the mass with a probe allows identification of the pathology, since cholesteatoma is tender. Postoperative cholesteatoma in the anterior angle can usually be removed in the outpatient clinic under local anesthesia via transcanal approach. Under an ear speculum, the sac is opened and the cholesteatoma is aspirated. It is advisable to place a plastic sheet in the EAC for ~3 weeks to prevent the formation of adhesions that could lead to reformation of cholesteatoma. In rare cases, cholesteatoma is formed posteriorly and destructs mastoid cells, requiring extirpation via retroauricular incision (see ▶ Fig. 3.71, ▶ Fig. 3.72, ▶ Fig. 3.73, ▶ Fig. 3.74, ▶ Fig. 3.75, ▶ Fig. 3.76, ▶ Fig. 3.77, ▶ Fig. 3.78, ▶ Fig. 3.79).

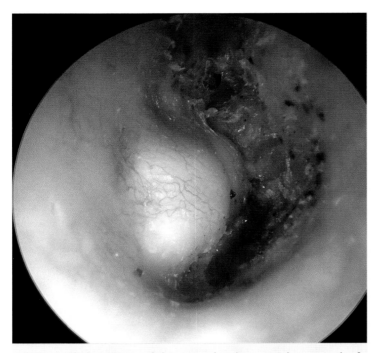

Fig. 3.71 Cholesteatoma of the external auditory canal, as a result of incorrect repositioning of skin flaps in a previous intact canal wall tympanoplasty. This condition has to be differentiated from exostosis. A probe is used to palpate the mass. If its consistency is tender and soft, cholestreatoma is diagnosed.

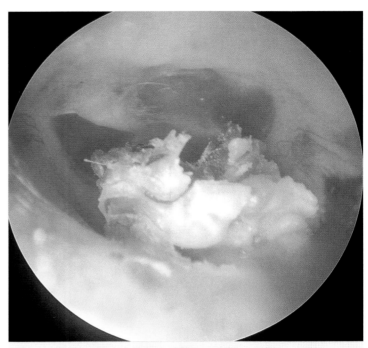

Fig. 3.72 Cholesteatoma of the inferior wall of the left external auditory canal being removed in the outpatient clinic. In this case, the squamous debris led to erosion of the underlying bone.

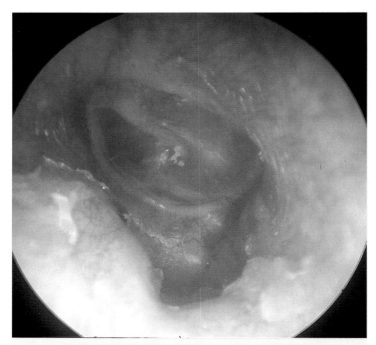

Fig. 3.73 Same patient, a few months later. Note the bone erosion caused by the cholesteatoma.

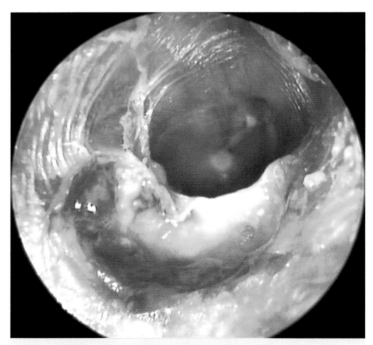

Fig. 3.74 Case similar to that of ▶ Fig. 3.73. Removal of cholesteatoma of the inferior wall of the external auditory canal. Note the bony erosion. Some cholesteatoma matrix is still present.

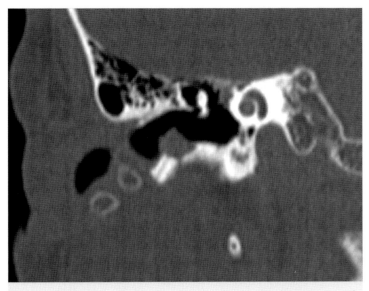

Fig. 3.75 CT scan, coronal view of the same case. Cholesteatoma and bony erosion of the inferior wall of the external auditory canal could be appreciated.

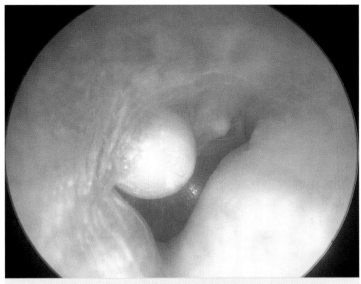

Fig. 3.76 Cholesteatoma of the external auditory canal. The external auditory canal is stenotic for the presence of exostosis of the anterior and inferior walls. The mass could be easily differentiated from a bony formation by gently pushing with a hook (see ▶ Fig. 3.77).

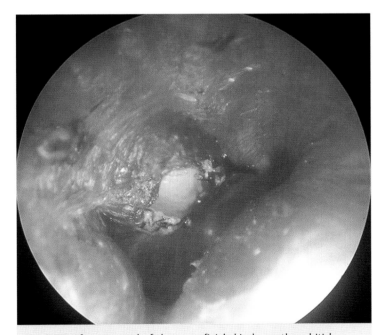

Fig. 3.77 After removal of the superficial skin layer, the whitish cholesteatoma mass could be appreciated.

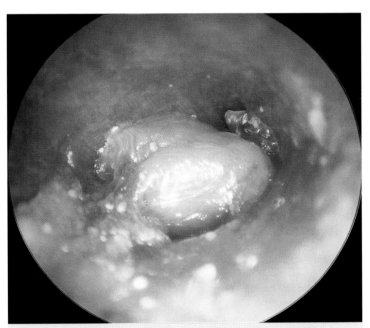

Fig. 3.78 A case similar to that in ▶ Fig. 3.71. The mass originating from the posterior canal wall inhibits the normal process of epithelial migration toward the outside.

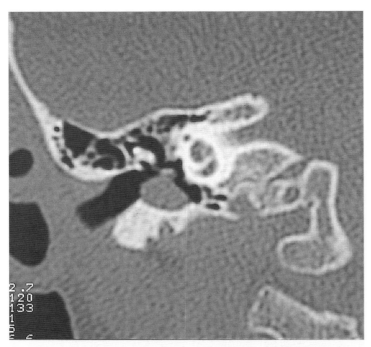

Fig. 3.79 CT of the same case, coronal view. The cholesteatoma is clearly seen in the anteroinferior portion of the external auditory canal with partial erosion of the underlying bone.

3.4 Pathologies Extending to the External Auditory Canal

Some middle ear and skull base pathologies can extend into the EAC (e.g., cholesteatoma, glomus tumors, meningiomas, neuromas, neurofibromas, carcinoid tumors, and histiocytosis X). These cases are discussed here to underline the importance of their inclusion in the differential diagnosis of polyps in the EAC. Moreover, taking a biopsy of these polyps in the outpatient clinic without proper radiological study is sometimes hazardous. For a detailed discussion of these pathologies, the reader is referred to the relevant chapters.

3.4.1 Carcinoid Tumors

A carcinoid tumor is an adenomatous neuroendocrinal tumor of ectodermal origin. It has the same histologic and histochemical characteristics as other carcinoid tumors that involve different parts of the body. A carcinoid tumor is suspected whenever an adenomatous tumor of the middle ear has acinic or trabecular histologic features. Clinically, they manifest as hearing loss, tinnitus, aural fullness, facial nerve paresis vertigo, and otalgia. The diagnosis is confirmed by electron microscopy and immunohistochemistry to demonstrate the presence of serotonin and argyrophilic granules. These tumors require functional surgery that entails removal of the tympanic membrane and ossicular chain together with the mass. The tympanic membrane is grafted at the same stage, whereas the ossicular chain is reconstructed in a second stage. This strategy ensures the pathology is completely eradicated (see ▶ Fig. 3.80, ▶ Fig. 3.81, ▶ Fig. 3.82, ▶ Fig. 3.83).

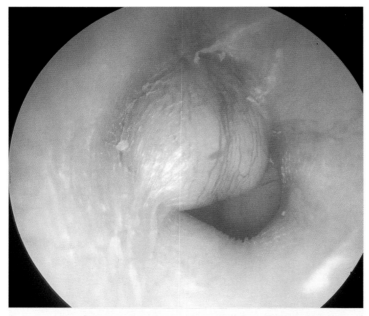

Fig. 3.80 This patient complained of hearing loss in the left ear and otalgia of 3 months' duration. Otoscopy revealed a mass occupying the external auditory canal and originating from its anterosuperior region. The inferior part of the tympanic membrane, which is the only visible part, appears whitish due to the presence of a mass in the middle ear. The audiogram (▶ Fig. 3.81) revealed the presence of conductive hearing loss. CT scan (▶ Fig. 3.82 and ▶ Fig. 3.83) demonstrated the presence of an isointense soft-tissue mass occupying the middle ear and mastoid with extension into the external auditory canal. No erosion of the ossicular chain, nor of the intercellular septa of the mastoid air cells, was noted. Intraoperatively, a glandular-like tissue was found and a frozen section obtained. The biopsy, confirmed by immunohistochemical and electronmicroscopic studies, proved the presence of a carcinoid tumor. A tympanoplasty was performed with total removal of the pathology and the involved malleus and incus.

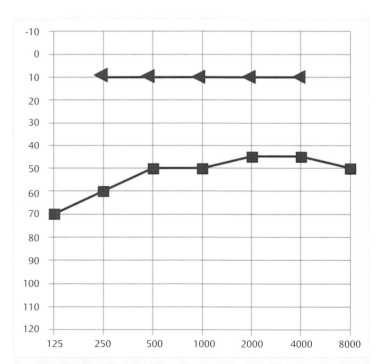

Fig. 3.81 The audiogram shows the presence of significant ipsilateral conductive hearing loss.

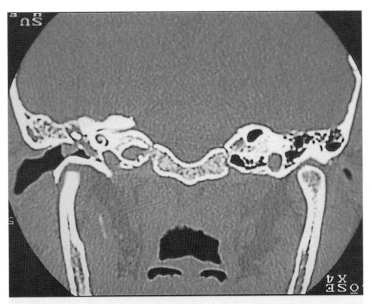

Fig. 3.82 The CT scan demonstrates a soft-tissue mass occupying the middle ear with extrusion through the tympanic membrane.

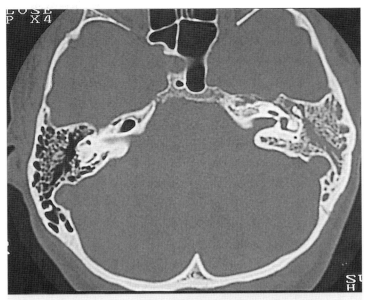

Fig. 3.83 CT scan, axial view. Presence of glue in the mastoid cells without erosion of the intercellular septa.

3.4.2 Histiocytosis X

Histiocytosis X refers to a group of disorders of the reticuloendothelial system characterized by proliferation of cytologically benign histiocytes. The disease can present in three clinical forms, the most benign of which is eosinophilic granuloma, which is usually monostotic. A moderately aggressive form is known as Hand-Shüller-Christian disease. It is characterized by multifocal lesions that are predominantly osteolytic. The most severe form, Letter-Siwe disease, occurs in children under 3 years of age and presents with diffuse multiorgan involvement. It has a mortality rate of ~40% despite therapy with cytotoxic drugs and corticosteroids. Survivors suffer from diseases such as diabetes insipidus, pulmonary fibrosis, and vertebral involvement (see ▶ Fig. 3.84, ▶ Fig. 3.85).

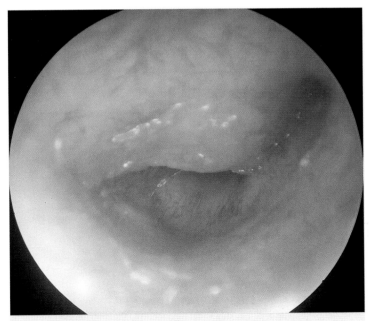

Fig. 3.84 A bulging of the posterosuperior wall of the external auditory canal in a 4-year-old child. A similar picture was also seen in the other ear (see CT scan in ▶ Fig. 3.85).

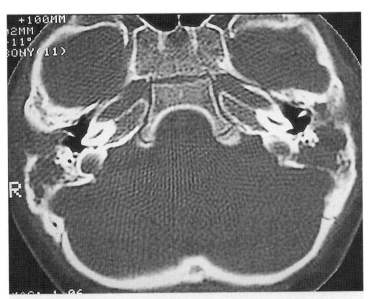

Fig. 3.85 CT scan of the same case as in ▶ Fig. 3.84. The middle ear and the mastoid are occupied by an isointense mass. A frozen section obtained during surgery revealed the presence of histiocytosis X. The patient was referred to a specialized center for appropriate staging and therapy with cytotoxic drugs and corticosteroids.

3.4.3 Meningiomas

Meningiomas are a diverse set of tumors arising from the meninges, the membranous layers surrounding the central nervous system. They arise from the arachnoid "cap" cells of the arachnoid villi in the meninges. These tumors are usually benign in nature; however, a small percentage are malignant. Many meningiomas are asymptomatic, producing no symptoms throughout a person's life, and require no treatment other than periodic observation. They constitute ~14 to 20% of all intracranial neoplasms, representing the second most common tumor of the cerebellopontine angle after vestibular schwannoma, accounting for 6 to 15% of all neoplasms at this site. Posterior fossa meningiomas could be classified according to their site of dural origin into five groups: cerebellar convexity, tentorium, posterior surface of the petrous bone, clivus, and foramen magnum. A further classification subdivided meningiomas of the posterior surface of the petrous bone on the basis of the exact site of implant in relation to the internal auditory canal (IAC): meningiomas located anterior to the IAC, tumors centered on the IAC, and tumors located posterior to the IAC.

Surgical treatment of these tumors must be individualized basing on patient's age, general health condition, tumor location and size, neurologic symptoms, and deficits caused by the tumor (see ▸ Fig. 3.86, ▸ Fig. 3.87, ▸ Fig. 3.88, ▸ Fig. 3.89, ▸ Fig. 3.90, ▸ Fig. 3.91, ▸ Fig. 3.92, ▸ Fig. 3.93, ▸ Fig. 3.94).

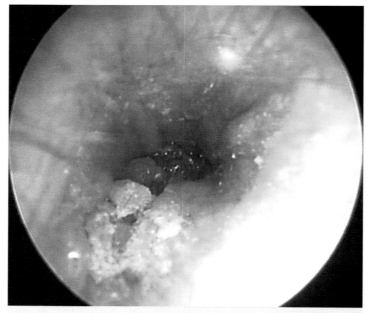

Fig. 3.86 Right ear. The external auditory canal is completely obliterated by an en-plaque meningioma (see ▸ Fig. 3.87, ▸ Fig. 3.88). The patient complained only of right hearing loss. The patient had a transcanal biopsy in an outpatient clinic elsewhere. The procedure was stopped due to excessive bleeding. Prior to do a biopsy, it's of utmost importance to assess radiological investigations such as HRCT scan of the temporal bone and brain MRI with contrast. A subtotal removal of the pathology with a subtotal petrosectomy was performed to preserve functions of the facial and lower cranial nerves.

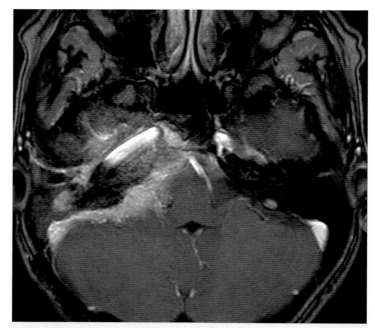

Fig. 3.87 MRI with gadolinium enhancement (T1W). The lesion has a diffuse and extensive posterior fossa dura involvement. A complete tumor resection in this case is usually not achievable due to the involvement of vital structures (carotid, basilar, and vertebral arteries).

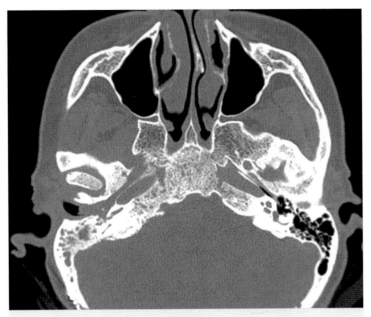

Fig. 3.88 CT scan of the temporal bone (axial section). The tumor extends to the external auditory canal, obliterating it.

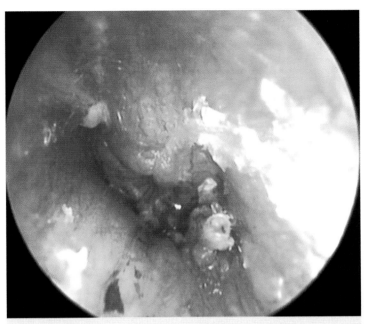

Fig. 3.89 Left ear. Another case similar to that in ▶ Fig. 3.86. An en-plaque meningioma protrudes outside the external auditory canal, which is completely filled by the tumor. The patient complained of hearing loss, tinnitus, dizziness, and intermittent otorrhea. After radiological investigations (see ▶ Fig. 3.90, ▶ Fig. 3.91), the patient was first managed with a biopsy under local anesthesia with histological confirmation of a meningioma. A subtotal petrosectomy with blind sac closure of the external auditory canal was performed to remove the pathology from the middle ear and mastoid and preserve functions of facial nerve and lower cranial nerves.

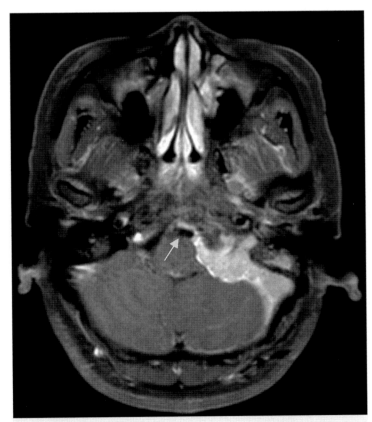

Fig. 3.90 MRI with gadolinium enhancement (T1W). The lesion has a broad posterior fossa dural attachment. The tumor surrounds the basilar artery (arrow).

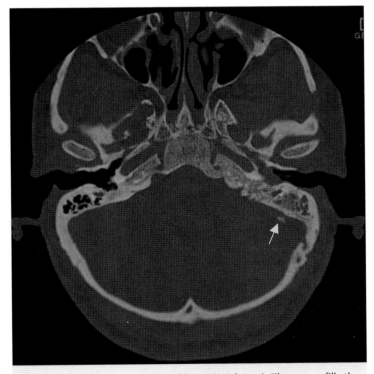

Fig. 3.91 CT scan of the temporal bone (axial view). The tumor fills the external auditory canal and the middle ear cleft. Hyperostosis (arrow) is common and frequently seen in en-plaque meningiomas.

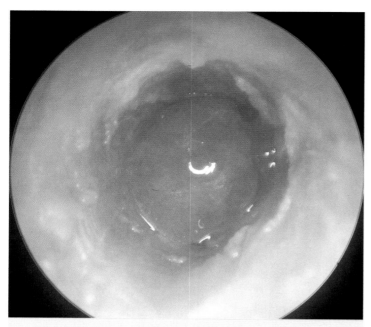

Fig. 3.92 Aural polyp in a patient with an en-plaque meningioma. An outpatient polypectomy in this case might lead to excessive bleeding.

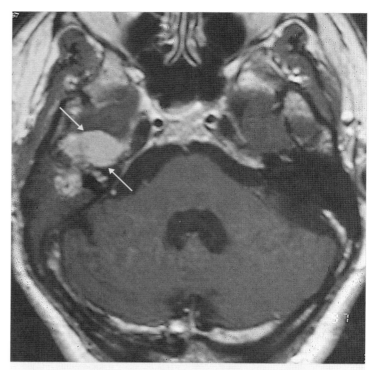

Fig. 3.93 MRI with gadolinium enhancement, axial view. The tumor (*arrows*) is located in the temporal fossa and reaches the area of the petrous apex and Meckel's cavity.

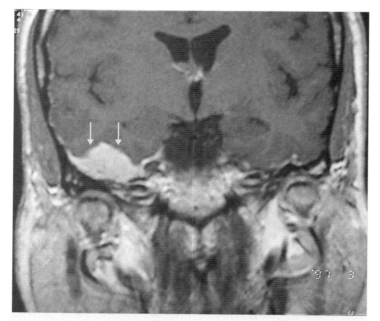

Fig. 3.94 MRI with gadolinium, coronal view. The meningioma displaces the temporal lobe upwards (*arrow*); pathognomonic tails of the dura are visible.

3.4.4 Facial Nerve Tumors

Tumors of the facial nerve are very rare. In the vast majority of cases, the tumor affecting the facial nerve is a schwannoma. In our series the rate of schwannoma was 72%; the next tumor in frequency is hemangioma at a rate of 18% followed by meningioma and neurofibroma at 5% each. Other pathologies, such as paraganglioma and neuroblastoma, are rarely encountered and are usually presented as case reports in literature. The commonest segment involved is the geniculate ganglion, for which the reported rate in the literature range from 50 to 75%, followed by the first and second segments with almost equal incidence of involvement. The presenting symptom of facial nerve tumors can be divided into facial nerve-related symptoms, hearing and equilibrium-related symptoms, and other sporadic symptoms. The vast majority of the patients present with facial nerve weakness. Treatment generally aims at total removal of the tumor, restoration or preservation of facial nerve function, and conservation of hearing. In case of good facial nerve function (Grade I House-Brackmann scale), a wait-and scan policy with yearly MRI could be adopted. Refer to ▶ Fig. 3.95, ▶ Fig. 3.96, ▶ Fig. 3.97, ▶ Fig. 3.98. For a deeper analysis of treatment choices, see Chapter 12.

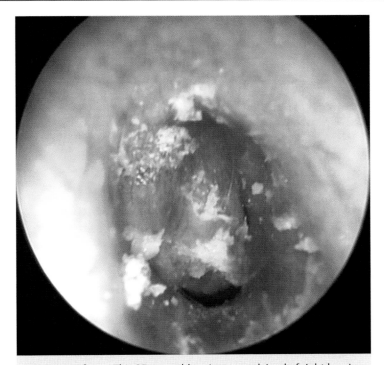

Fig. 3.95 Left ear. This 25-year-old patient complained of right hearing loss and hemifacial spasm. However, facial nerve function was normal (Grade I House-Brackmann scale). The otoscopy shows a mass obliterating the external auditory canal. After proper radiological investigations (see ▶ Fig. 3.93, ▶ Fig. 3.94), which were suggestive of a facial nerve schwannoma, we proposed an MRI scan after 1 year. However, surgical treatment of this case should be taken into account considering the extension of the disease outside the external auditory canal (e.g., subtotal petrosectomy even without tumor removal).

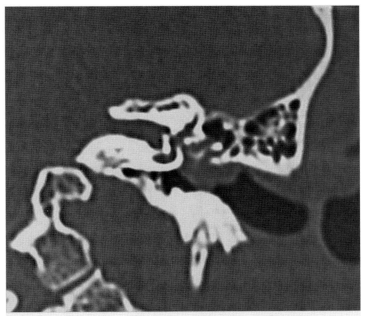

Fig. 3.96 CT scan of the temporal bone (coronal view). The tumor can be seen as a soft-tissue mass originating from the tympanic segment of the facial nerve and eroding the fallopian canal. The mass protrudes outside the external auditory canal.

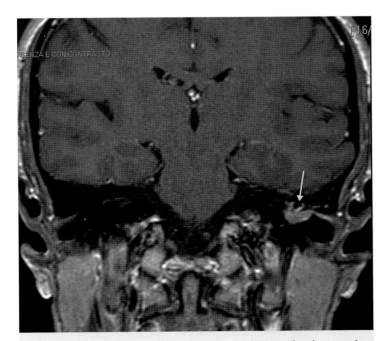

Fig. 3.97 MRI with gadolinium enhancement (T1-weighted, coronal view). The tumor (arrow) shows contrast enhancement; the second portion and even the area of the geniculate ganglion seem affected (see ▶ Fig. 3.98).

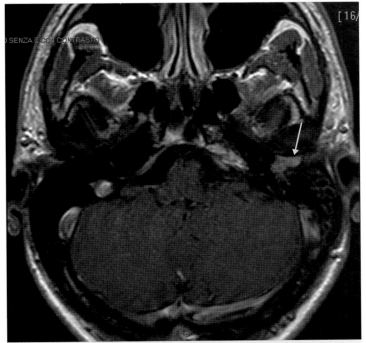

Fig. 3.98 MRI with gadolinium enhancement (T1-weighted, axial view). Even the area of the geniculate ganglion shows contrast enhancement (arrow).

3.4.5 Lower Cranial Nerves Schwannoma

Jugular foramen schwannomas arising from cranial nerves IX, X, and XI are rare, slowly growing benign tumors that constitute ~2.9 to 4% of all intracranial schwannomas. It has been hypothesized that these tumors may originate from the ganglia of cranial nerves IX and X, which are all situated close to the jugular foramen. However, the exact nerve of origin remains for the most part unknown. Following the path of least resistance, these tumors may expand through the perijugular skull base, superiorly into the posterior fossa cistern, or inferiorly into the parapharyngeal space. The dumbbell-shaped tumors have both intracranial and cervical extension with a component in the jugular foramen. The ideal primary treatment of these tumors is total tumor removal, even if the risk of lower cranial nerve deficits after surgery is very high. So, in case of normal function of lower cranial nerves we recommend surgery only in patients under 65 years old. The petro-occipital-trans-sigmoid approach (POTS) is the ideal surgical approach for these tumors, allowing preservation of the hearing and facial nerve functions (see ► Fig. 3.99, ► Fig. 3.100, ► Fig. 3.101, ► Fig. 3.102).

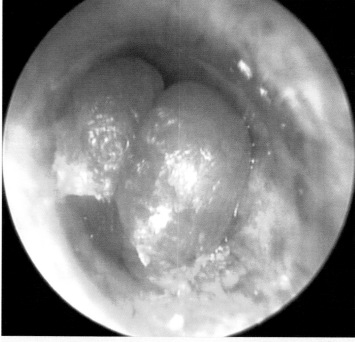

Fig. 3.99 Left ear. A bilobulated mass obliterates the external auditory canal. Radiological investigations (► Fig. 3.100, ► Fig. 3.101, ► Fig. 3.102) showed a tumor arising from the jugular foramen, suggestive for a lower cranial nerve schwannoma. A biopsy under local anesthesia confirmed the diagnosis of schwannoma. The patient underwent total tumor removal through a POTS approach with preservation of facial and cochlear functions. The patient had already left vocal fold paralysis that slightly worsened after the operation. After speech therapy, he correctly compensated with no need of further interventions.

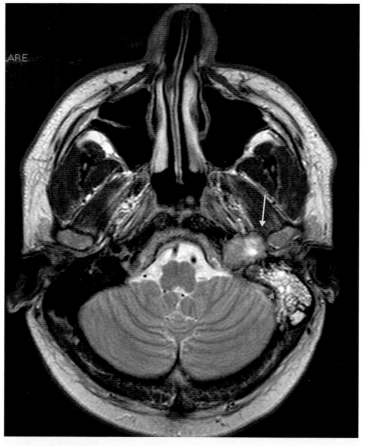

Fig. 3.100 MRI (T2W), axial view. The tumor (*yellow arrow*) causes obstruction of the Eustachian tube, with subsequent accumulation of fluid in the mastoid (*green arrow*).

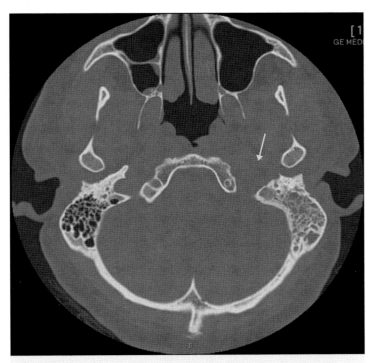

Fig. 3.101 CT scan (axial view). The tumor enlarges the jugular foramen area (*arrow*). The jugulo-carotic spine is not visible.

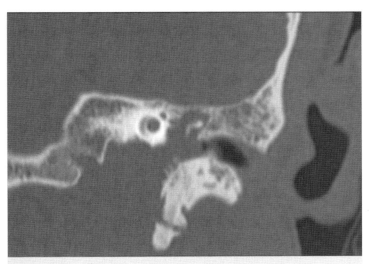

Fig. 3.102 CT scan (coronal view). From the jugular foramen the tumor extends to the middle and external ear, eroding the hypotympanic plate and the infralabyrinthine cells.

3.4.6 Other Pathologies

See ▶ Fig. 3.103, ▶ Fig. 3.104, ▶ Fig. 3.105, ▶ Fig. 3.106, ▶ Fig. 3.107, ▶ Fig. 3.108, ▶ Fig. 3.109, ▶ Fig. 3.110, ▶ Fig. 3.111.

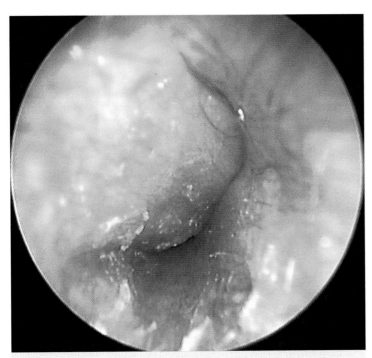

Fig. 3.103 Left ear. A soft mass arising from the anterior wall of the external auditory canal completely obliterates the meatus. The patient complained of subjective hearing loss. The MRI (▶ Fig. 3.101) confirmed the presence of a lesion suggestive for a neuroma. The patient underwent surgical removal of the lesion through a retroauricular approach; the histology confirmed the diagnosis of schwannoma of the external auditory canal. The auriculo-temporal branch of V3, which is responsible for the sensory innervation of the superior and anterior walls of the meatus, could be the origin of the tumor.

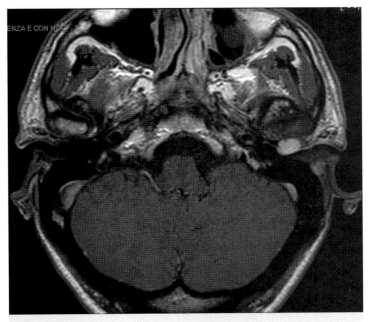

Fig. 3.104 MRI (axial view, T1 W sequence + Gd enhancement). The lesion has an oval shape and shows enhancement after gadolinium administration. It is in close proximity with the temporomandibular joint. Neuromas of the external auditory canal are very rare lesion but can be suspected performing proper radiological investigation before any surgical intervention.

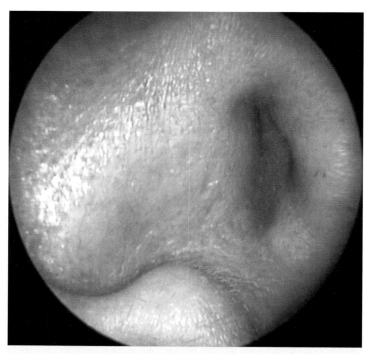

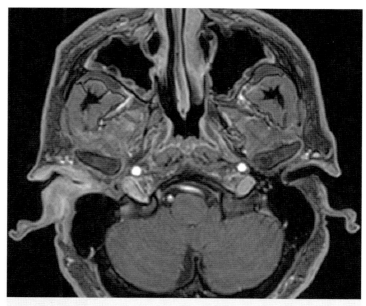

Fig. 3.106 MRI (axial view, T1 W sequence + Gd enhancement). Neurofibroma of the right external auditory canal. The lesion enhances after gadolinium administration.

Fig. 3.105 Right ear. Both the anterior and posterior walls of the external auditory canal show an increasing of the soft tissue volume, which obliterates the meatus. This 20-year-old patient suffers from neurofibromatosis type 1 and referred to fluctuating subjective right hearing loss. The MRI reveals the presence of a diffuse impairment of the soft tissue of the external ear, which is consistent with a *neurofibroma*. A biopsy conducted under local anesthesia confirmed the diagnosis.

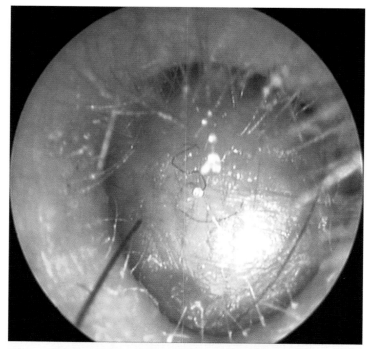

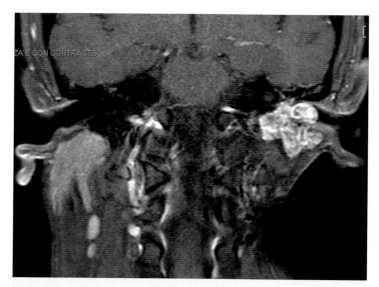

Fig. 3.108 MRI of the same case, showing invasion of the external auditory canal by the tumor.

Fig. 3.107 Left ear. *Pleomorphic adenoma* with extension into the external auditory canal. This pluri-operated patient showed a recurrent tumor from the residual portion of the parotid gland that had spread into the external auditory meatus (see ► Fig. 3.108).

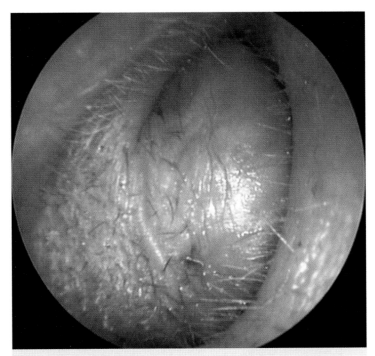

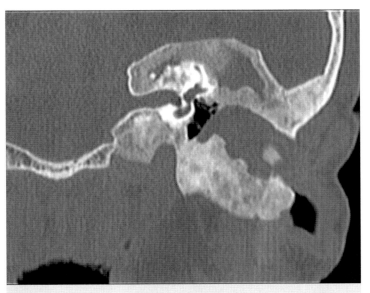

Fig. 3.110 CT scan (coronal view). The pathology completely obliterates the external auditory canal with no involvement of the otic capsule. The tympanic bone is remodeled and there is a loss of the normal cortico-medullary definition.

Fig. 3.109 Left ear. *Fibrous dysplasia* of the temporal bone. The lesion completely obliterates the external auditory canal causing conductive hearing loss. The lesion also involves the mastoid (see ▶ Fig. 3.110, ▶ Fig. 3.111). Fibrous dysplasia is a disorder of the bone metabolism, consisting in abnormal production of weak immature bone intermixed with fibrous stroma in a disorganized fashion. This patient only complained of hearing loss, but ear deformities, recurrent otitis, and cholesteatoma could be present. Occasionally, facial nerve palsy or other cranial nerves impairment can occur. Management depends on the extension of the disease and symptoms and can vary from a simple radiological follow-up to surgical treatment (generally, canalplasty or tympanoplasty). In case of a rapid growth of the disease in a long-standing fibrous dysplasia, a malignant transformation should be taken into account.

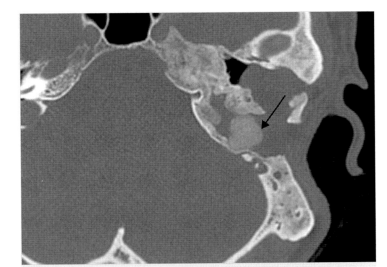

Fig. 3.111 CT scan (axial view). Ground-glass pattern (*black arrow*) is pathognomonic for fibrous dysplasia. MRI appearance is less characteristic and it can be difficult in some cases to differentiate fibrous dysplasia from chondrosarcoma, chordoma, or other malignant diseases using MRI alone.

3.5 Temporal Bone Fractures

Temporal bone fractures have been classified as longitudinal or transverse depending on the overall axis of the fracture related to the long axis of the petrous pyramid. Longitudinal fracture is most common, representing from 70 to 90% of temporal bone fractures. Complications of temporal bone fractures include hearing loss of any type, vertigo, facial palsy, and CSF leak. Occasionally, impairment of other cranial nerves (X and XI) could occur in case of involvement of the jugular foramen. Thrombosis of the jugular vein or sigmoid sinus could rarely occur and can be visible after proper radiological examination. Cases of rupture of the internal petrosal carotid artery after a temporal bone fracture are anecdotal.

Cholesteatoma is another potential complication of temporal bone fracture due to the migration of the skin corresponding to the fracture line toward the middle ear and mastoid.

The presence of hemotympanum is particularly common after temporal bone fracture and sometimes may be the initial sign of a subtle fracture. Presence of middle ear effusion or air-fluid levels after a temporal bone trauma, especially if unilateral, could lead to the suspect of a temporal bone fracture with CSF leakage into the middle ear. Fractures with involvement of the external auditory canal may displace some bone fragments, reducing the lumen of the external ear canal (see ▶ Fig. 3.112, ▶ Fig. 3.113, ▶ Fig. 3.114).

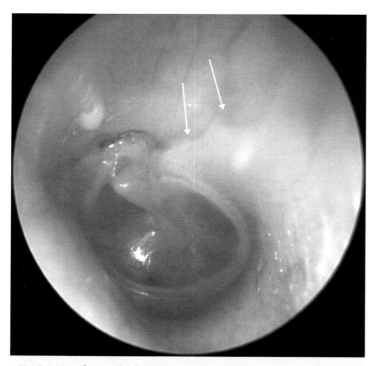

Fig. 3.112 Left ear. The fracture line is visible (*arrows*). The patient had temporal bone fracture 10 years before our evaluation, for a left facial palsy (Grade VI). The CT scan showed a supralabyrinthine petrous bone cholesteatoma (see Chapter 10), which could be secondary to skin migration from the area of the fracture line.

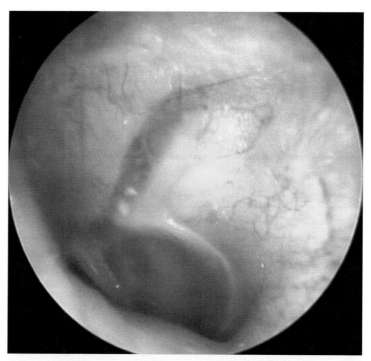

Fig. 3.113 Left ear. Posttraumatic fracture of the temporal bone. A posterosuperior fissure is seen in the posterior canal wall.

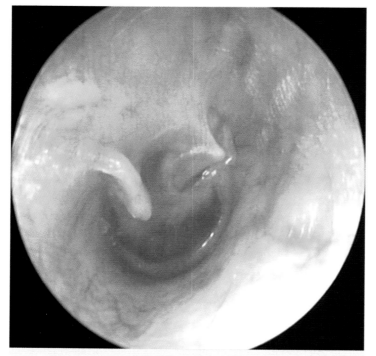

Fig. 3.114 Left ear. Posttraumatic dated fracture of the temporal bone with bone displacement of the posterior wall of the external auditory canal. The meatal skin now completely covers the protruding bone.

3.6 Carcinoma of the External Auditory Canal

Malignant neoplasms of the temporal bone are rare, accounting for ~0.2% of all head and neck malignancies. Squamous cell carcinoma is the most common histologic subtype to occur in the temporal bone (¾ of cases) followed by basal cell carcinoma, adenocarcinoma, adenoid cystic carcinoma, mucoepidermoid carcinoma, ceruminoma, melanoma, and sarcoma. Carcinomas of the temporal bone may arise from every part of the temporal bone, including the EAC, middle ear, mastoid, endolymphatic sac, petrous apex, and the IAC (► Table 3.2). These tumors can be locally aggressive due to the presence of numerous pathways in the temporal bone along which the tumor can spread from the site of origin. In ~11% of cases, cervical lymph node metastases are present at the time of diagnosis.

Staging of the disease is of utmost importance for determining the ideal surgical treatment and for defining outcomes and prognosis. Even though there is no universally accepted staging system for carcinomas of the temporal bone, the Pittsburgh staging system has been adopted in many centers for a correct classification of squamous cell carcinoma of the EAC (► Table 3.3; ► Fig. 3.115, ► Fig. 3.116, ► Fig. 3.117).

The most common symptoms of carcinoma of the EAC include otorrhea, otalgia, hearing loss, facial nerve paralysis, and vertigo. An accurate microscopic examination is important for proper evaluation of the lesion extension. Frequently, an exfoliative lesion is

Table 3.2 Classification of malignancies that arise within the temporal bone

Subsites of temporal bone carcinoma	Tumors
External auditory canal	Squamous cell carcinoma Verrucous carcinoma Adenoid cystic carcinoma Acinic cell carcinoma Mucoepidermoid carcinoma Merkel cell carcinoma Malignant cylindroma Ceruminous carcinoma Ductal carcinoma Metastasis
Tympanic membrane	Squamous cell carcinoma Lymphoma Metastasis
Middle ear	Squamous cell carcinoma Adenocarcinoma Amelanotic melanoma Lymphoepithelial carcinoma Hemangiopericytoma Carcinoid Malignant inverting papilloma Langherans cell histiocytosis Metastasis
Mastoid	Endolymphatic sac tumors Langherans cell histiocytosis Plasmacytoma Lymphoma Sarcoma Metastasis
Facial nerve	Malignant schwannoma Metastasis
Petrous apex	Chondrosarcoma Langherans cell histiocytosis Metastasis
Internal auditory canal	Squamous cell carcinoma Epidermoid carcinoma Metastasis
Labyrinth	Metastasis

Table 3.3 Modified Pittsburg staging system for squamous cell carcinoma of the external auditory canal

Factor	Description
T status	
T1	Tumor limited to the EAC without bony erosion or evidence of soft tissue involvement
T2	Tumor limited to the EAC with bone erosion (not full thickness) or limited soft tissue involvement (< 5 mm)
T3	Tumor eroding the osseous EAC (full thickness) with limited soft tissue involvement (< 5 mm) or tumor involving the middle ear and/or mastoid
T4	Tumor eroding the cochlea, petrous apex, medial wall of the middle ear, carotid canal, jugular foramen, or dura; or tumor with extensive soft tissue involvement (> 5 mm), such as involvement of temporomandibular joint or styloid process; or with evidence of facial paresis
N status	
N0	No regional nodes identified
N1	Single ipsilateral regional node < 3 cm in size
N2a	Single ipsilateral regional node 3–6 cm in size
N2b	Multiple ipsilateral nodes
N2c	Bilateral or contralateral nodes
N3	Node > 6 cm
Overall stage	
I	T1N0
II	T2N0
III	T3N0
IV	T4N0 and T1–T4 N +

Abbreviation: EAC, external auditory canal.

noted, whereas an ulcer is present in other cases. Carcinoma should be suspected when there is a persistent otitis externa characterized by pain and otorrhea that does not resolve adequately with medical treatment. A biopsy of the lesion will clear up any doubts. It is important to perform an accurate examination of the upper deep cervical, postauricular, and parotid lymph nodes (anterior extension of the tumor). The cranial nerves have to be evaluated. The facial nerve is the most frequently involved. Involvement of the mandibular nerve indicates tumor extension toward the glenoid fossa. A high-resolution CT scan (bone window) is the most important radiological investigation as it permits the evaluation of bone erosion at the level of the EAC and middle ear. MRI with gadolinium allows evaluation of tumor extension into the soft tissues. Surgery is the primary treatment of choice in temporal bone malignancies. Radiotherapy is used as an adjuvant treatment to surgery except in advanced tumors requiring palliation. The surgical procedures employed for the resection are:

- *Lateral temporal bone resection (LTBR):* This is the primary surgery of choice in T1 and T2 tumors. The approach entails a complete canal wall up mastoidectomy with an extended facial recess opening. The EAC is resected en bloc along with the tympanic membrane, the malleus after disarticulation, and removal of the incus, with the medial limit defined at the level of the incudostapedial joint. Superficial parotidectomy can be done with LTBR, especially in T2 tumors.
- *Subtotal temporal bone resection (STBR):* This is used in T3 and T4 tumors and it is an extension of the LTBR. After the steps of LTBR are performed, this procedure extends medially in a piecemeal fashion and includes IAC identification, facial nerve exposure, and removal of the otic capsule with preservation of the petrous apex. The capsule of the temporomandibular joint and, if necessary, the condyle of the mandible is resected when found involved. If the tumor extends into the mastoid and dural involvement is suspected, middle and posterior fossa craniotomies might be necessary to achieve adequate exposure. If the dura is found infiltrated, its incision is undertaken and it is excised until free margins are reached. If the facial nerve is invaded by the tumor, it should be included in the specimen. The sigmoid sinus and jugular bulb are preserved unless infiltrated.

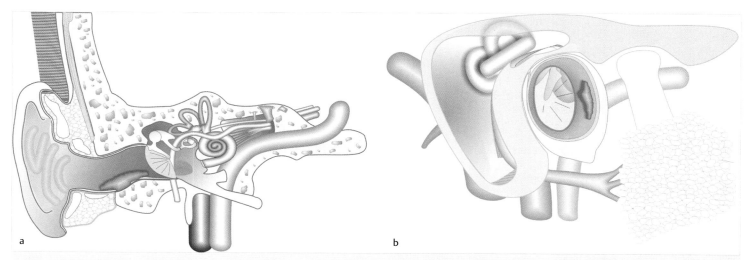

Fig. 3.115 (a,b) Schematic Illustration of a T1 tumor (red). The tumor is limited to the external auditory canal without bony erosion. In case of a T2 tumor, there is bony erosion (not full-thickness) or limited soft tissue involvement.

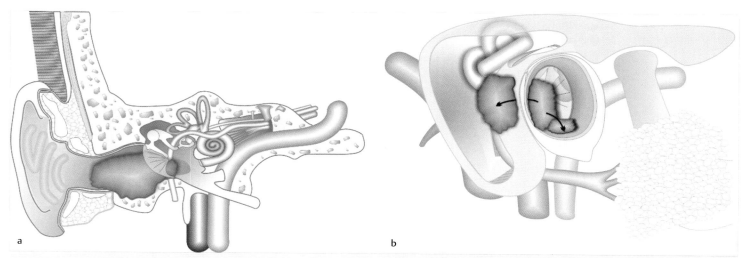

Fig. 3.116 (a,b) Schematic Illustration of a T3 tumor (red). The tumor involves the osseous external auditory canal (full thickness) or the middle ear/mastoid **(b)**.

- *Total temporal bone resection (TTBR):* This procedure is used in advanced T4 tumors. It may be performed with or without resection of the pinna. Bone is resected superiorly for 3 cm above the temporal line to expose the middle fossa dura and behind the sigmoid sinus by a similar amount to leave a residual margin of healthy bone. Medial dissection extends through the labyrinth and exposes the intrapetrous carotid artery. Inferiorly, the sigmoid sinus and jugular bulb are mobilized from surrounding bone. The sternocleidomastoid and digastric muscles are freed from the mastoid tip. At this stage in the procedure, the ascending ramus of the mandible is transected with a Gigli saw or a drill, and this and the head and coronoid process are dissected free and removed. A total parotidectomy is completed, and the specimen is removed en bloc. The residual tip of the petrous bone is then removed with a high-speed drill. Resection of the carotid artery can also be accomplished if the contralateral cerebral blood supply has been proven to be adequate by angiography and preoperative balloon occlusion.

For further details, refer to ▶ Table 3.4, ▶ Fig. 3.118, ▶ Fig. 3.119, ▶ Fig. 3.120, ▶ Fig. 3.121, ▶ Fig. 3.122, ▶ Fig. 3.123, ▶ Fig. 3.124, ▶ Fig. 3.125, ▶ Fig. 3.126, ▶ Fig. 3.127, ▶ Fig. 3.128, ▶ Fig. 3.129, ▶ Fig. 3.130, ▶ Fig. 3.131, ▶ Fig. 3.132, ▶ Fig. 3.133, ▶ Fig. 3.134, ▶ Fig. 3.135, ▶ Fig. 3.136, ▶ Fig. 3.137, ▶ Fig. 3.138, ▶ Fig. 3.139, ▶ Fig. 3.140, ▶ Fig. 3.141, ▶ Fig. 3.142, ▶ Fig. 3.143, ▶ Fig. 3.144, ▶ Fig. 3.145, ▶ Fig. 3.146, ▶ Fig. 3.147, ▶ Fig. 3.148, ▶ Fig. 3.149.

Table 3.4 Gruppo Otologico's series in the treatment of SSC of the temporal bone (1993–2011, 45 cases, published data); survival rates are reported

T status	Patients (%)	Disease-specific survival rate (5 years) (%)	Recurrence-free survival rate (5 years) (%)
T1	11.1	100	100
T2	13.3	100	100
T3	31.1	86.2	79
T4	42.2	48.7	45.2

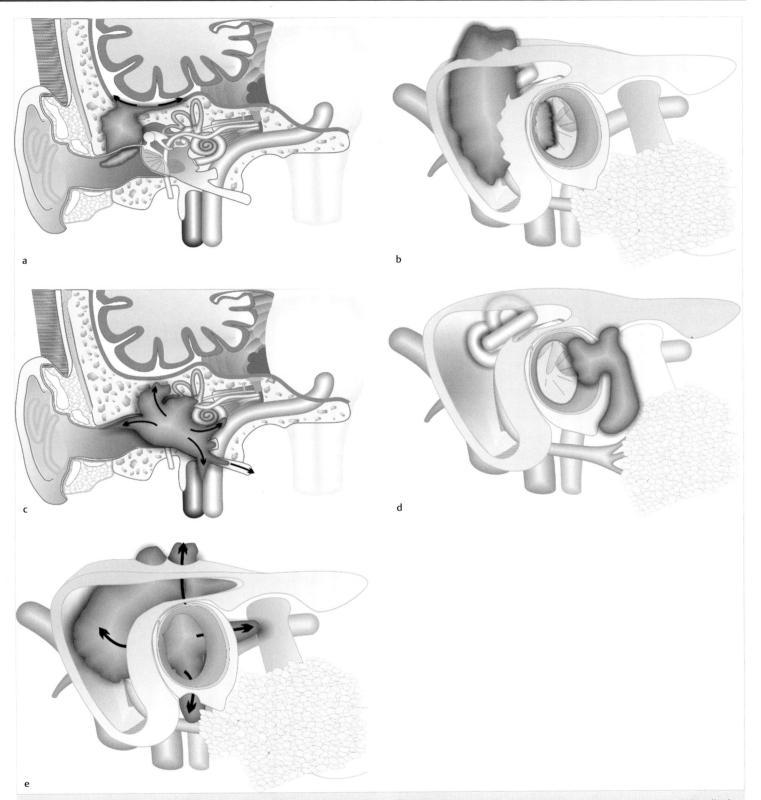

Fig. 3.117 (a–e) Schematic Illustration of a T4 tumor (red). The tumor involves the middle fossa dura **(a)**, middle fossa dura and medial wall of middle ear and mastoid **(b)**, otic capsule, jugular foramen, and infralabyrinthine-apical compartment **(c)**, temporomandibular joint **(d)**, and the whole temporal bone **(e)**.

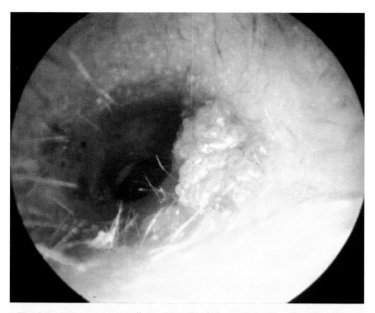

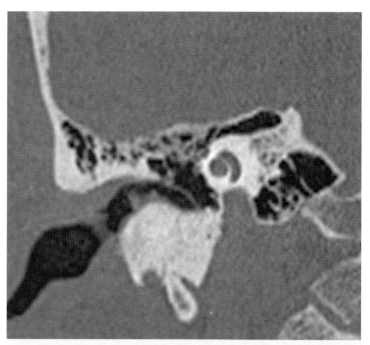

Fig. 3.118 Squamous cell carcinoma of the right external auditory canal. Patient complained of occasional bloody otorrhea. A biopsy was undertaken and pathologic examination revealed the presence of carcinoma. The CT scan (see ▶ Fig. 3.119) demonstrated a T1 tumor arising from the anterior–inferior wall of the external auditory canal. Lateral temporal bone resection was performed. After 4 years, the patient has no recurrence of the disease.

Fig. 3.119 CT scan, coronal view. The lesion arises from the anterior–inferior wall of the external auditory canal without bony erosion (T1 stage).

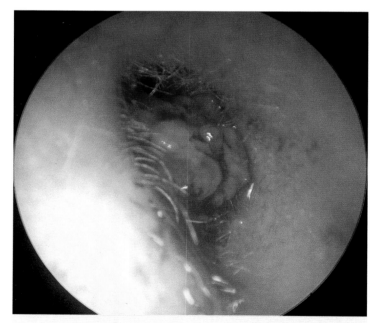

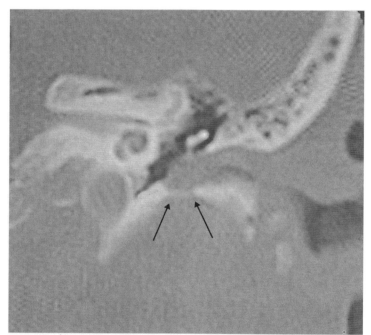

Fig. 3.120 An exfoliative neoplasm that occupies the left external auditory canal. The patient complained of otalgia and attacks of bloody otorrhea of 1-month duration. A biopsy was taken and pathologic examination revealed the presence of squamous cell carcinoma. A CT scan (▶ Fig. 3.116) demonstrated erosion of the external auditory canal, particularly its anterior–inferior wall, without invasion into the glenoid fossa. En bloc removal of the tumor was performed, together with superficial parotidectomy. Radiotherapy was performed postoperatively.

Fig. 3.121 CT scan demonstrated erosion of the anteroinferior wall of the external auditory canal (not full thickness-T2 stage). The glenoid fossa is not involved.

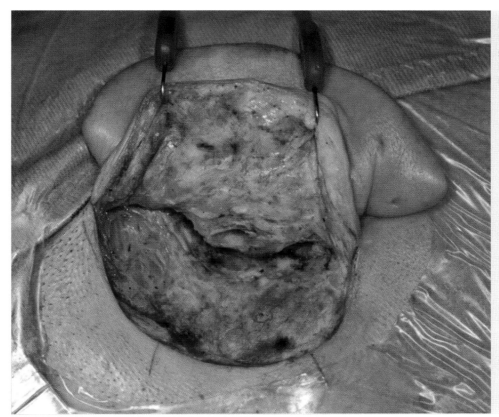

Fig. 3.122 Same patient as in ▶ Fig. 3.118. Example of lateral temporal bone resection. The skin incision starts 3 cm behind the retroauricular sulcus. The external auditory canal has to be transected laterally to the tumor.

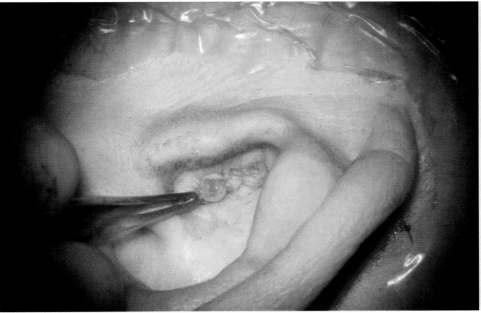

Fig. 3.123 Cul-de-sac closure of the external auditory canal.

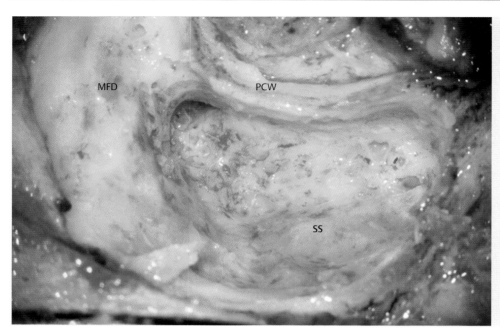

Fig. 3.124 Mastoidectomy with identification of middle fossa dura and sigmoid sinus. MFD, middle fossa dura; SS, sigmoid sinus; PCW, posterior canal wall.

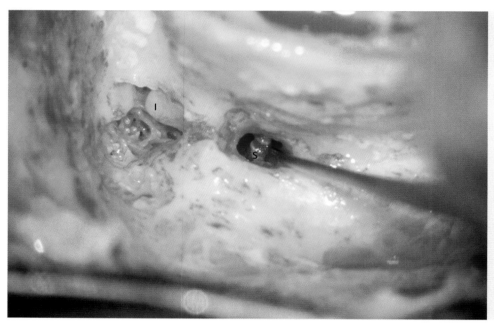

Fig. 3.125 Facial recess tympanotomy. I, incus; S, stapes.

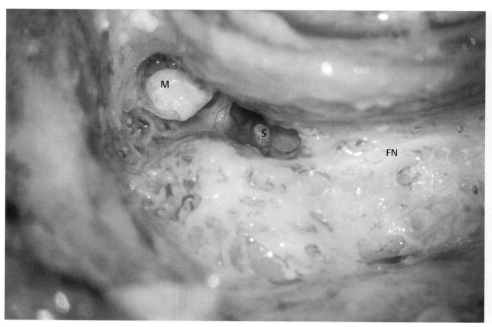

Fig. 3.126 Dislocation of the incudo-stapedial joint. FN, facial nerve; M, malleus (head); S, stapes.

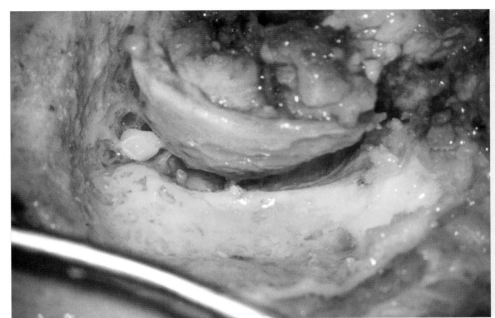

Fig. 3.127 Epi- and hypotympanotomy.

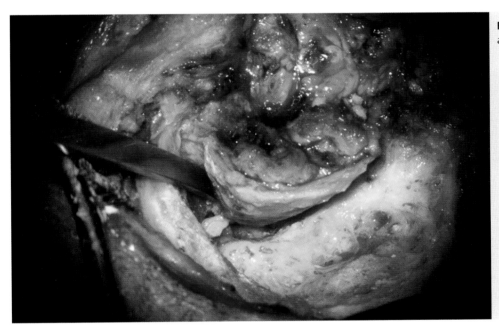

Fig. 3.128 En-bloc resection of the external auditory canal.

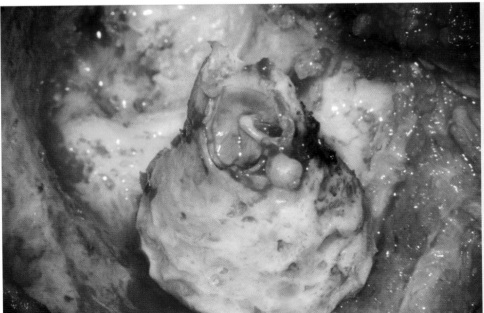

Fig. 3.129 En-bloc specimen including malleus, tympanic membrane, and external auditory canal.

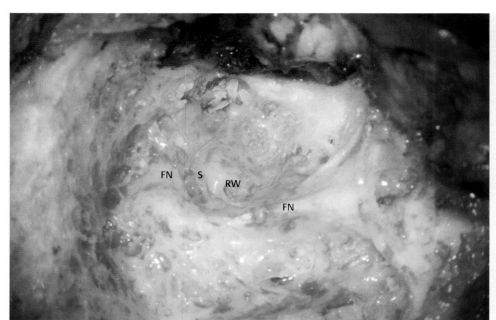

Fig. 3.130 Temporal bone cavity after tumor removal. S, stapes; RW, round window; FN, facial nerve.

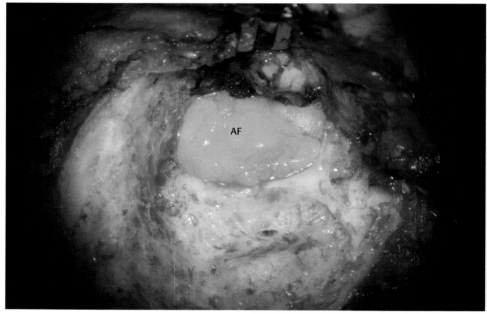

Fig. 3.131 Closure of the cavity with abdominal fat. AF, abdominal fat.

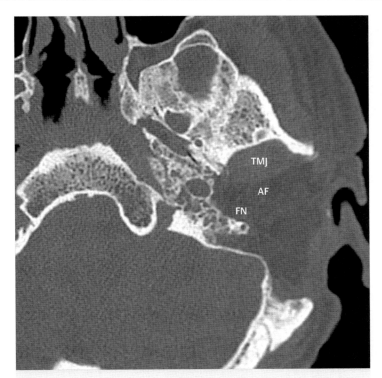

Fig. 3.132 Postoperative CT scan. The cavity is completely obliterated with abdominal fat. All the anterior tympanic bone has been removed. The facial nerve has been left in place. AF, abdominal fat; FN, facial nerve; TMJ, temporomandibular joint.

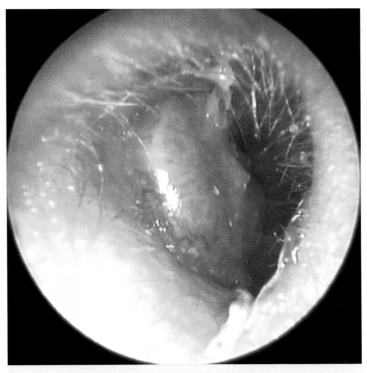

Fig. 3.133 Squamous cell carcinoma of the left external auditory canal. The lesion completely obliterates the meatus and the tympanic membrane is not viewable. The patient complained of hearing loss, persistent otorrhea, otalgia, and pain in the temporomandibular joint. CT and MRI scans (▶ Fig. 3.118, ▶ Fig. 3.119, ▶ Fig. 3.120) revealed extension of the pathology to the glenoid fossa with limited soft tissue involvement (T3 stage). A subtotal temporal bone resection with parotidectomy plus postoperative radiotherapy were performed.

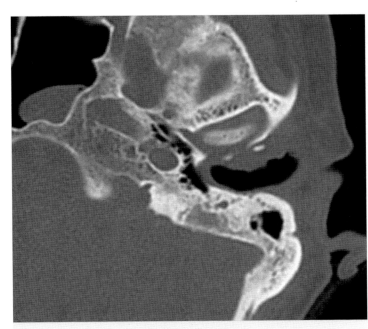

Fig. 3.134 CT scan (axial view). The anterior wall of the external auditory canal is eroded by the tumor, which extends toward the temporomandibular joint.

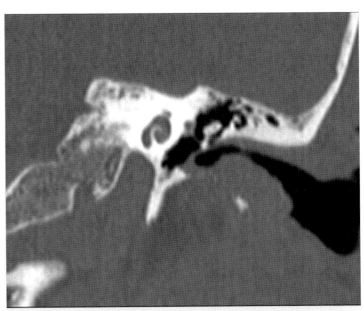

Fig. 3.135 CT scan (axial view). The inferior wall of the external auditory canal is eroded by the tumor, which seems to protrude into the glenoid fossa.

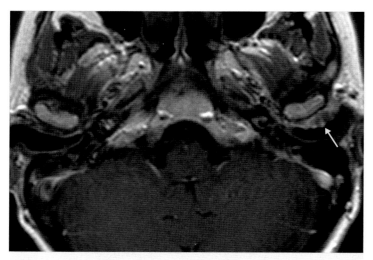

Fig. 3.136 MRI scan (axial view, T1W + Gd). The tumor (*arrow*) arises from the anterior wall of the external auditory canal without involvement of the mandibular condyle.

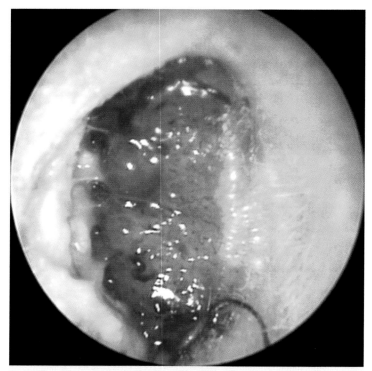

Fig. 3.137 Squamous cell carcinoma of the right external auditory canal. The patient complained of hearing loss and persistent bloody otorrhea. The lesion, involving the middle ear, was removed through a subtotal temporal bone resection. Postoperative radiotherapy followed the surgical procedure.

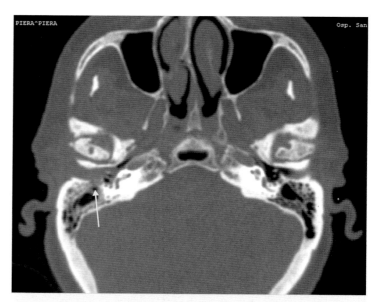

Fig. 3.138 CT scan (axial view). The tumor involves the middle ear and erodes the posterior wall of the external auditory canal (*arrow*), extending toward the mastoid (T3 stage).

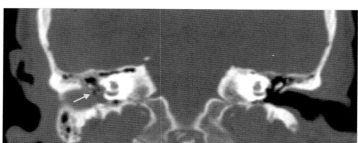

Fig. 3.139 CT scan (coronal view). The tumor involves the middle ear with erosion of the incudo-stapedial joint (*arrow*).

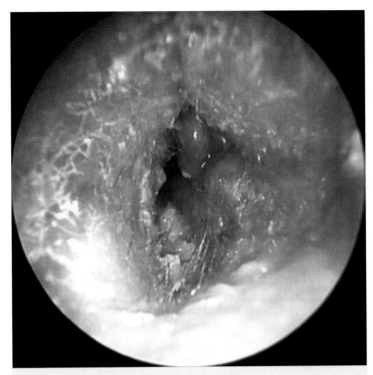

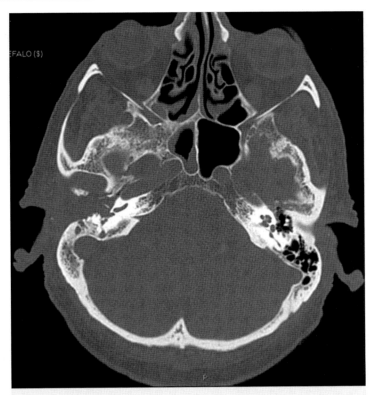

Fig. 3.140 Squamous cell carcinoma of the right external auditory canal in a 70-year-old patient. The patient complained of recurrent otitis and facial palsy with no improvement after prolonged antibiotic therapies. Biopsy under local anesthesia and proper radiological investigations confirmed the provisional diagnosis. The tumor (stage T4) involved even the middle fossa dura and extended anteriorly. In cases like this prognosis is poor, so the adoption of an extensive surgical approach (i.e., total temporal bone resection with dural excision) could be questionable, because it does not influence the survival rate. Considering patient's age we performed a subtotal temporal bone resection with facial nerve resection, total parotidectomy, and dura preservation and coagulation. Radiotherapy followed the surgical procedure.

Fig. 3.141 CT scan of the same case (axial view). The tumor involves the middle ear and extends toward the temporomandibular joint.

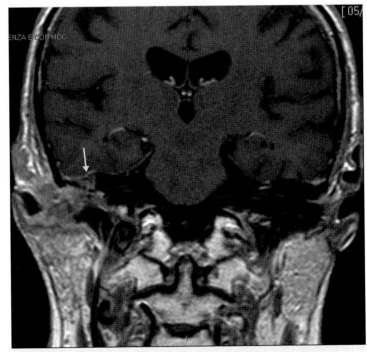

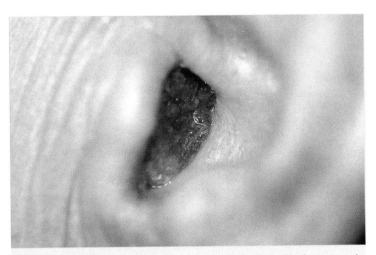

Fig. 3.143 Squamous cell carcinoma protruding through the external auditory canal with extension into the glenoid fossa and infiltration of the middle fossa dura (see CT scan, ▶ Fig. 3.144 and MRI, ▶ Fig. 3.145). Palliative surgery was performed, followed by radiotherapy.

Fig. 3.142 MRI (coronal view). The tumor involves the middle fossa dura (*arrow*).

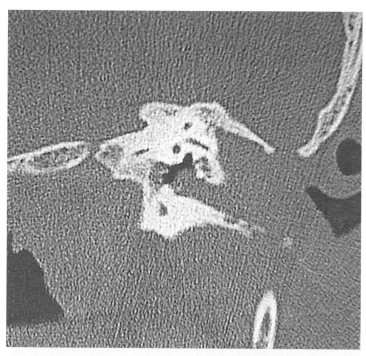

Fig. 3.144 CT scan. The carcinoma occupies all of the middle ear and mastoid. The glenoid fossa and the middle fossa plate are eroded.

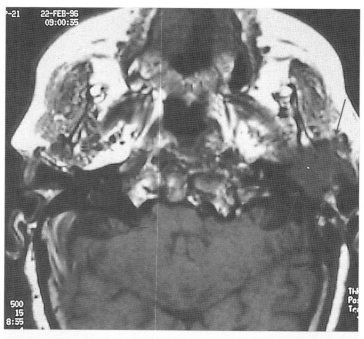

Fig. 3.145 MRI shows marked anterior extension of the tumor into the infratemporal fossa (*arrows*).

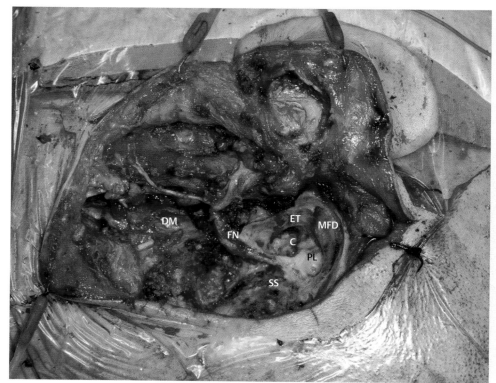

Fig. 3.146 Example of subtotal temporal bone resection with total parotidectomy and neck dissection (level II). The facial nerve has been preserved, as well as the cochlea and the posterior labyrinth. FN, facial nerve; MFD, middle fossa dura; SS, sigmoid sinus; PL, posterior labyrinth; C, cochlea; DM, digastric muscle; ET, Eustachian tube.

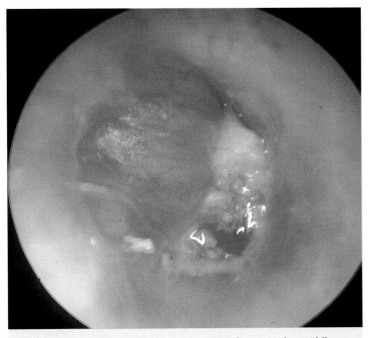

Fig. 3.147 Nasopharyngeal carcinoma extending into the middle ear and external auditory canal. A polypoid mass infiltrates the tympanic membrane and partially fills the external auditory canal (see CT scan, ▶ Fig. 3.148 and MRI, ▶ Fig. 3.149). The patient was considered inoperable and was referred for radiotherapy.

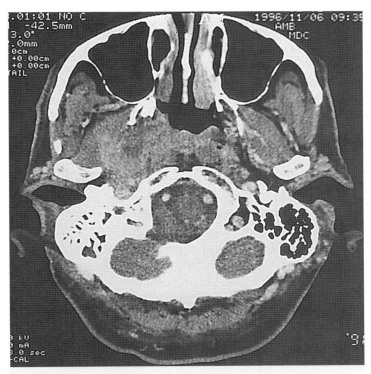

Fig. 3.148 The CT scan demonstrates marked infiltration of the nasopharynx, the pterygoid muscles, and the petrous apex.

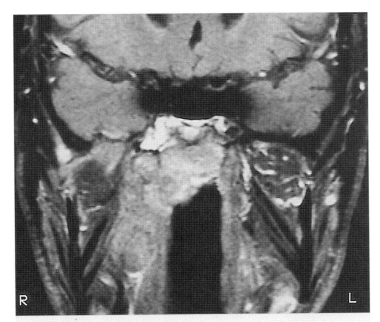

Fig. 3.149 MRI with gadolinium confirms the infiltration.

Summary

A carcinoma arising from the external auditory canal is frequently confused with suppurative otitis. Because of the high incidence of otitis externa and media and because these pathologies are frequently chronic, the diagnosis of carcinoma of the external auditory canal is almost always late. Diagnosis is made through biopsy. A high-resolution CT scan and MRI are necessary for proper evaluation. A high-resolution CT scan determines the osseous erosion caused by the tumor, whereas MRI is superior to CT for the evaluation of soft tissues. MRI shows the presence of dural invasion, intracranial extension, as well as extracranial soft-tissue involvement. The Pittsburg staging system has been adopted in many centers for classification of squamous cell carcinoma of the external auditory canal, which is the most frequent tumor of the temporal bone. Therapy for carcinoma of the external auditory canal is almost always surgical. For T1 and T2 tumors, lateral temporal bone resection is the ideal surgical management. It entails excision of the external auditory canal (bone and soft tissues), tympanic membrane, and ossicular chain with preservation of the facial nerve. Anteriorly, bone removal extends up to the level of the temporomandibular joint. The cavity is then obliterated with abdominal fat and the external auditory canal closed as a cul-de-sac. When indicated, the resection can include a superficial parotidectomy. In case of T3-T4 tumors, a subtotal temporal bone resection is indicated. In such cases, a middle and posterior fossa craniotomy is necessary. Bone removal is performed up to the level of the medial third of the petrous apex and the internal carotid artery. Usually, the facial nerve and the middle ear are sacrificed. If there is dural involvement, dural removal and reconstruction should be done in young patients. Neck dissection, total parotidectomy, and resection of the mandibular condyle have to be done depending on the extent of the disease. For more advanced T4 tumors, palliative surgery with postoperative radiotherapy are indicated. Adjuvant radiotherapy has an undisputed role for T2, T3, and T4 tumors.

Chapter 4

Otitis Media

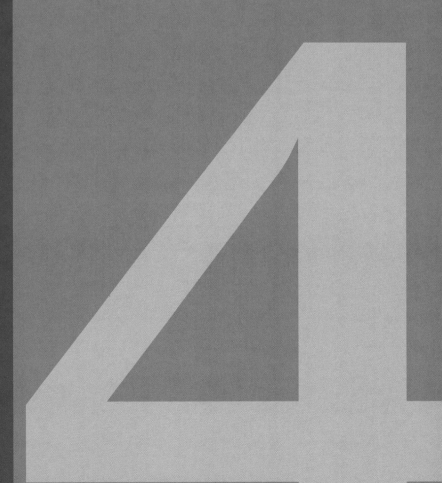

4 Otitis Media

Abstract

Otitis media can be classified into two different types. *Secretory otitis media* is characterized by the presence of middle ear effusion behind an intact tympanic membrane; the tympanic membrane is retracted, immobile, dark yellowish, bluish, or it may be transparent with a hairline (liquid level) or air bubbles visible through it. It is usually caused by Eustachian tube dysfunction. In case of unilateral disease, the nasopharynx has to be explored to exclude the presence of a tumor. *Acute otitis media* is the consequence of an upper airway infection with blockage of the Eustachian tube and effusion in the middle ear, when the fluid in the middle ear gets additionally infected with bacteria. The tympanic membrane is bulged, and shows signs of cloudiness and redness. In severe or untreated cases, the tympanic membrane may rupture, allowing the pus in the middle ear space to drain into the ear canal. A simple medical treatment is required in most of the cases.

Keywords: secretory otitis media, acute otitis media

4.1 Secretory Otitis Media (Otitis Media with Effusion)

Secretory otitis media is characterized by the presence of middle ear effusion composed of a transudate/exudate of the mucosa of the middle ear cleft that is formed behind an intact tympanic membrane. Classically, the tympanic membrane is retracted, immobile, dark yellowish or bluish, and thickened. At times, it may be transparent with a hairline (liquid level) or air bubbles visible through it.

The causes are generally: Eustachian tube obstruction secondary to mucosal edema due to infection (sinusitis, nasopharyngitis) or allergy; extrinsic pressure on the cartilaginous portion of the Eustachian tube due to hyperplasia of glandular or lymphoid tissue or, rarely, due to tumors; and malfunction of the tubal muscles, as in children with cleft palate, or malformation of the tube itself, as in Down syndrome. Other factors that may contribute include: bacteriologic, immunologic, genetic, socioeconomic status, seasonal variation, as well as lack of transmission of specific immunoglobulins in nonbreast-fed infants. All these factors cause tubal dysfunction or occlusion, leading to negative middle ear pressure due to oxygen absorption by the mucosa of the middle ear cleft. Normally, the tendency of the tubal walls to collapse at the level of the isthmus can be overcome by an increase in the nasopharyngeal pressure. A negative middle ear pressure up to –25 mm Hg can be thus corrected. On the other hand, with edema of the tubal mucosa, the same increase in the nasopharyngeal pressure cannot overcome a negative middle ear pressure less than –5 mm Hg. In children, hyperplasia of the adenoid tissue is the most common predisposing factor, and nasopharyngitis is the most frequent cause of secretory otitis media. In adults, the condition is much less common and the presence of persistent unilateral otitis media with effusion can be due to a nasopharyngeal tumor that occludes the tubal opening, or a neoplasm that compresses or infiltrates the tube along its course.

In cases that do not resolve despite proper medical treatment (nasal and systemic decongestants, mucolytics, and antibiotics) or in cases with persistent conductive hearing loss (see ► Fig. 4.1, ► Fig. 4.2), the insertion of a ventilation tube is indicated. In children, adenoidectomy is also performed. Surgery aims at alleviating the conductive hearing loss, avoiding the sequelae of otitis media with effusion. Sequelae include recurrent otitis media, tympanosclerosis, adhesive otitis media, retraction pockets with eventual cholesteatoma formation, and, in some long-standing cases, the formation of cholesterol granuloma (see Chapter 5). In this chapter, some typical cases of otitis media with effusion are shown. Refer to ► Fig. 4.3, ► Fig. 4.4, ► Fig. 4.5, ► Fig. 4.6, ► Fig. 4.7, ► Fig. 4.8, ► Fig. 4.9, ► Fig. 4.10, ► Fig. 4.11, ► Fig. 4.12. For the surgical treatment (myringotomy and ventilation tube insertion), the reader is referred to Chapter 14 on postsurgical conditions.

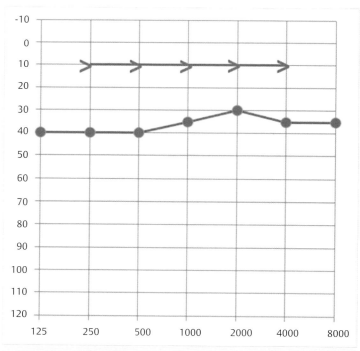

Fig. 4.1 Conductive hearing loss. Bone conduction is normal. Air conduction is on average of 35 dB.

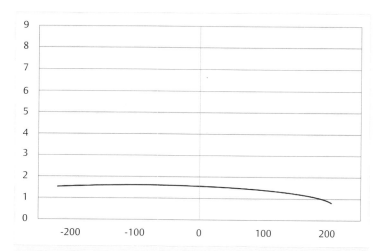

Fig. 4.2 Tympanogram type B, typical of middle ear effusion.

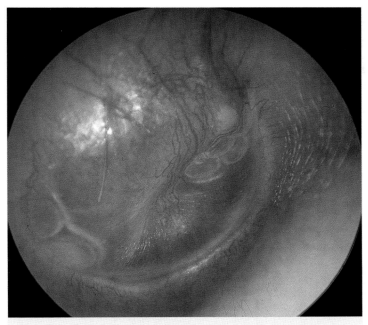

Fig. 4.3 Right ear. Secretory otitis media. Air bubbles can be seen anterior to the handle of the malleus and also in the posteroinferior quadrant.

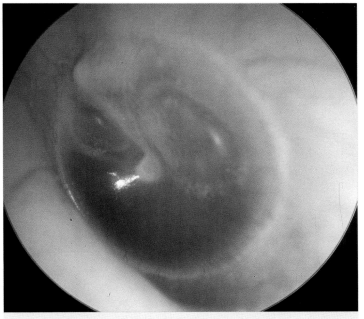

Fig. 4.4 Left ear. Secretory otitis media. Middle ear effusion having a reddish color inferiorly and a yellowish color superiorly. In this case, the differential diagnosis includes glomus tympanicum. If doubts still exist after microscopic examination, medical treatment is administered for several weeks and the patient is reexamined.

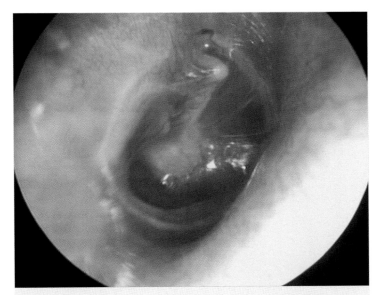

Fig. 4.5 Right ear. Secretory otitis media with middle ear effusion and air bubbles visible in the anterosuperior quadrant. The tympanic membrane is retracted toward the promontorium. This case reflects usually a chronic condition that should be managed with the insertion of a ventilation tube.

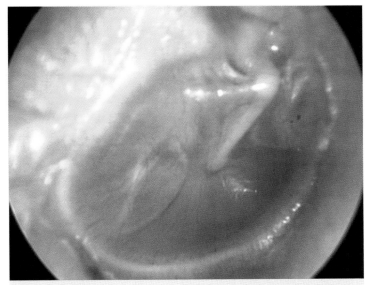

Fig. 4.6 Right ear. Secretory otitis media with middle ear effusion and air bubbles visible in the posterior quadrants. The patient has also a cholesteatoma in the contralateral ear (see Fig. 8.22). The CT scan shows the presence of fluid trapped in the mastoid (see ▶ Fig. 4.7).

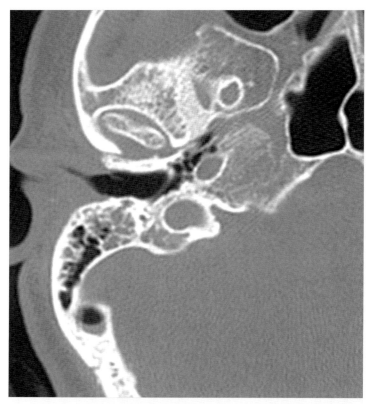

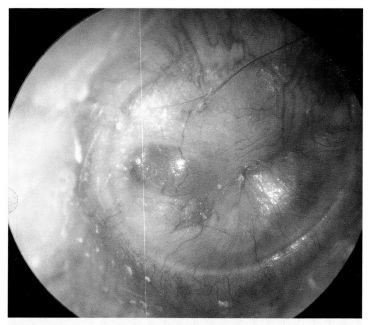

Fig. 4.8 Right ear. The presence of glue in the middle ear leads to bulging of the tympanic membrane. In the posterior quadrant, a thinned area of the drum is visualized, through which the yellowish color of the effusion is visible. The area would probably be the site of a future perforation.

Fig. 4.7 CT scan, axial view of case in ▶ Fig. 4.6. The fluid is trapped in the mastoid air cells. The septa between the pneumatized cells are preserved.

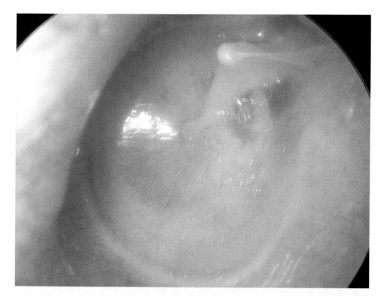

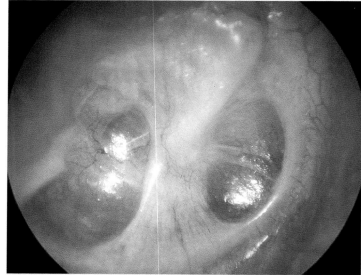

Fig. 4.9 Left ear. Secretory otitis media. The tympanic membrane is thickened. Catarrhal fluid can be seen through the relatively thinner anteroinferior quadrant.

Fig. 4.10 Right ear. Secretory otitis media. The effusion is visible through two thinned areas of the tympanic membrane lying anterior and posterior to the handle of the malleus.

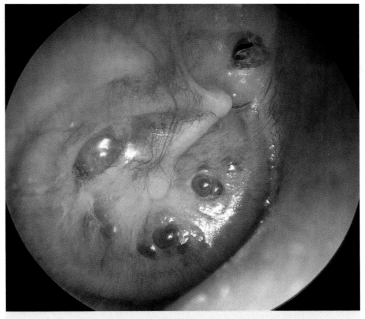

Fig. 4.11 Right ear. Secretory otitis media with tympanosclerosis and epitympanic erosion. The tympanic membrane shows areas of tympanosclerosis alternating with areas of atrophy. Glue is present in the middle ear.

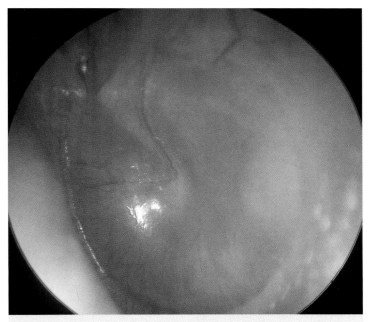

Fig. 4.12 Left ear. Otitis media with effusion and a whitish retrotympanic mass in the posterior quadrant at 3 o'clock can be observed. The presence of congenital cholesteatoma was considered in the differential diagnosis. Exploratory tympanotomy showed only "glue" in the middle ear that was particularly dense in the posterior mesotympanum.

4.2 Secretory Otitis Media Secondary to Neoplasm

See following figures (▶ Fig. 4.13, ▶ Fig. 4.14, ▶ Fig. 4.15, ▶ Fig. 4.16, ▶ Fig. 4.17, ▶ Fig. 4.18, ▶ Fig. 4.19, ▶ Fig. 4.20, ▶ Fig. 4.21, ▶ Fig. 4.22, ▶ Fig. 4.23, ▶ Fig. 4.24, ▶ Fig. 4.25, ▶ Fig. 4.26, ▶ Fig. 4.27, ▶ Fig. 4.28, ▶ Fig. 4.29, ▶ Fig. 4.30).

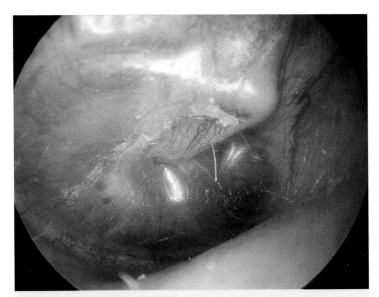

Fig. 4.13 Right ear. Seromucoid effusion in the middle ear. Air bubbles can be seen in the anterior quadrants of the tympanic membrane. The patient is a 53-year-old woman who presented with signs of right otitis media with effusion causing conductive hearing loss and ipsilateral paresthesia of the maxillary and mandibular nerves, followed by episodes of trigeminal neuralgia and diplopia in the last few months. Computed tomography (CT) scan and magnetic resonance imaging (MRI) with gadolinium (see subsequent figures) revealed the presence of a tumor (later proven to be a trigeminal neurinoma) with an intra- and extracranial extensions. The tumor compressed the Eustachian tube and resulted in middle ear effusion. Total removal of the tumor was performed in a single-stage operation using an infratemporal fossa type B approach with orbitozygomatic extension (see ▶ Fig. 4.16).

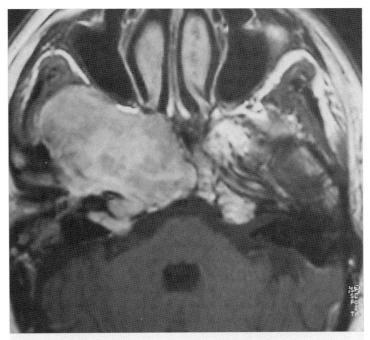

Fig. 4.14 MRI, axial view, showing the extension of the giant trigeminal neuroma.

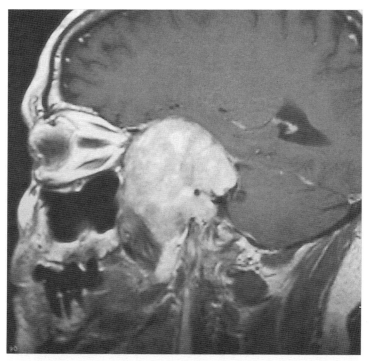

Fig. 4.15 MRI, sagittal view, confirms the intra- and extracranial extensions of the tumor.

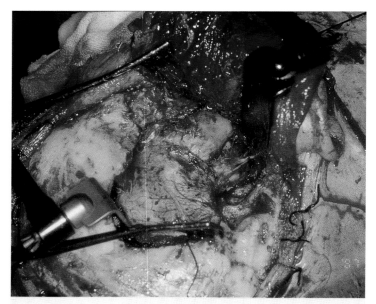

Fig. 4.16 Trigeminal neurinoma removal using an infratemporal type B approach with orbitozygomatic extension.

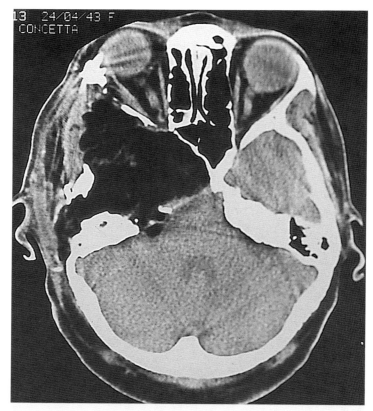

Fig. 4.17 Postoperative CT scan showing total tumor removal.

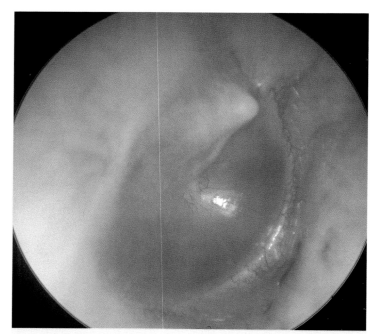

Fig. 4.18 A different case similar to the one in ▶ Fig. 4.11. This 64-year-old woman complained of right nasal obstruction and a sensation of right ear fullness of 1-year duration. One month before presentation, the patient began to suffer from neuralgic pain in the region of the maxillary nerve. The tympanic membrane looks yellowish due to the presence of middle ear effusion (see subsequent figures).

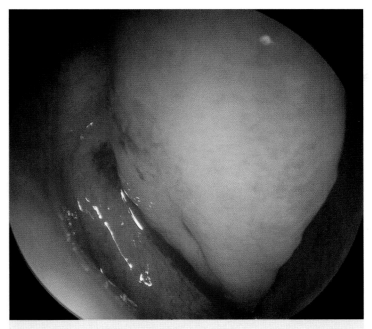

Fig. 4.19 Right nasal cavity, same case. A mass is visualized in the middle meatus. A biopsy proved it to be a neurinoma.

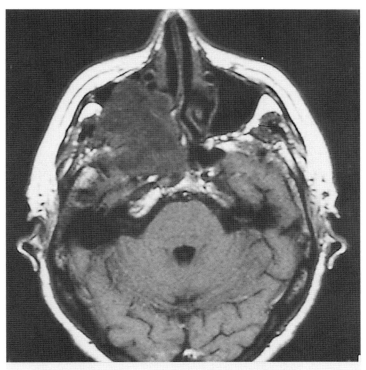

Fig. 4.20 MRI of the same case. A huge trigeminal neurinoma with intra- and extracranial extensions can be seen.

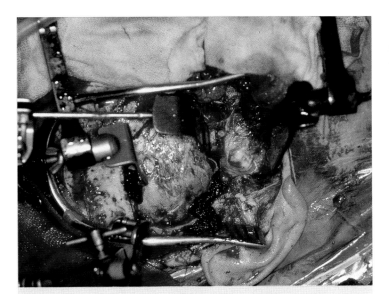

Fig. 4.21 A single-stage, total removal was accomplished using a preauricular infratemporal subtemporal orbitozygomatic approach.

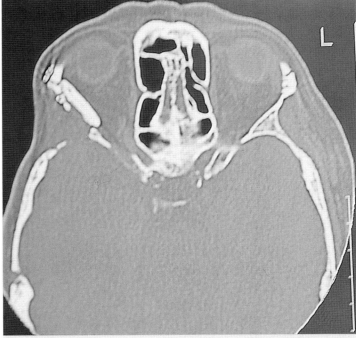

Fig. 4.22 Postoperative CT scan showing total tumor removal. The floor and the lateral wall of the orbit have been reconstructed.

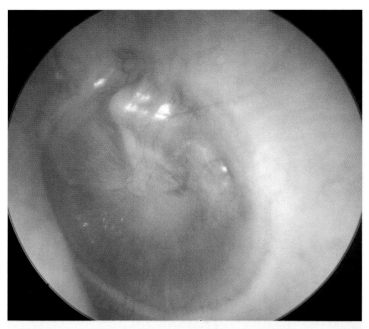

Fig. 4.23 Left ear. An air-fluid level is seen in a young patient with a juvenile nasopharyngeal angiofibroma.

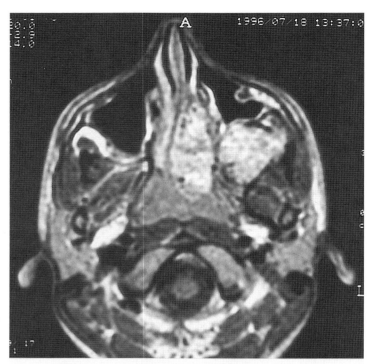

Fig. 4.24 MRI of the same case. The angiofibroma occupies the nasopharynx, pterygopalatine fossa, and infratemporal fossa on the left side. Removal was accomplished using a Fisch type C infratemporal fossa approach.

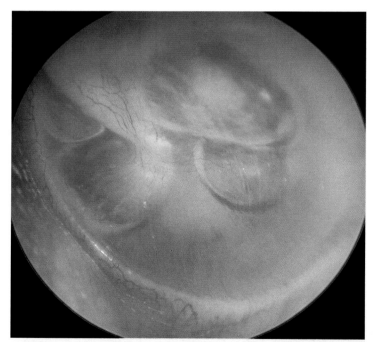

Fig. 4.25 Left ear showing a pulsating air-fluid level in a patient operated 1 year previously to remove a lower cranial nerve neurinoma using a petro-occipital trans-sigmoid approach (POTS) (see preoperative MRI, ▶ Fig. 4.26; postoperative CT scan, ▶ Fig. 4.27). The patient complained of a sensation of ear blockage and watery rhinorrhea on leaning forward. The middle ear is full of cerebrospinal fluid (CSF) passing through open hypotympanic air cells that communicate with the subarachnoid space. The CSF rhinorrhea was treated by obliterating the Eustachian tube and middle ear with the temporalis muscle and by closure of the external auditory canal as a cul-de-sac.

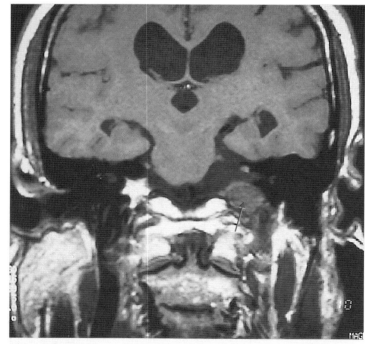

Fig. 4.26 MRI of the same case showing a schwannoma of the lower cranial nerves (arrow).

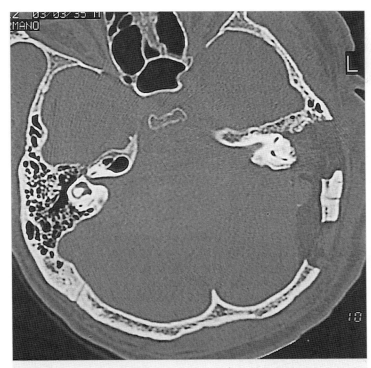

Fig. 4.27 Postoperative CT scan shows the petro-occipital craniotomy and the surgical cavity with preservation of the inner ear.

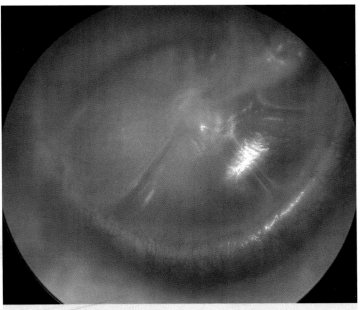

Fig. 4.28 Right ear. Otitis media with effusion in a 47-year-old female patient who complained of right hearing loss and a sensation of ear fullness of 1-year duration. Nasopharyngeal examination was doubtful. MRI (see ▶ Fig. 4.29, ▶ Fig. 4.30) demonstrated the presence of a neoplasm at the level of the right Rosenmüller fossa. A biopsy was performed in this region and revealed the presence of an adenoid cystic carcinoma. The patient was operated and then referred for radiotherapy. Small nasopharyngeal carcinomas can miss detection on MRI. Therefore, adults with unilateral otitis media with effusion, even with normal radiologic examination, should undergo biopsy of the nasopharynx under local anesthesia.

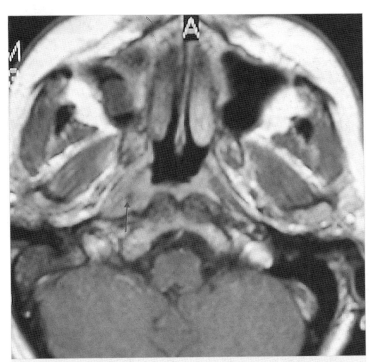

Fig. 4.29 MRI. Small neoplasm at the level of the Rosenmüller fossa (*arrow*).

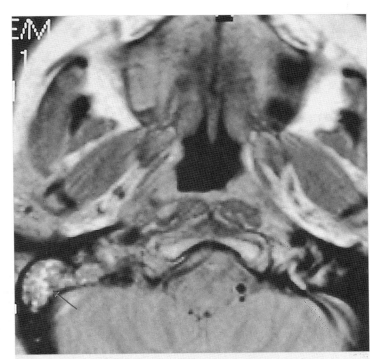

Fig. 4.30 MRI. Effusion in the ipsilateral mastoid is clearly visible (*arrow*).

4.3 Acute Otitis Media

Acute otitis media is usually developing on the basis of a (viral) upper respiratory infection with blockage of the Eustachian tube and effusion in the middle ear, when the fluid in the middle ear gets additionally infected with bacteria. The most common bacteria found in this case are *Streptococcus pneumoniae*, *Haemophilus influenzae*, and *Moraxella catarrhalis*.

In severe or untreated cases, the tympanic membrane may rupture, allowing the pus in the middle ear space to drain into the ear canal. Even though the rupture of the tympanic membrane suggests a highly painful and traumatic process, it is almost always associated with the dramatic relief of pressure and pain.

In a simple case of acute otitis media in an otherwise healthy person, the body's defenses are likely to resolve the infection and the ear drum nearly always heals.

To confirm the diagnosis, middle ear effusion and inflammation of the eardrum have to be identified; signs of these are fullness, bulging, cloudiness, and redness of the eardrum.

Complications of acute otitis media consist in perforation of the ear drum, infection of the mastoid space behind the ear, or bacterial meningitis in rare cases.

Oral and topical analgesics are effective to treat the pain caused by otitis media; the first line antibiotic treatment, if warranted, is amoxicillin (see ▶ Fig. 4.31, ▶ Fig. 4.32, ▶ Fig. 4.33).

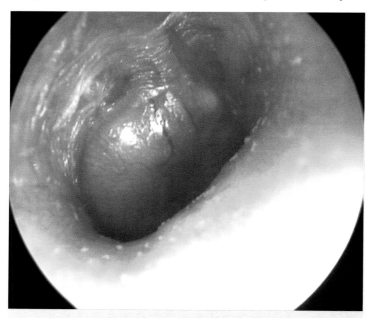

Fig. 4.31 Right ear. Acute otitis media in a 10-year-old boy with upper respiratory infection. The tympanic membrane is bulged on the posterior quadrants and the patient complains of acute pain.

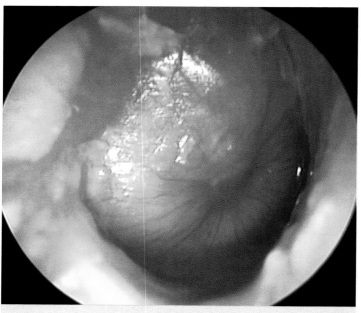

Fig. 4.32 Right ear. Another case of acute otitis media with posterior bulging of the tympanic membrane. The eardrum is close to being ruptured (see ▶ Fig. 4.33).

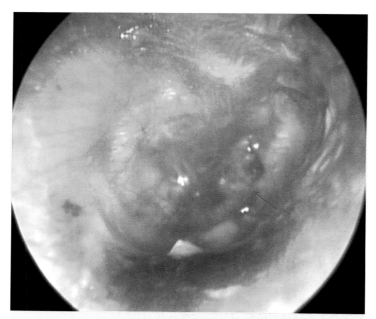

Fig. 4.33 Right ear. Same case of ▶ Fig. 4.32. After few days from the first observation, the patient refers only otorrhea. This stage is characterized by the relief of the ear pain. The eardrum is not bulged and there's fluid in the external auditory canal. A small anterior perforation of the eardrum is visible (*arrow*).

Summary

Otitis media with effusion in children is generally bilateral. If it does not resolve despite appropriate medical treatment for a sufficient period, a myringotomy and the insertion of ventilation tubes are indicated. If necessary, adenoidectomy is also performed in the same session.

In all adult cases of unilateral prolonged otitis media with effusion, nasopharyngeal examination is obligatory to exclude nasopharyngeal carcinoma. In these cases, it is often advisable to take a biopsy under local anesthesia. Biopsy is still indicated even if the radiologic examination has proven normal. A biopsy should not be attempted, however, during endoscopic examination of the nasopharynx if the mass appears macroscopically vascular. Profuse hemorrhage can occur and may be difficult to control.

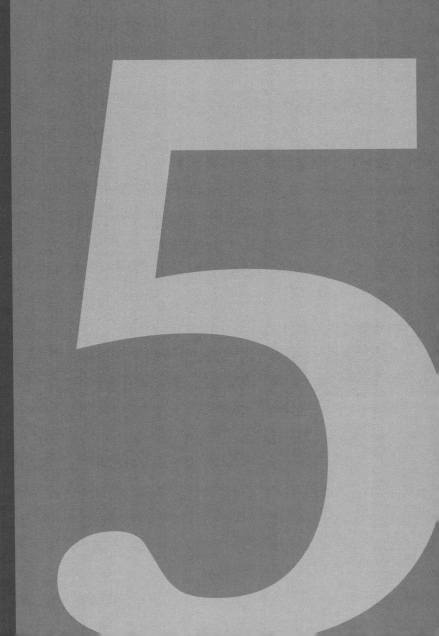

Chapter 5

Cholesterol Granuloma

5 Cholesterol Granuloma

Abstract

In case of a cholesterol granuloma of the temporal bone, the tympanic membrane could appear bluish in color due to hemosiderin crystals in the middle ear. Cholesterol granuloma is thought to arise from obstructed drainage and insufficient aeration of cellular compartments of the temporal bone. Surgical treatment with mastoidectomy is usually performed, even though in the initial phases it may be sufficient to insert a ventilation tube.

Keywords: cholesterol granuloma, hemosiderin, temporal bone drainage

Cholesterol granuloma is a histologic term used to describe a foreign body, giant cell reaction to cholesterol crystals, and hemosiderin derived from ruptured erythrocytes. Cholesterol granuloma is thought to arise from obstructed drainage and insufficient aeration of cellular compartments of the temporal bone. This leads to reabsorption of air, negative pressure, mucosal edema, and hemorrhage. It can be present in the middle ear, mastoid, or petrous apex. Generally, patients with tympanomastoid cholesterol granuloma have a long history of recurrent otitis media or otitis media with effusion. They also complain of conductive hearing loss, and on otoscopy the tympanic membrane appears bluish in color. In some cases, where granulation tissue is more prevalent, cholesterol granuloma can present as a retrotympanic reddish-brown mass that may cause bulging of the tympanic membrane, thus mimicking a glomus tumor. In these cases, a computed tomography (CT) scan is sufficient to clear up any doubts. A cholesterol granuloma rarely causes bone erosion. On the contrary, bone erosion is characteristic of glomus tumors causing destruction of the jugular hypotympanic septum with an irregular "moth-eaten" contour.

Hemotympanum is a different condition due to the presence of blood in the tympanic cavity. The most common causes include head trauma with or without skull base fracture, nasal packing, epistaxis, or clotting disorders.

In the initial phases, before cholesterol granuloma is formed, it might be sufficient to insert a ventilation tube, thus preventing further development of the granuloma. When the granuloma has already formed, it is necessary to perform a tympanoplasty with mastoidectomy that opens the intercellular septa, with subsequent aeration of the middle ear and mastoid.

Refer to the figures presented in this chapter (▶ Fig. 5.1, ▶ Fig. 5.2, ▶ Fig. 5.3, ▶ Fig. 5.4, ▶ Fig. 5.5, ▶ Fig. 5.6, ▶ Fig. 5.7, ▶ Fig. 5.8, ▶ Fig. 5.9, ▶ Fig. 5.10, ▶ Fig. 5.11, ▶ Fig. 5.12, ▶ Fig. 5.13, ▶ Fig. 5.14, ▶ Fig. 5.15, ▶ Fig. 5.16, ▶ Fig. 5.17, ▶ Fig. 5.18).

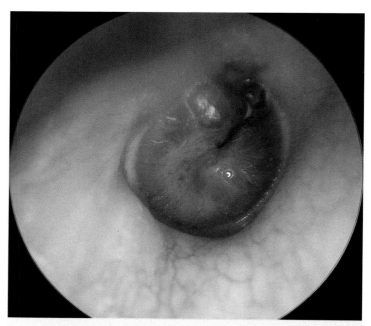

Fig. 5.1 Right ear. Typical blue tympanum caused by cholesterol granuloma. The blue color is due to hemosiderin crystals. The granuloma not only involves the middle ear but also generally extends into the mastoid air cells.

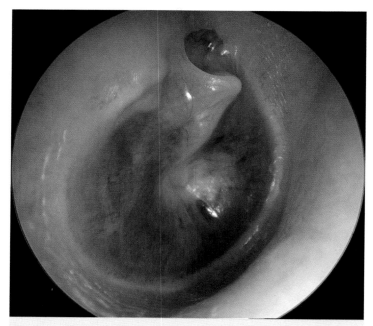

Fig. 5.2 Blue tympanum caused by cholesterol granuloma. An epitympanic retraction due to Eustachian tube dysfunction is also present.

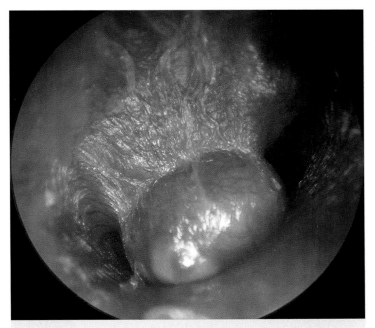

Fig. 5.3 Cholesterol granuloma associated with an inflammatory polyp that leads to bulging of the tympanic membrane.

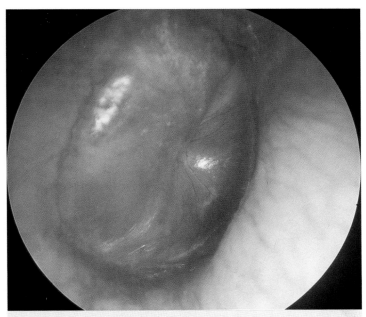

Fig. 5.4 Characteristic blue color of the tympanic membrane caused by a cholesterol granuloma.

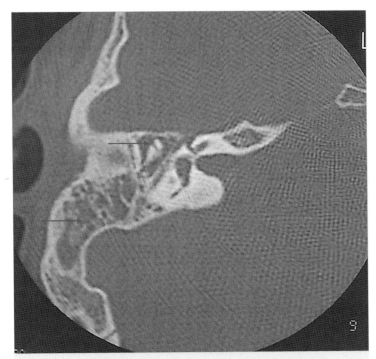

Fig. 5.5 Axial CT of the case shown in ▶ Fig. 5.4. The granuloma and effusion are present in the middle ear and mastoid without causing any bony erosion. The ossicular chain (malleus and incus) is intact and the intercellular septa in the mastoid are preserved.

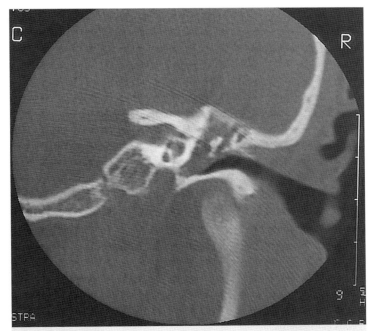

Fig. 5.6 Coronal CT scan of the same patient.

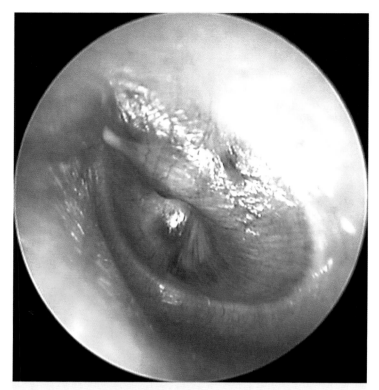

Fig. 5.7 Another case of cholesterol granuloma in a left ear.

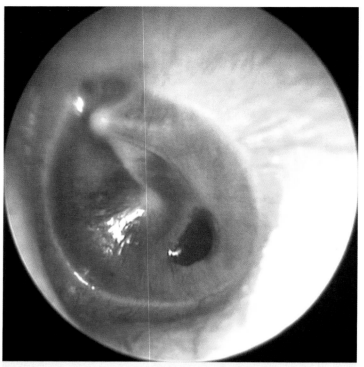

Fig. 5.8 Left ear. Cholesterol granuloma. The tympanic membrane shows a posteroinferior atrophic area, which could be the site of a previous perforation.

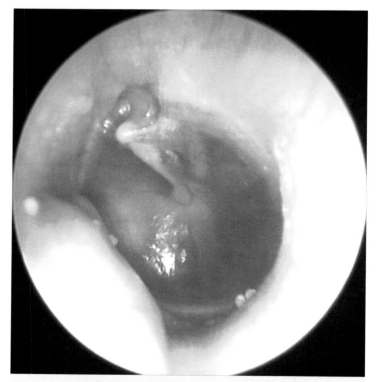

Fig. 5.9 Left ear. Granuloma of the petrous apex extended in the area of the Eustachian tube. A brownish retro-tympanic mass can be seen in the anterosuperior quadrant. The closure of the Eustachian tube leads to accumulation of fluids in the tympanic cavity and mastoid (see ▶ Fig. 5.9, ▶ Fig. 5.10). The patient has conductive hearing loss with fullness and hemifacial pain. In this case, an infra- or retrolabyrinthine approach could be used for the drainage of the granuloma.

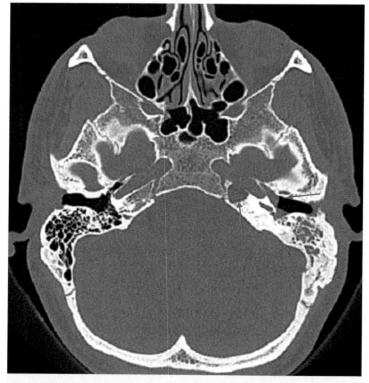

Fig. 5.10 CT scan, axial view of the case in ▶ Fig. 5.9. Granuloma of the petrous apex extended in the tubal region (arrows). Effusion is present in the mastoid and middle ear.

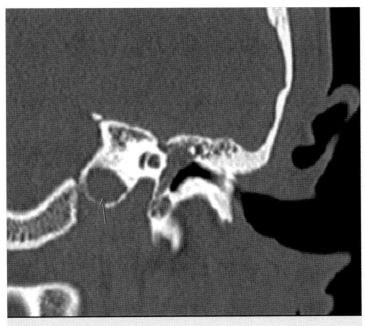

Fig. 5.11 CT scan, coronal view.

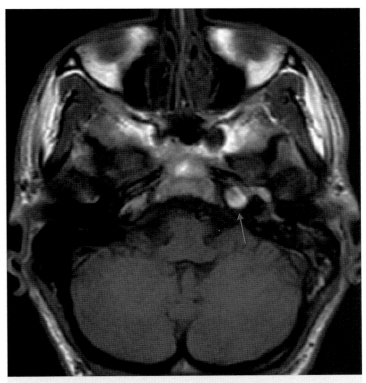

Fig. 5.12 MRI, axial view, T1 W sequence. Cholesterol granuloma shows a typical hyperintense signal in both T1 and T2 weighted sequences (*arrow*).

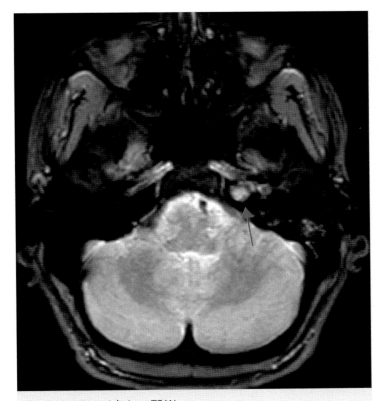

Fig. 5.13 MRI, axial view, T2 W sequence.

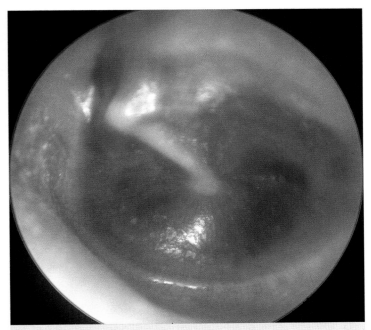

Fig. 5.14 Left ear. A 17-year-old male patient complained of conductive hearing loss of 1 year's duration accompanied by left nasal obstruction. Otoscopy revealed the presence of a left cholesterol granuloma. Rhinoscopy showed the presence of a nasopharyngeal swelling that extended into the left nasal cavity. The swelling was suggestive of a juvenile nasopharyngeal angiofibroma.

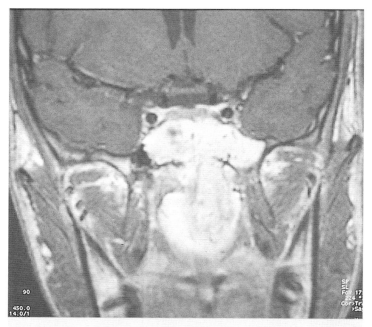

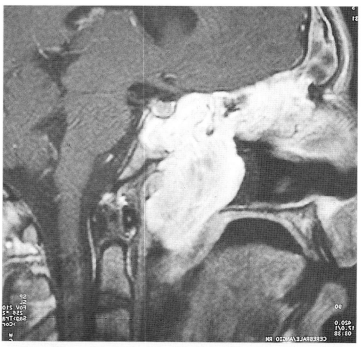

Fig. 5.15 Magnetic resonance imaging (MRI) of the same case, coronal view, showing the extension of the angiofibroma in the nasopharynx and sphenoid sinus.

Fig. 5.16 MRI of the same case, sagittal view, showing the extension of the tumor from the ethmoid to the rhinopharynx pushing the soft palate.

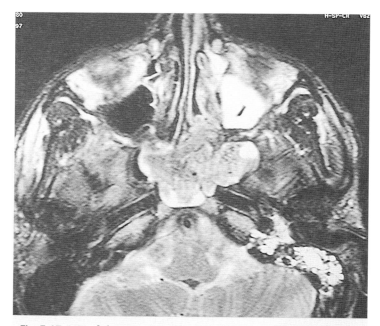

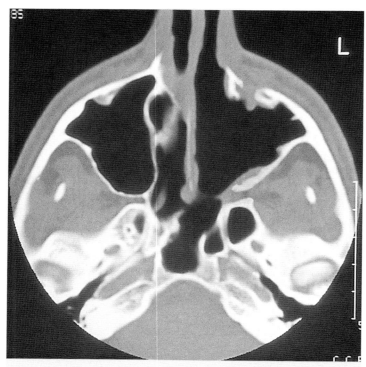

Fig. 5.17 MRI of the same case, axial view. Involvement of the middle ear and mastoid by the cholesterol granuloma can be observed.

Fig. 5.18 Postoperative CT (1 year) confirming the total tumor removal.

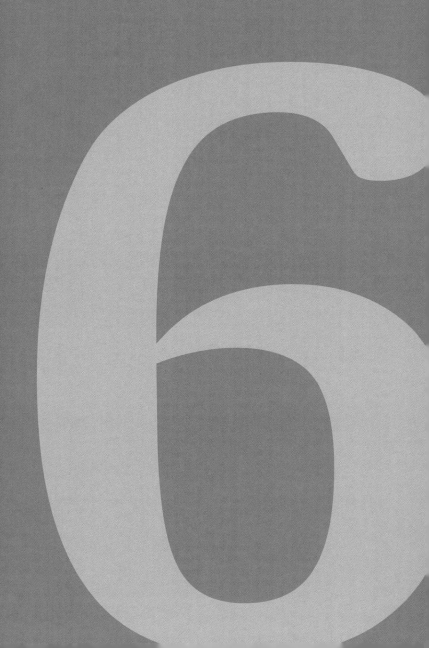

Chapter 6

Atelectasis, Adhesive Otitis Media

6 Atelectasis, Adhesive Otitis Media

Abstract

Adhesive otitis media is characterized by retraction of the thin and atrophic tympanic membrane to the medial wall of the middle ear due to the negative middle ear pressure caused by Eustachian tube dysfunction or persistent secretory otitis media. Different grades of atelectasis can be distinguished, based on Sadè classification: Grade I corresponds to a mild retraction, while Grade IV is a complete atelectasis of the tympanic membrane. Treatment depends on the grade of retraction and hearing function. Each grade of atelectasis with the relative management will be discussed in this chapter.

Keywords: adhesive otitis media, retraction pocket, Sadè classification, ventilation tube

Adhesive otitis media is characterized by complete or partial adhesions between the thin retracted and atrophic pars tensa and the medial wall of the middle ear. Necrosis of the long process of the incus or the stapes suprastructure can also occur, with a resultant natural myringostapedopexy. It should be differentiated from atelectasis and from simple drum retraction, in which the tympanic membrane is mobile with the Valsalva or Toynbee maneuvers.

Sadè (1979) distinguished five grades of atelectasis (▶ Fig. 6.1): Grade I is characterized by a mild retraction of the tympanic membrane; in grade II, the retracted tympanic membrane comes in contact with the incus or the stapes; in Grade III, the tympanic membrane touches the promontory; Grade IV is adhesive otitis media; and, in Grade V, there is a spontaneous perforation of the atelectatic ear drum with otorrhea and polyp formation.

Nakano (1993) proposed two types of adhesive otitis: type A, in which the retracted and atrophic tympanic membrane adheres completely to the promontory, and, type B, in which retraction and adhesion affect mainly the posterior part of the tympanic membrane, usually without retraction of its anterior half. Histologically, the tympanic membrane is atrophic due to thinning or even absence of the lamina propria. It can be hypothesized that the negative middle ear pressure caused by Eustachian tube dysfunction or persistent secretory otitis media leads to atrophy of the elastic fiber of the pars tensa. An occasional episode of acute suppurative otitis media might form adhesions between the mucosa of the promontory and the retracted tympanic membrane.

The figures in this chapter present different grades of atelectasis and types of adhesive otitis media (▶ Fig. 6.2, ▶ Fig. 6.3, ▶ Fig. 6.4, ▶ Fig. 6.5, ▶ Fig. 6.6, ▶ Fig. 6.7, ▶ Fig. 6.8, ▶ Fig. 6.9, ▶ Fig. 6.10, ▶ Fig. 6.11, ▶ Fig. 6.12, ▶ Fig. 6.13, ▶ Fig. 6.14, ▶ Fig. 6.15, ▶ Fig. 6.16, ▶ Fig. 6.17, ▶ Fig. 6.18, ▶ Fig. 6.19, ▶ Fig. 6.20, ▶ Fig. 6.21, ▶ Fig. 6.22, ▶ Fig. 6.23, ▶ Fig. 6.24, ▶ Fig. 6.25, ▶ Fig. 6.26, ▶ Fig. 6.27, ▶ Fig. 6.28, ▶ Fig. 6.29, ▶ Fig. 6.30, ▶ Fig. 6.31, ▶ Fig. 6.32, ▶ Fig. 6.33, ▶ Fig. 6.34, ▶ Fig. 6.35, ▶ Fig. 6.36, ▶ Fig. 6.37, ▶ Fig. 6.38).

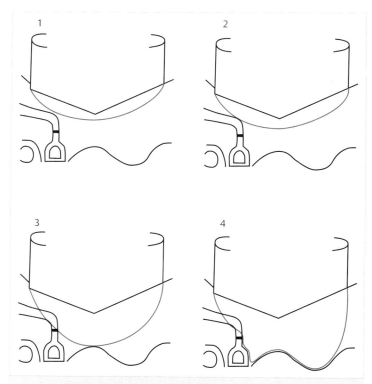

Fig. 6.1 Sadè classification of atelectasis (modified) (see text).

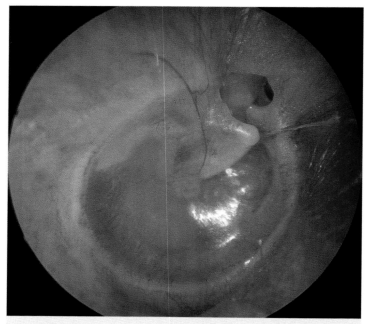

Fig. 6.2 Right ear. Sadè Grade I atelectasis. The tympanic membrane is retracted but does not come into contact with the middle ear structures. A mild retraction of the pars flaccida, through which the head of the malleus is visible, is also noted. The base of the retraction pocket is under control, with no sign of cholesteatoma. It is also possible in this case to assume that the drum is mobile on Valsalva or Toynbee maneuvers. This patient presented with very mild conductive hearing loss and a normal tympanogram (type A) (see ▶ Fig. 6.3 and ▶ Fig. 6.4).

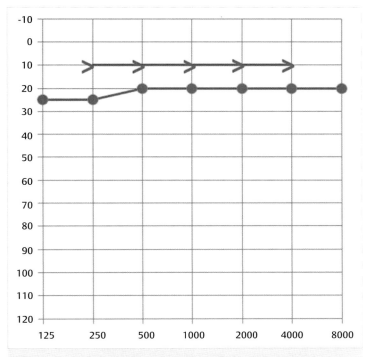

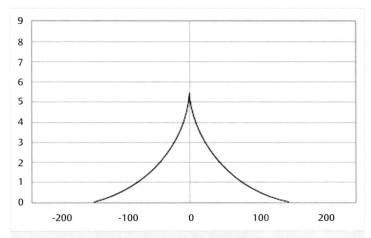

Fig. 6.4 Tympanogram of the same case. Normal or type A.

Fig. 6.3 Audiogram of the same case. Mild conductive hearing loss.

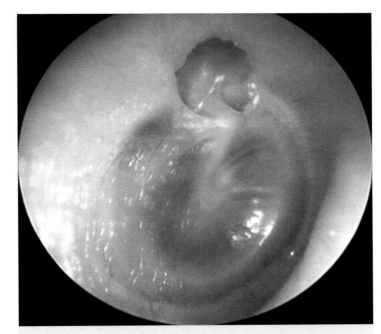

Fig. 6.5 Right ear. Grade I atelectasis. This case could represent an evolution of that in ▶ Fig. 6.2. There is a deeper retraction pocket with erosion of the scutum. Even if it is a self-cleaning retraction pocket and the base seems under control, it is better to perform a CT scan to exclude an epitympanic cholesteatoma or strictly follow-up the patient with proper otoscopic evaluations. The hearing function is the same as in ▶ Fig. 6.3.

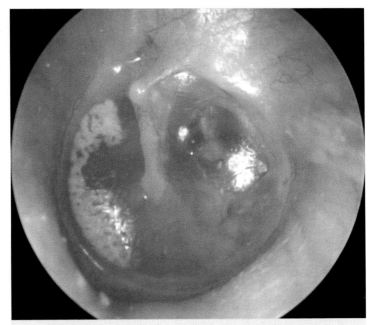

Fig. 6.6 Left ear. Another case of Grade I atelectasis. There is an erosion of the long process of the incus, resulting in mild conductive hearing loss (within 20 dB). A myringosclerosis of the anterior quadrants of the tympanic membrane is also visible. Considering the hearing function and the absence of other symptoms, the patient could be just followed up with otoscopic examinations. In case of worsening of hearing function, ossiculoplasty with autologous remodeled incus and a posterior reinforcement of the tympanic membrane with tragal cartilage should be considered.

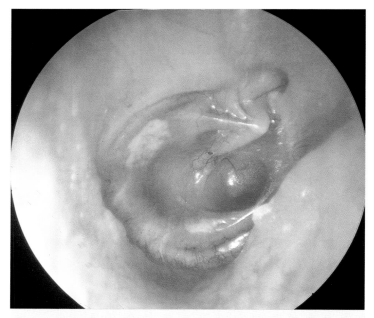

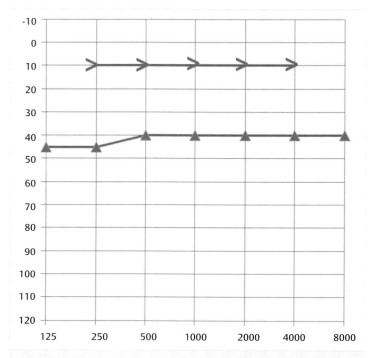

Fig. 6.7 Right ear. Grade I atelectasis with the malleus slightly medialized. An epitympanic retraction pocket is also seen. A yellowish middle ear effusion can be appreciated. Pure tone audiogram revealed a 40-dB conductive hearing loss (▶ Fig. 6.8), whereas the tympanogram was type B, i.e., typical of middle ear effusion (▶ Fig. 6.9). In this case, the insertion of a ventilation tube is indicated to avoid further retraction of the tympanic membrane, to aerate the middle ear, and to improve hearing.

Fig. 6.8 Audiogram of the same case, showing a 40-dB conductive hearing loss.

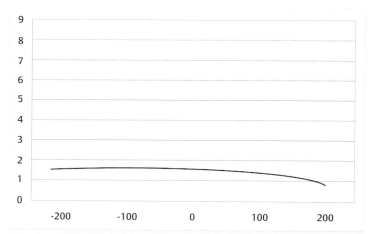

Fig. 6.9 Type B tympanogram of the same case, typical of middle ear effusion.

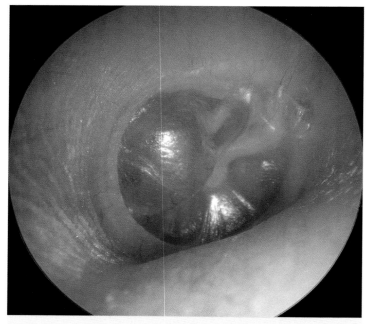

Fig. 6.10 Right ear. Grade I atelectasis. The tympanic membrane is markedly thinned due to partial resorption of the lamina propria. The incus is seen in transparency. Pure tone audiogram is normal (▶ Fig. 6.11), whereas the tympanogram has a very high compliance (▶ Fig. 6.12). As the tympanic membrane is mobile with the Valsalva maneuver, insertion of a ventilation tube is not indicated.

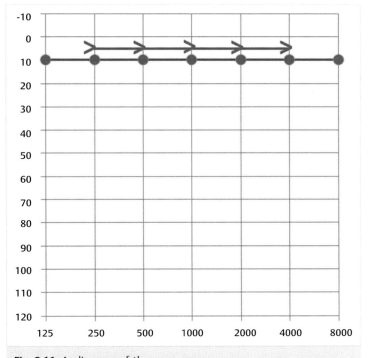

Fig. 6.11 Audiogram of the same case.

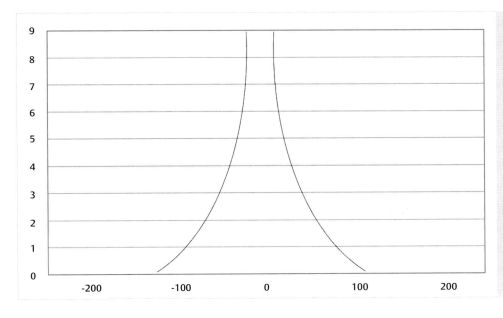

Fig. 6.12 Tympanogram of the same case, type Ad according to the classification of Liden-Jerger, 1976.

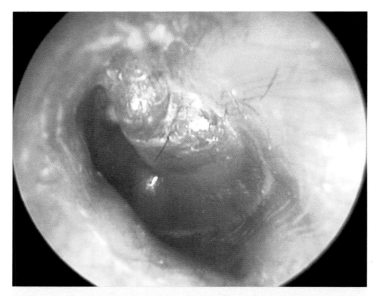

Fig. 6.13 Another case similar to that in ▶ Fig. 6.10. Note the hyperectasis of the posterior quadrants of the tympanic membrane. The hearing function is close to normal.

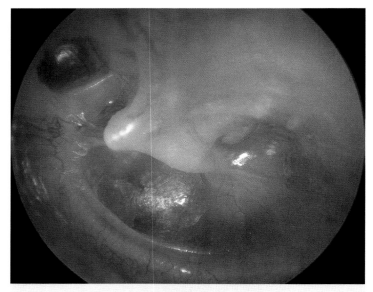

Fig. 6.14 Left ear. Grade II atelectasis with marked epitympanic retraction. The tympanic membrane touches the incus. The malleus is medialized. Air-fluid level is seen in the anteroinferior quadrant. The insertion of a ventilation tube is necessary to restore normal conditions.

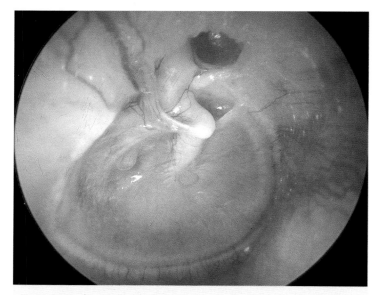

Fig. 6.15 Right ear. Grade II atelectasis. A condition similar to the previous case, but with the onset of thickening of the tympanic membrane.

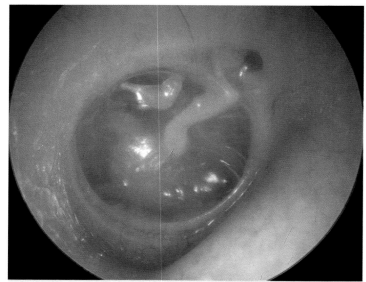

Fig. 6.16 Right ear. Grade II atelectasis. The tympanic membrane is very thin due to the absence of the fibrous layer. The membrane adheres to the incudostapedial joint and the tensor tympani tendon. Insertion of a ventilation tube is indicated.

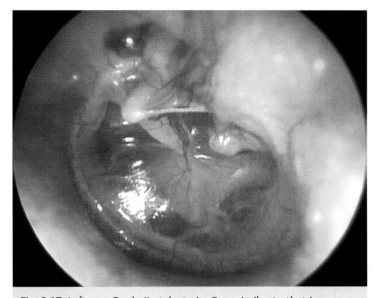

Fig. 6.17 Left ear. Grade II atelectasis. Case similar to that in ▶ Fig. 6.16. The tympanic membrane is very thin and adheres to the incudostapedial joint (long process of the incus partially eroded). There is an attical retraction pocket with erosion of the scutum. The body, the neck, and part of the head of the malleus are visible. Audiometry shows a mild conductive hearing loss. In this case insertion of a ventilation tube is indicated, but the patient should be strictly followed up to exclude evolution of both the attical and mesotympanic retractions into cholesteatoma.

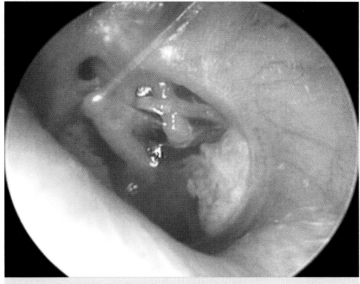

Fig. 6.18 Left ear. Grade II atelectasis. The tympanic membrane is completely adherent to the incudostapedial joint. The chorda tympani is visible. Myringosclerosis in both the posterior and anterior quadrants is present. A ventilation tube should be placed to prevent further retraction and erosion of the ossicular chain.

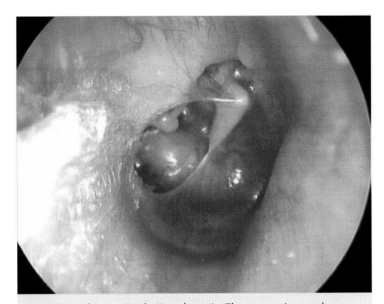

Fig. 6.19 Right ear. Grade III atelectasis. The tympanic membrane, being adherent to the long process of the incus, caused erosion of the latter with subsequent conductive hearing loss (see ▶ Fig. 6.20). Part of the tympanic membrane adheres to the promontorium, so the round window is visible in transparency. The patient referred to occasional otorrhea. A tympanoplasty should be performed with reinforcement of the tympanic membrane and incus interposition between the handle of the malleus and the stapes.

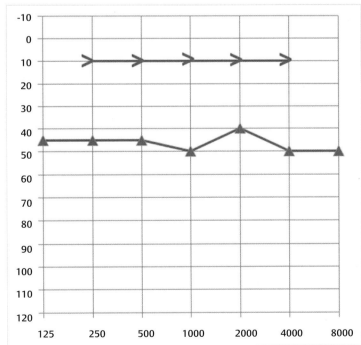

Fig. 6.20 Audiogram in the same case showing conductive hearing loss.

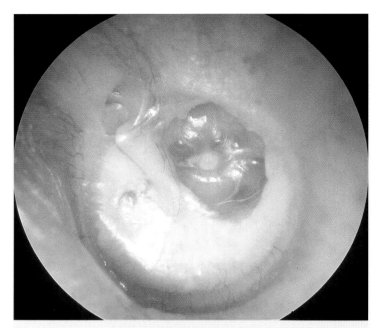

Fig. 6.21 Left ear. Posterior retraction pocket. The tympanic membrane remains adherent to the stapes even after Valsalva maneuver (myringostapedopexy). The remaining part of the tympanic membrane is thick and shows tympanosclerosis. Audiometry revealed normal hearing. Patients with myringostapedopexy generally have good hearing; therefore, surgery is not indicated except if conductive hearing loss develops and/or a posterior retraction pocket is associated with frequent otorrhea. Surgery varies from simple myringoplasty (when the tympanic membrane needs reinforcement) to tympanoplasty (in which the ossicular chain is eroded and needs ossiculoplasty).

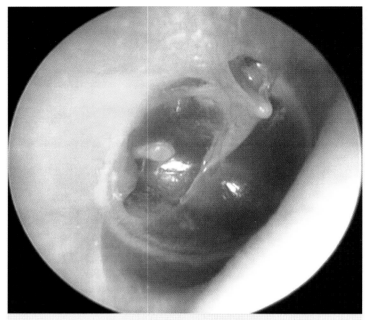

Fig. 6.22 Right ear. Grade III atelectasis. The long process of the incus is absent. The tympanic membrane is thin and adheres to the head of the stapes and slightly to the promontorium. Hearing function is normal, so surgery is not indicated.

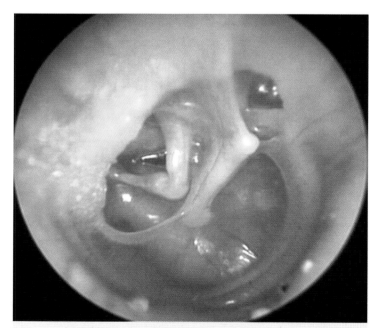

Fig. 6.23 Right ear. Grade III atelectasis. The tympanic membrane completely adheres to the long process of the incus (slightly eroded) and the stapes. The second portion of the facial nerve is visible under the incus. There is also a retraction pocket of the anterosuperior quadrant. In this case, placement of a ventilation tube is indicated to prevent further erosion of the ossicular chain and the formation of a cholesteatoma.

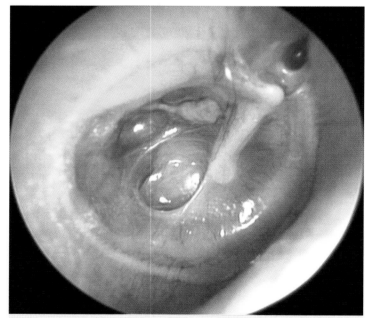

Fig. 6.24 Right ear. Grade III atelectasis. Myringostapedopexy with normal hearing. The long process of the incus is absent.

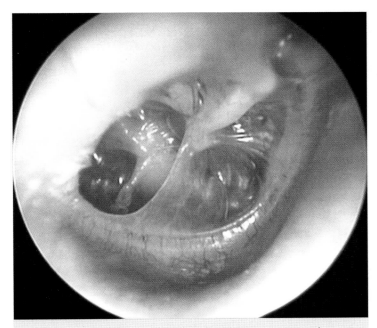

Fig. 6.25 Right ear. Grade III atelectasis. The tympanic membrane is adherent to the oval window (myringoplatinopexy). The long process of the incus is eroded. The round window is visible too. Hearing is normal even in this case, so surgery is indicated only in case of otorrhea or destabilization of the mesotympanic retraction pocket.

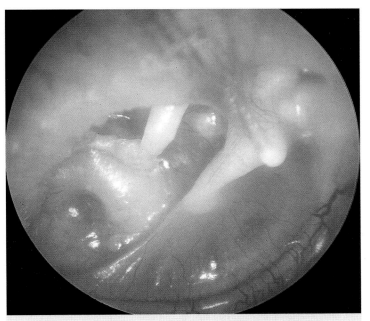

Fig. 6.26 Right ear. Posterior retraction pocket. The tympanic membrane adheres to the promontory, the round window, the partially eroded long process of the incus, the head of the stapes, and the stapedius tendon. The processus cochleariformis is clearly visible between the malleus and the long process of the incus. Middle ear effusion can be observed anterior to the malleus and in the region of the oval window. In this case, ventilation tube insertion is indicated in an attempt to prevent further erosion of the ossicular chain and the formation of mesotympanic cholesteatoma.

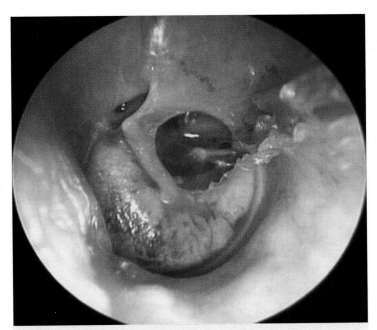

Fig. 6.27 Left ear. Posterior retraction pocket with myringostapedopexy. The patient complained of recurrent otorrhea. Hearing function is normal. The retraction pocket is not under control with skin migration toward the mesotympanic area. The suspect of a mesotympanic cholesteatoma is high, so a CT scan is recommended in this case, even for a correct surgical management.

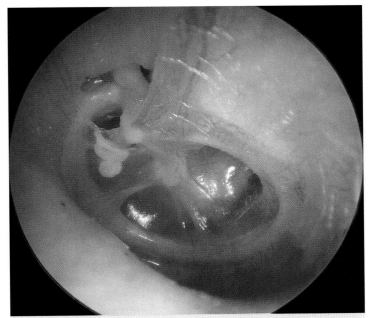

Fig. 6.28 Left ear. Grade III atelectasis. The thin and atrophic tympanic membrane is in contact with the promontory. Middle ear effusion is seen. A tympanosclerotic plaque is present in the anterosuperior quadrant. The head of the malleus is visible through an epitympanic retraction pocket. The insertion of a ventilation tube is indicated.

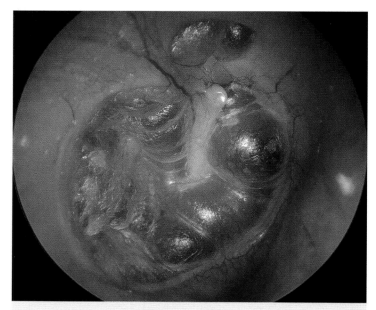

Fig. 6.29 Right ear. Adhesive otitis media or Grade IV atelectasis associated with a mild epitympanic retraction pocket. The thin and atrophic tympanic membrane completely covers the promontory. The tympanic membrane retraction has caused erosion of the long process of the incus, with a subsequent spontaneous myringostapedopexy. As the patient has no hearing loss, surgery is not indicated.

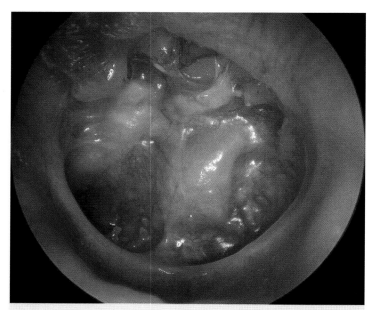

Fig. 6.30 Left ear. Adhesive otitis media. This case represents the long-term sequelae of persistent secretory otitis media with chronic Eustachian tube dysfunction. The fibrous and mucosal layers of the tympanic membrane have been resorbed, whereas the epidermal layer is completely adherent to the medial wall of the middle ear. The promontory, round and oval windows, as well as residue of the ossicular chain are all visible. The handle of the malleus is completely medialized and partially eroded. The long process of the incus is eroded whereas the stapes suprastructure is completely absent. As the patient is not suffering from otorrhea, surgery is not advised.

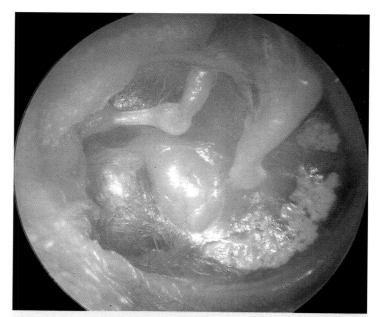

Fig. 6.31 Right ear. The thin and atrophic tympanic membrane adheres to the promontory, incudostapedial joint, pyramidal process, and stapedius tendon. The long process of the incus is partially eroded. Calcifications are present in the anterior quadrants. As hearing is normal, surgery is not indicated.

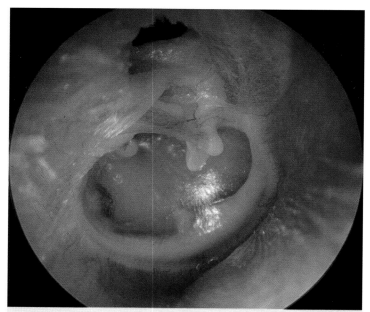

Fig. 6.32 Right ear. Atelectasis associated with marked epitympanic erosion through which the head of the malleus and the body of the incus are seen covered with epithelial squamae. The tympanic membrane is thin and transparent due to absence of the fibrous layer. The handle of the malleus is amputated. The long process of the incus is eroded, and a natural myringostapedopexy is seen. The promontory, round window, head of the stapes, and oval window can be seen through the thin tympanic membrane. Despite the attic epithelialization, a true cholesteatoma has not yet formed. Regular follow-up of such patient is vital. Should the disease progress with cholesteatoma formation, surgery in the form of an open tympanoplasty is indicated.

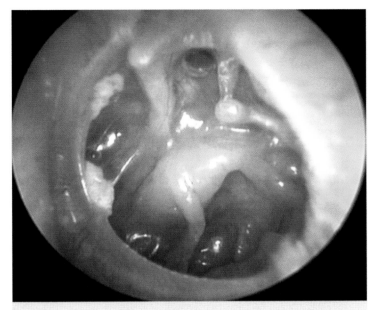

Fig. 6.33 Right ear. Adhesive otitis media. Similar to the case in ▶ Fig. 6.18, the fibrous and mucosal layers of the tympanic membrane have been resorbed, whereas the epidermal layer is completely adherent to the medial wall of the middle ear. The handle of the malleus is medialized, while the long process of the incus is eroded. The contralateral ear has a similar aspect, with the same hearing function. Considering that the patient suffered from bilateral moderate conductive hearing loss (see ▶ Fig. 6.34) and the clinical condition had been stable since years, the application of a right bone anchored hearing aid was performed.

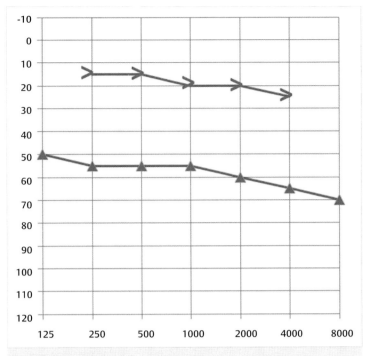

Fig. 6.34 Audiogram of the same case.

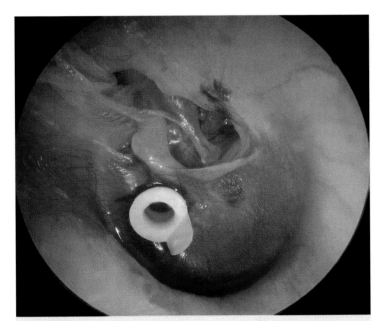

Fig. 6.35 Left ear. Meso- and epitympanic retraction pockets that adhere to the head of the malleus, the partially eroded long process of the incus, and the incudostapedial joint. A ventilation tube has been inserted in the anterior quadrant to avoid further retraction that might lead to cholesteatoma.

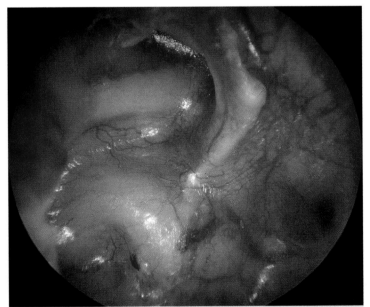

Fig. 6.36 Right ear. Large mesotympanic retraction pocket that caused erosion of the incus and stapes suprastructure. The second portion of the facial nerve passing superior to the oval window, the promontory, and the round window can all be seen in transparency. In patients with good social hearing and no otorrhea, surgery is not indicated.

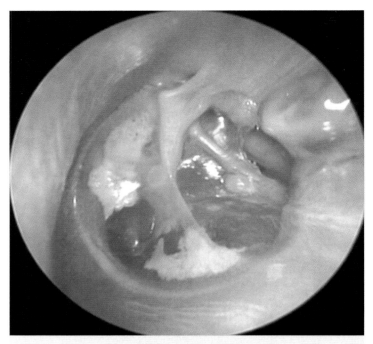

Fig. 6.37 Left ear. Grade V atelectasis. There is a mesotympanic retraction pocket with myringostapedopexy and skin migration on the medial surface of the perforation. The long process of the incus is absent. The second portion of the facial nerve is clearly visible under the tympanic perforation. Tympanoplasty is recommended in such condition.

Summary

In Grades I to III atelectasis, a long-term ventilation tube is usually inserted to prevent further retraction of the tympanic membrane. However, in cases with marked conductive hearing loss that denotes erosion of the incus or the superstructure of the stapes, ossiculoplasty is performed after extraction and sculpturing of the eroded incus. A large disk of tragal cartilage is used to reinforce the tympanic membrane. Indications for surgery in adhesive otitis media include cases with tympanic membrane perforation (Grade V according to Sadè 1979), with or without polyps, granulation or otorrhea, those cases with a large infected retraction pocket causing frequent otorrhea, or those with conductive hearing loss due to ossicular chain erosion. In all these cases, a tympanoplasty is performed using a postauricular incision. A disk of tragal cartilage is used with the perichondrium adherent to its lateral surface. If the handle of the malleus is present, it is incorporated into the cartilaginous disk after a triangular defect has been created to accommodate it. This technique has the advantage of preventing retraction and adhesions between the tympanic membrane and the promontory. At the same time, it enables repair of the tympanic membrane perforation with the tragal perichondrium. It can be concluded that there is no single treatment for the atelectatic ear. The milder the degree of atelectasis, the more conservative the treatment is. It should be noted, however, that in the long term conservative treatment (e.g., ventilation tube) has not been found to modify the further evolution of atelectasis. As atelectasis results from Eustachian tube dysfunction, the ideal solution would be correction of this defect. At present, there is no acceptable "functional" surgery for the Eustachian tube. Individual treatment should be administered according to the consequences of this dysfunction in each case. Such a strategy, however, requires a flexible approach and versatile surgical techniques.

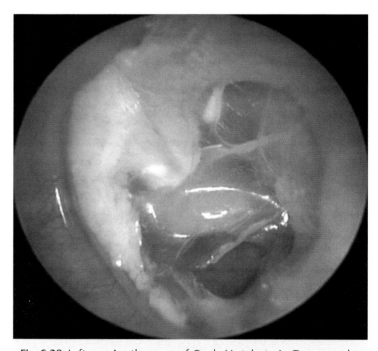

Fig. 6.38 Left ear. Another case of Grade V atelectasis. Tympanosclerosis of the anterior quadrant is present with malleus fixation. The long process of the incus is amputated and the stapes suprastructure is absent. The tympanic perforation corresponds to the area of the round window. This patient suffered from severe conductive hearing loss. Cartilage tympanoplasty was performed with incus reposition between the handle of the malleus and the oval window.

Chapter 7

Noncholesteatomatous Chronic Otitis Media

7

7 Noncholesteatomatous Chronic Otitis Media

Abstract

Chronic otitis media corresponds to a tympanic membrane perforation that does not heal spontaneously. The most commonly encountered forms are active chronic suppurative otitis media, characterized by otorrhea, and inactive chronic suppurative otitis media, in which the ear is dry. Tympanic perforations could also be classified depending on the quadrant involved. In the majority of cases, this condition represents an anatomical and functional defect that needs surgical correction (myringoplasty). Tympanosclerosis represents a worst clinical condition characterized by fibroblastic invasion of the middle ear due to chronic inflammation. As a result, calcium deposits could stiffen the tympanic membrane and/or the ossicular chain with hearing loss. Surgical management of this condition is still controversial.

Keywords: chronic otitis media, tympanic perforation, otorrhea, myringoplasty, tympanosclerosis

The difference between acute and chronic otitis media is not the duration of the disease but rather the anatomopathological characteristics. Untreated acute otitis media persisting for months is still a process that tends essentially to return to normality. On the other hand, a chronic otitis, even if the ear stops discharging, has anatomopathological sequelae of clinical importance. The most common encountered forms are active chronic suppurative otitis media, characterized by otorrhea, and inactive chronic suppurative otitis media, in which the ear is dry. Naturally, the active form may become quiescent either spontaneously or following treatment. The ear becomes dry and the condition is designated inactive. A dry perforation, however, may be infected, leading to ear discharge. In this latter case, the mucosa may be hyperplastic and thick due to interstitial edema, fibrosis, or cellular infiltration. In other cases, persistence of suppuration can lead to ulceration of the mucosa, formation of granulation tissue, and even bone resorption. The anatomical sequelae of chronic otitis media vary. They may be in the form of a simple central tympanic membrane perforation, erosion of the ossicular chain, or formation of tympanosclerosis. Both the active and inactive forms cause functional alterations such as conductive or mixed hearing loss (very rarely sensorineural). The absence of squamous epithelium in the middle ear has led to the designation of this form as a "safe type" of otitis media. This is to distinguish it from cholesteatoma, which is considered "unsafe" due to the potential complications that may arise from the presence of keratinized squamous epithelium in the middle ear.

7.1 General Characteristics of Tympanic Membrane Perforations

Tympanic membrane perforations are usually present at the pars tensa. Pars flaccida perforations are generally associated with epitympanic cholesteatoma.

If a tympanic membrane perforation does not heal spontaneously, the epithelial and mucosal layers creep and meet along the borders of the perforation. This pathological communication between the middle and external ear can be considered a true "air fistula." In the presence of a tympanic membrane perforation, the patient is subjected to recurrent infections and ear discharge. Whenever tympanic membrane perforations are diagnosed, the following three assessments must be performed: (1) at the level of the perforation, the site, size, and state of the remainder of the tympanic membrane around the perforation should be determined; (2) at the level of the middle ear, the state of the mucosa, the condition of the ossicular chain (if possible), and the presence or absence of epithelialization should be evaluated; (3) the otoscopic examination has to be complemented with pure tone audiometry to obtain a better understanding of the ossicular chain (possible erosion of the incus, fixity of the chain).

Pars tensa perforations can be either central or marginal. Marginal perforations lie at the periphery of the tympanic membrane with absence of the fibrous annulus. Marginal perforations are considered "unsafe" because the skin of the external auditory canal, in the absence of the annulus, can easily advance toward the middle ear, giving rise to cholesteatoma.

Otoscopic examination can often define the junction between the skin and the mucosa at the borders of the tympanic membrane perforation. At this junction, the squamous epithelium has a "velvety" appearance. The presence of a red de-epithelialized ring along the perforation rim indicates the evagination of the mucosa toward the external surface of the tympanic membrane residue.

However, invagination of the skin toward the inner surface of the tympanic membrane residue is more difficult to diagnose. This inward skin migration is favored by the atrophy of the mucosa which occurs as a result of the perforation. At the time of myringoplasty, freshening of the edge of the perforation not only promotes the attachment of the graft but also greatly reduces the risk of leaving entrapped skin on the undersurface of the drum, which may lead to iatrogenic cholesteatoma.

Conductive hearing loss caused by tympanic membrane perforation has two main causes: (1) reduction of the tympanic membrane surface area on which the acoustic pressure exerts its action and (2) reduction of the vibratory movements of the cochlear fluids, because sound reaches both windows at nearly the same time without dampening and phase-changing effect of the intact tympanic membrane.

The site of the perforation cannot be correlated to a particular audiometric pattern. However, it is generally observed that hearing loss occurs more in the low frequencies and that, for perforations of the same size, hearing loss occurs more in the posterior perforations than in anterior ones.

The majority of posttraumatic and postotitic perforations heal spontaneously. When large portions of the tympanic membrane are lost or when chronic or recurrent infections occur, the perforation may become permanent. In these cases, the tympanic membrane must be repaired (myringoplasty) to restore the normal physiology of the ear.

7.2 Posterior Perforations

These type of perforations have been shown in ► Fig. 7.1, ► Fig. 7.2, ► Fig. 7.3, ► Fig. 7.4, ► Fig. 7.5, ► Fig. 7.6, ► Fig. 7.7, ► Fig. 7.8, ► Fig. 7.9, ► Fig. 7.10.

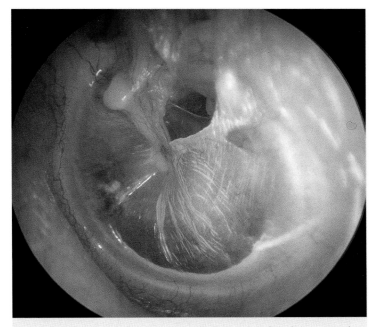

Fig. 7.1 Left ear. The tympanic membrane is very thin due to atrophy of the fibrous layer. A posterosuperior marginal perforation is seen. This perforation is risky because the skin of the external auditory canal can easily advance into the middle ear, forming a cholesteatoma. In this case, a myringoplasty using an endomeatal approach is indicated.

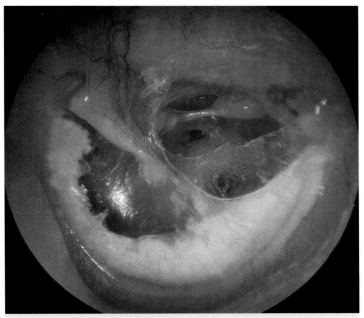

Fig. 7.2 Left ear. Perforation of the posterosuperior quadrant of the tympanic membrane. Visualized through the perforation are the incudostapedial joint, the stapes, the stapedius tendon, the pyramidal process, the promontory, and the round window. The residue of the tympanic membrane is very thin due to absence of the fibrous layer. Tympanosclerosis can be seen in the marginal part of the drum residue. From the surgical point of view, posterior perforations are the easiest to repair, especially when partial reconstruction of the tympanic membrane is all that is required. When the residue of the tympanic membrane is transformed into a rigid tympanosclerotic plaque, it is advisable to remove it, conserving the epidermal layer to be laid over the graft.

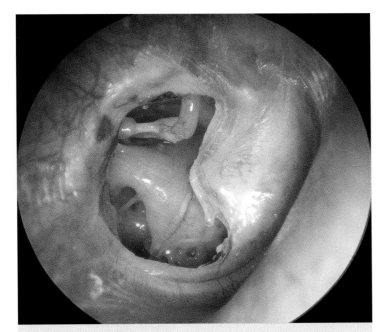

Fig. 7.3 Right ear. Large perforation of the posterior quadrants. Normal middle ear mucosa. The incudostapedial joint is intact. The oval window with the annular ligament surrounding the footplate can be seen. The pyramidal eminence, the stapedius tendon, the round window, and Jacobson's nerve running on the promontory are also visible. The remaining anterior quadrants of the tympanic membrane are tympanosclerotic and rigid, blocking the mobility of the malleus.

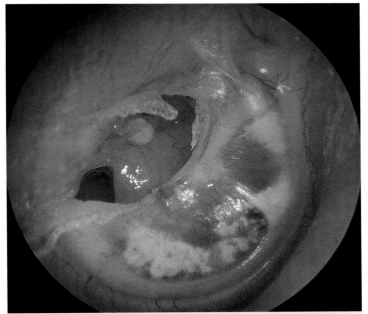

Fig. 7.4 Right ear. Presence of chronic otitis media. Dry perforation of the posterior quadrants of the tympanic membrane, through which the head of the stapes and the round window are visible. The long process of the incus is necrosed. The middle ear mucosa is normal. The tympanic membrane residue shows tympanosclerosis with alternating areas of calcification and areas of thinned membrane due to atrophy of the fibrous layer. The operation, performed through a postauricular incision, will also include the reconstruction of the ossicular chain using the autologous incus.

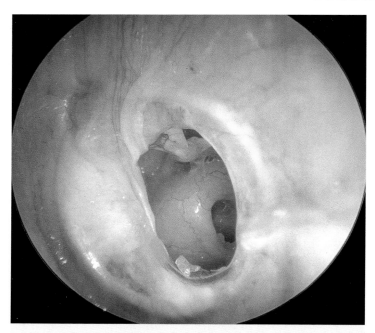

Fig. 7.5 Left ear. Posterior nonmarginal perforation. The incudosta-pedial joint, the promontory, and the round window are all discernible.

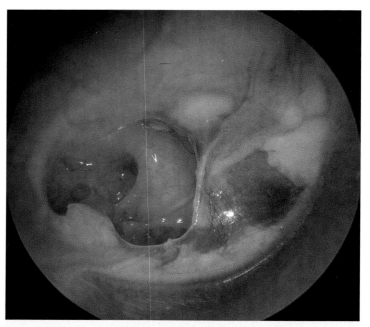

Fig. 7.6 Right ear. Presence of a simple chronic otitis media; a posteroinferior drum perforation. The middle ear mucosa is normal. The round window and Jacobson's nerve running on the promontory are seen. The incus can also be appreciated posterior to a retromalleolar tympanosclerotic plaque. The tympanic membrane residue shows areas of atrophy alternating with areas of tympano-sclerosis.

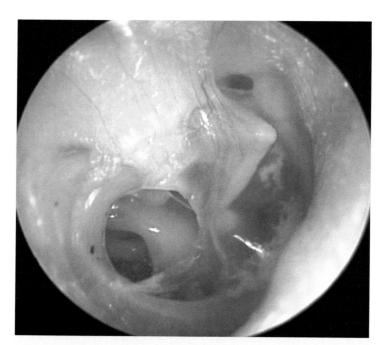

Fig. 7.7 Right ear. Perforation of the posteroinferior quadrant of the tympanic membrane. The anterior quadrants show slight myringo-sclerosis. The oval window and the promontorium are visible. Middle ear mucosa is normal. In this case, underlay myringoplasty with endocanalar approach is indicated.

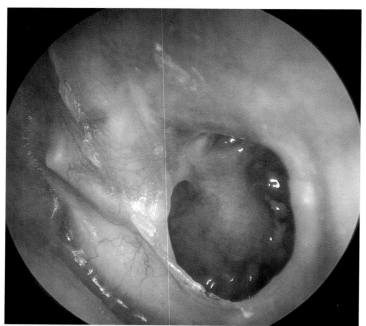

Fig. 7.8 Left ear. Perforation of the posterior quadrants of the tympanic membrane. The skin advances along the posterosuperior border of the perforation toward the incudostapedial joint. The middle ear mucosa appears hypertrophic. Mucoid discharge is also present. A tympanosclerotic plaque can be seen in the residue of the tympanic membrane.

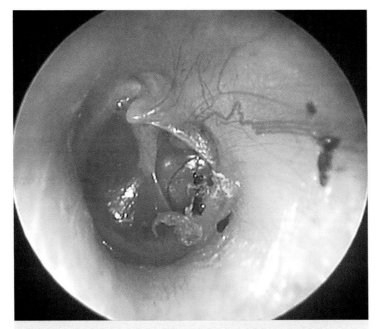

Fig. 7.9 Left ear. Perforation of the posterior quadrants of the tympanic membrane. The perforation borders are irregular with epithelialization toward the middle ear. A small mesotympanic cholesteatoma could be suspected. In this case, retroauricular-approach myringoplasty with mastoid exploration is the treatment of choice.

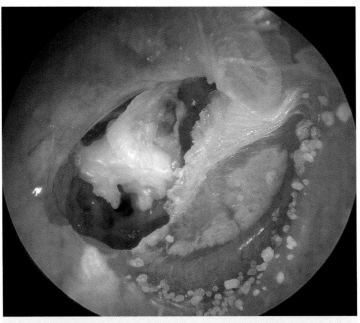

Fig. 7.10 Right ear. Marked posterior marginal perforation through which the skin penetrates into the middle ear. The incudostapedial joint is not visible.

7.3 Anterior Perforations

These type of perforations have been shown in ► Fig. 7.11, ► Fig. 7.12, ► Fig. 7.13, ► Fig. 7.14, ► Fig. 7.15, ► Fig. 7.16, ► Fig. 7.17.

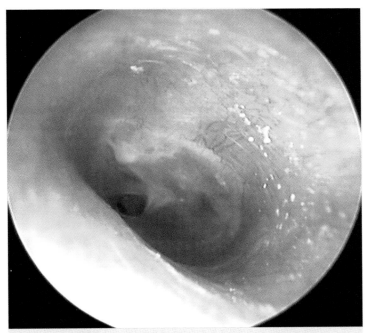

Fig. 7.11 Left ear. Small anterior perforation of the tympanic membrane. Hearing function is normal. Surgical treatment of this case depends on patient's symptoms (i.e., recurrent otorrhea). Anterior hump of the external auditory canal can be seen, preventing total visualization of the annulus. In this case, myringoplasty should be performed with canalplasty.

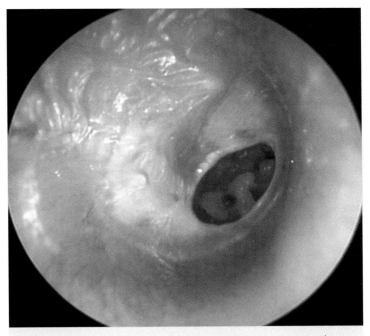

Fig. 7.12 Right ear. Anterior perforation of the tympanic membrane. Middle ear mucosa is normal and the tubal orifice is visible. The rest of the tympanic membrane is tympanosclerotic, resulting in moderate conductive hearing loss (see ► Fig. 7.13). In this case, mobility of the ossicles should be checked during the myringoplasty.

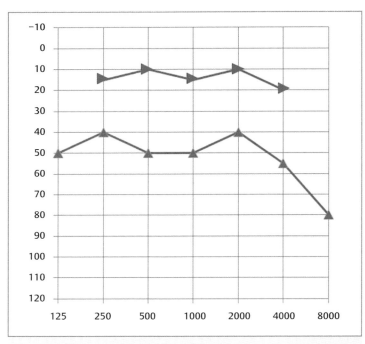

Fig. 7.13 Audiometry of the previous case.

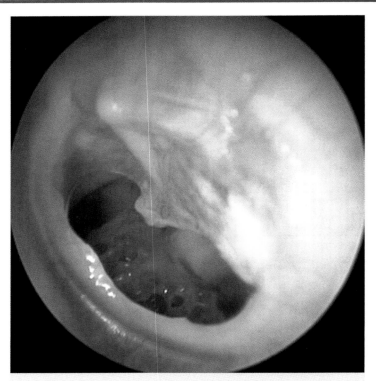

Fig. 7.14 Left ear. Anterior perforation of the tympanic membrane with inferior and posterior extension. The tubal orifice, as well as Jacobson's nerve and inferior tympanic artery, is clearly visible. Posteriorly, a tympanosclerotic plaque is present. The mass can be confused with a cholesteatoma. Testing the consistency of the mass using an instrument under the microscope could be useful: in case of cholesteatoma, the mass is soft and will break, whereas tympanosclerosis is generally hard.

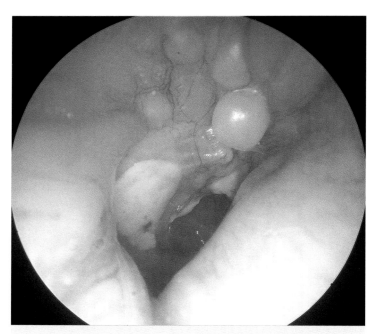

Fig. 7.15 Right ear. Anterior perforation in a patient with anterior and posterior humps of the external auditory canal as well as osteoma of the superior canal wall. In this case, canalplasty should be performed at the same time as myringoplasty.

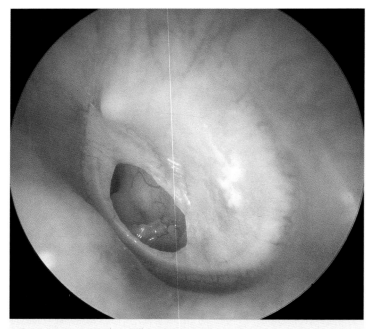

Fig. 7.16 Case similar to that in ▶ Fig. 7.12. Left ear. Dry anteroinferior perforation. The middle ear mucosa is normal. The tympanic membrane residue shows tympanosclerosis, giving it a white appearance. The tubal orifice can be seen from the anterior margin of the perforation.

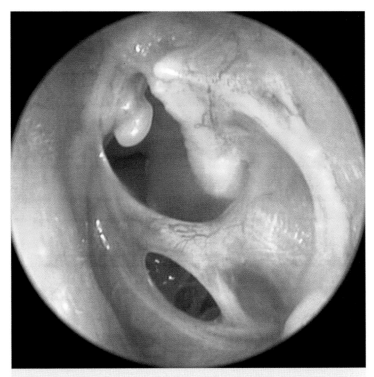

Fig. 7.17 Left ear. Perforations of the anterior quadrants of the tympanic membrane. A small bridge of intact membrane separates the two perforations. The tubal orifice, as well as the supratubal recess and the hypotympanic area, is visible. The malleus handle is amputated with medial epithelialization. A mass similar to a small cholesteatoma is visible medial to the anterosuperior border of the perforation. In this case, careful examination of the middle ear should be performed.

7.4 Inferior Perforations

These type of perforations have been shown in ► Fig. 7.18, ► Fig. 7.19, ► Fig. 7.20, ► Fig. 7.21.

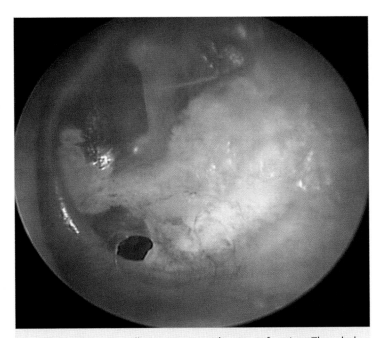

Fig. 7.18 Left ear. Small tympanic membrane perforation. The whole tympanic membrane is tympanosclerotic, mainly on its posterior quadrants. Audiometry showed moderate conductive hearing loss, maybe due to ossicular fixation. Even in this case, myringoplasty should be performed with careful inspection of the ossicular mobility.

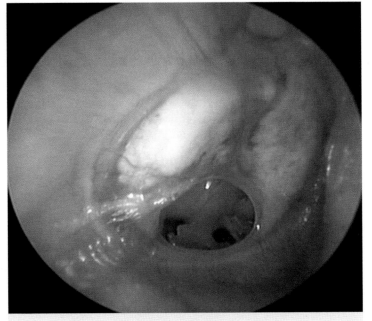

Fig. 7.19 Right ear. Inferior perforation. The posterior and anterior residues of the tympanic membrane show tympanosclerosis. The hypotympanic cells are also visible.

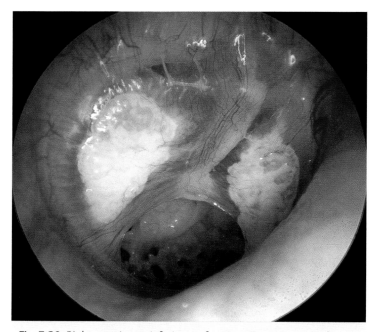

Fig. 7.20 Right ear. Anteroinferior perforation. Two tympanosclerotic plaques are observed: one anteromalleolar and the other retromalleolar. The middle ear mucosa is normal. The hypotympanic air cells are seen through the perforation.

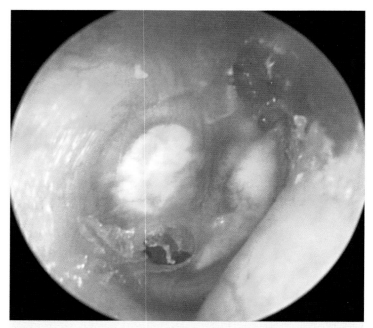

Fig. 7.21 Right ear. Inferior perforation. Even in this case the rest of the tympanic membrane is tympanosclerotic. The marginal tympanic perforation is unsafe, with epithelialization toward the inner surface of the tympanic membrane and the middle ear.

7.5 Subtotal and Total Perforations

These type of perforations have been shown in ▶ Fig. 7.22, ▶ Fig. 7.23, ▶ Fig. 7.24, ▶ Fig. 7.25, ▶ Fig. 7.26, ▶ Fig. 7.27, ▶ Fig. 7.28, ▶ Fig. 7.29.

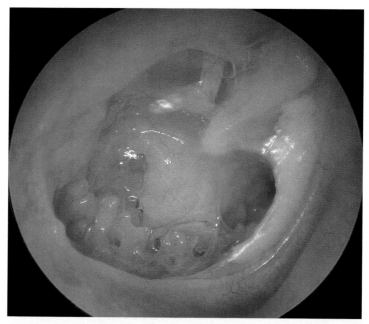

Fig. 7.22 Right ear. Large tympanic membrane perforation. The tubal orifice, the hypotympanic air cells, the promontory, the round and oval windows, and the intact stapes can be viewed. An onset of necrosis of the incus can be distinguished.

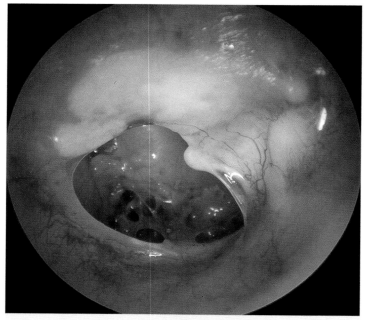

Fig. 7.23 Right ear. Perforation of the inferior quadrants of the tympanic membrane. All the tympanic membrane residue shows dense tympanosclerosis. Removal of these sclerotic plaques during myringoplasty assures an adequate vascularity to the graft and thus a high success rate for the operation.

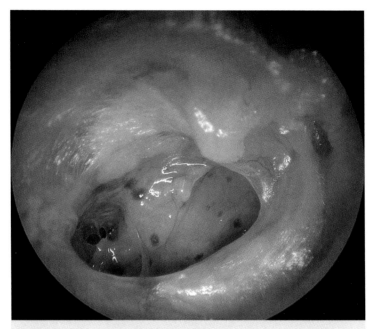

Fig. 7.24 Right ear. Similar case. The promontory and the round window are visible. A tympanosclerotic plaque that engulfs the ossicular chain is seen at the level of the posterosuperior border of the perforation.

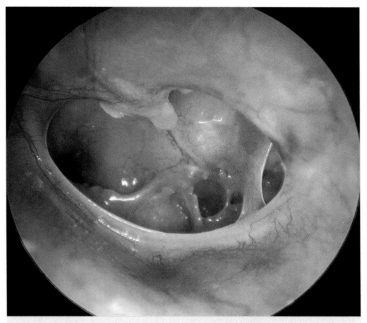

Fig. 7.25 Left ear. Subtotal perforation. The annulus as well as a fibrous rim is visualized along the inferior border of the perforation. The handle of the malleus is medialized. The tubal orifice, the hypotympanic air cells covered with mucosa, Jacobson's nerve on the promontory, and the long process of the incus are visible. The residue of the tympanic membrane is thickened. In cases in which only a small anterior residue of the tympanic membrane is found, an overlay technique in which the graft is put over the annulus is used, thus preventing detachment of the anterior part of the graft leading to reperforation.

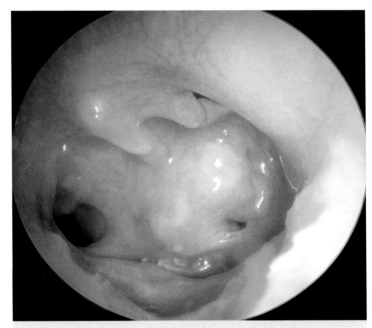

Fig. 7.26 Left ear. Total perforation of the tympanic membrane through which evolving tympanosclerotic plaques are visible. The long process of the incus is partially eroded. The handle of the malleus is medialized and adherent to the promontory. The tubal orifice and the hypotympanic air cells are also noted.

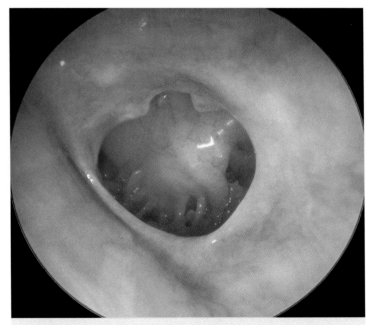

Fig. 7.27 Left ear. Subtotal perforation of the tympanic membrane. The middle ear mucosa is normal. The tympanic membrane residue is de-epithelialized. The incudostapedial joint, the medialized handle of the malleus, and the hypotympanic air cells are visible.

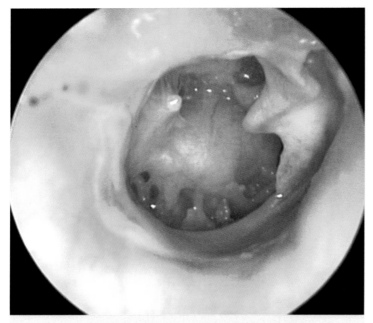

Fig. 7.28 Right ear. Subtotal perforation of the tympanic membrane. The anterior residue of the tympanic membrane is tympanosclerotic. The long process of the incus is absent. The handle of the malleus is eroded and medialized. The suprastructure of the stapes is visible and covered by mucosa. The cochleariform process, the second portion of the facial nerve, the promontorium, the round window, and the hypotympanic air cells are also visible.

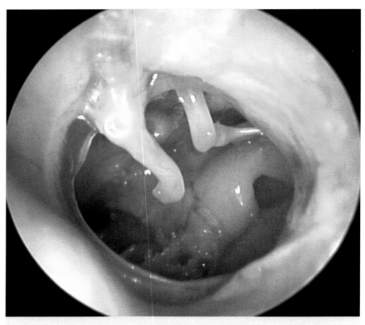

Fig. 7.29 Left ear. Total perforation of the tympanic membrane. All the structures of the middle ear are visible, including the tubal orifice. The anterior, inferior, and posterior annulus are under view.

7.6 Posttraumatic Perforations

These type of perforations have been shown in ▶ Fig. 7.30, ▶ Fig. 7.31, ▶ Fig. 7.32, ▶ Fig. 7.33, ▶ Fig. 7.34, ▶ Fig. 7.35, ▶ Fig. 7.36.

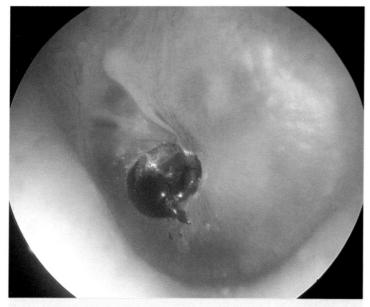

Fig. 7.30 Left ear. Posttraumatic perforation of the tympanic membrane in the region of the cone of light. The blood clot over the perforation has not been removed. This clot helps to guide spontaneous healing of the drum.

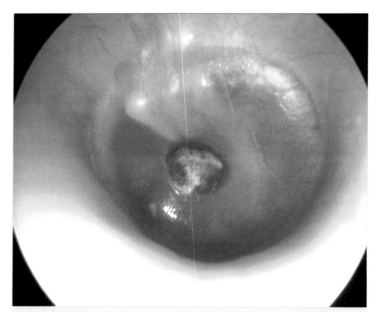

Fig. 7.31 Left ear. Similar case to that in ▶ Fig. 7.30.

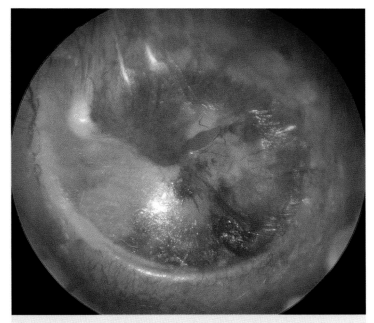

Fig. 7.32 Left ear. Posttraumatic perforation in the posterosuperior quadrant. The characteristic radial tear, running in the same direction as the fibers of the tympanic membrane, is apparent. Hemorrhagic points separating the epidermal layer from the fibrous layer are visible. These tiny hemorrhages are typical of posttraumatic perforations. The type of tympanic membrane perforation has a very high incidence of spontaneous healing.

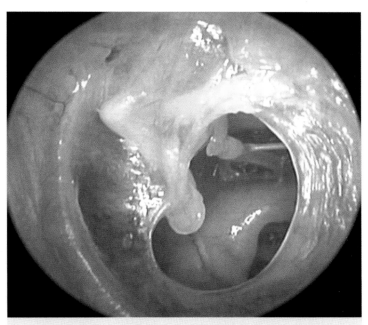

Fig. 7.33 Left ear. Long-lasting posttraumatic perforation (cotton swab) of the posterior quadrants. The edges of the perforation are sharp. The long process of the incus is eroded and slightly curved but in contact with the stapes suprastructure. The handle of the malleus seems broken but in contact with the tympanic membrane. All the stapes, stapedial tendon, and the oval window niche are visible. The round window and the second portion of the facial nerve are also under view. Fortunately, the patient had conductive hearing loss of only 10 to 15 dB. In this case, myringoplasty through a retroauricular approach is indicated.

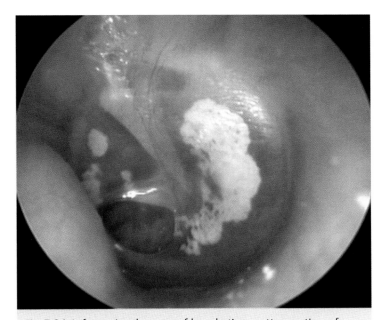

Fig. 7.34 Left ear. Another case of long-lasting posttraumatic perforation (cotton swab) of the anteroinferior quadrant. The tubal orifice is partially under view. Posterior quadrants of the tympanic membrane are myringosclerotic. In this case, myringoplasty should be performed with canalplasty due to the anterior hump of the external auditory canal.

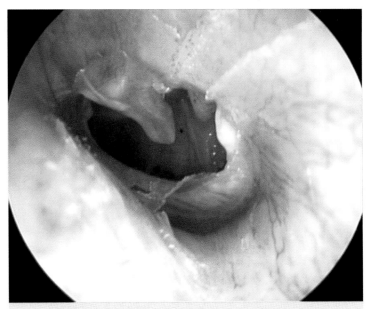

Fig. 7.35 Left ear. Subtotal perforation of the tympanic membrane (after a slap). The mucosal layer of the anterior portion of the tympanic membrane is everted. The tubal orifice and the incudostapedial joint are visible. There is a hump of the anterior wall of the external auditory canal which impedes visualization of the whole anterior annulus. Unfortunately, the patient developed a decreasing of the bone conduction, as a result of an injury even on the inner ear (see ▶ Fig. 7.36).

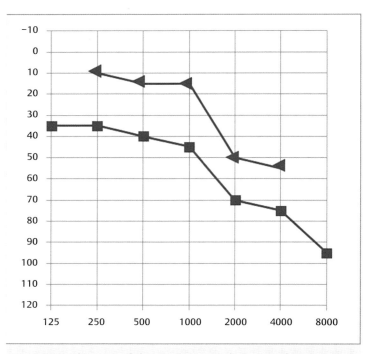

Fig. 7.36 Audiometry of the previous case shows mixed hearing loss.

Summary

The presence of a tympanic membrane perforation that does not heal spontaneously, as in chronic otitis media, represents an anatomical and functional defect that needs surgical correction in the majority of cases. Myringoplasty is indicated in cases with and without otorrhea, with a small or a large air–bone gap, and with no age limit. It is a contraindication when the tympanic membrane perforation is present in the only hearing ear. Myringoplasty is generally performed using a postauricular incision under local anesthesia—except for children in whom general anesthesia is used. The tympanic membrane is repaired by an autologous temporalis fascia graft. We prefer the underlay technique in the majority of cases because it gives better results both anatomically and functionally. The overlay technique is used in selected cases when the anterior residue of the tympanic membrane is pathologic or absent. When properly performed, the overlay technique gives optimal results in these cases. Canalplasty is done whenever bony humps of the external auditory canal are present, limiting control of the perforation borders. If reperforation occurs after myringoplasty (in ~5% of cases), a revision operation is indicated after a few months. The result of the first and second operation in terms of graft take and reperforation are generally comparable.

7.7 Perforations Complicated or Associated with Other Pathologies

See ► Fig. 7.37, ► Fig. 7.38, ► Fig. 7.39, ► Fig. 7.40, ► Fig. 7.41, ► Fig. 7.42, ► Fig. 7.43, ► Fig. 7.44, ► Fig. 7.45, ► Fig. 7.46, ► Fig. 7.47.

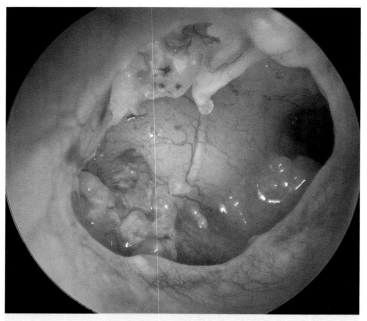

Fig. 7.37 Right ear. Exacerbation of chronic otitis with otorrhea in a patient with a small tympanic membrane perforation. After proper local therapy, the patient should be revaluated and eventually programmed for a myringoplasty.

Fig. 7.38 Right ear. Total perforation. Epidermization is present in the regions of the mesotympanum and the ossicular chain. The round window, hypotympanic air cells with thickened mucosa, Jacobson's nerve running on the promontory, and the tubal orifice are well visualized. This case is an example of chronic otitis media complicated by the presence of skin in the middle ear. Tympanoplasty should be staged. In the first stage, the skin is removed without traumatizing the ossicular chain, and the tympanic membrane is reconstructed. In the second stage, the middle ear is checked for any residual skin, and the ossicular chain is reconstructed.

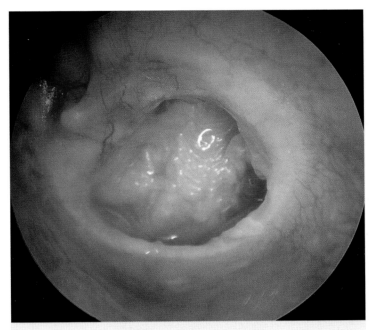

Fig. 7.39 Left ear. Large perforation with diffuse epidermization of the middle ear associated with purulent otorrhea. In these cases, even if the ossicular chain proves intact, mastoid exploration should be done. A second stage is performed 1 year after the first operation to check for any skin residues.

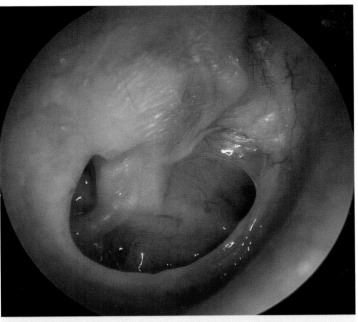

Fig. 7.40 Right ear. Perforation of the inferior quadrants of the tympanic membrane, the residues of which show tympanosclerosis. Epidermization is evident over the promontory. As epidermization is limited in this case, a single-stage tympanoplasty can be performed.

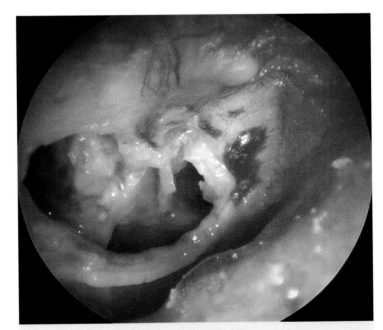

Fig. 7.41 Right ear. Another example of chronic otitis media complicated with diffuse epidermization of the middle ear. Surgery follows the same rules as for cholesteatomas.

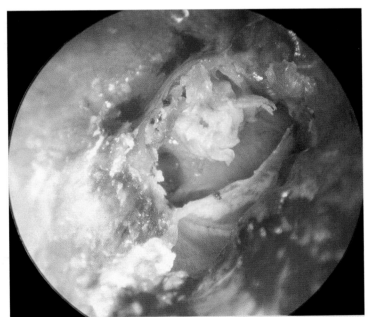

Fig. 7.42 Right ear. Large tympanic membrane perforation. The anterior drum residue shows tympanosclerosis. The ossicular chain is difficult to identify because of the presence of epidermization at this level. The round window is visible. A staged tympanoplasty is also indicated in this case.

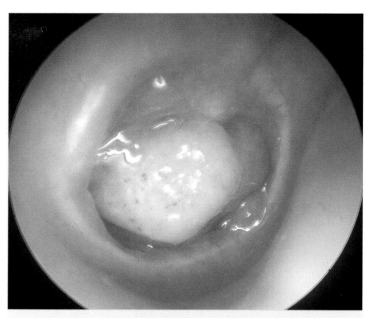

Fig. 7.43 Granulomatous otitis media. A roundish mass fills the middle ear. Serous otorrhea is present.

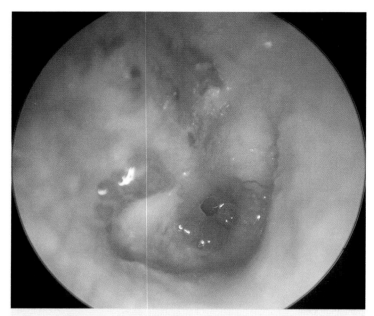

Fig. 7.44 Right ear. Small perforation of the inferior quadrants of the tympanic membrane, with eversion of the mucosa onto the outer layer of the membrane. Tympanosclerosis, both antero- and posteromalleolar, can be observed.

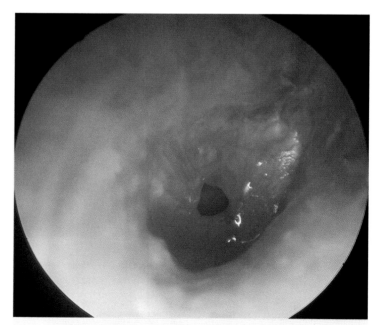

Fig. 7.45 Right ear. Case similar to that in ▶ Fig. 7.44. The mucosa has replaced the epithelial layer. Ear discharge is also present. During myringoplasty, curettage of the everted mucosa is necessary until the fibrous layer of the tympanic membrane is reached.

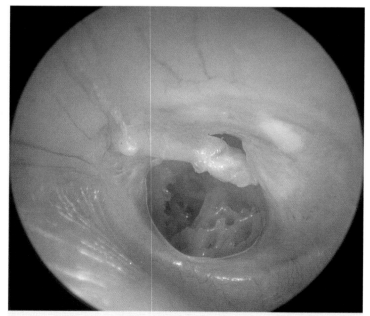

Fig. 7.46 Left ear. Perforation of the anterior quadrants. Skin envelopes the handle of the malleus. During myringoplasty, curettage of the skin is necessary before reconstruction.

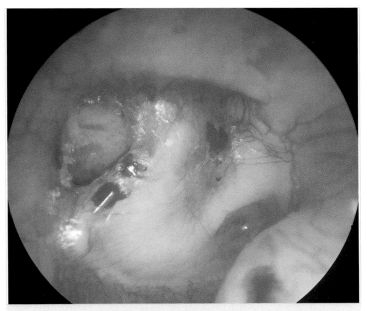

Fig. 7.47 Right ear. Posterior perforation. The residues of the tympanic membrane appear whitish and bulging. During surgery, the middle ear was occupied by granulomatous tissue that proved to be a tuberculosis (TB) on histopathological examination. This patient had a past history of pulmonary TB. Tuberculosis otitis media should be suspected in cases of pulmonary TB presenting with otorrhea.

7.8 Tympanosclerosis

Tympanosclerosis is characterized by fibroblastic invasion of the submucosal spaces of the middle ear followed by thickening, hyalinization, and fusion of collagen fibers into a homogenous mass with calcium deposits and phosphate crystals. Though the pathogenesis is not yet clear, it seems that chronic otitis media is a predisposing factor. There is accumulating evidence attributing the pathogenesis of tympanosclerosis to abnormal immune reaction. Tympanosclerosis also limits mobilization of the tympanic membrane and/or the ossicular chain, requiring appropriate surgical management. Simple reconstruction of the tympanic membrane without managing such pathologies results in unsatisfactory postoperative hearing. The status of the tympanic membrane and ossicular chain therefore needs to be checked before myringoplasty. However, tympanosclerosis may advance after surgery.

Two distinct forms are recognized, as discussed next.

7.8.1 Tympanosclerosis Associated with Tympanic Membrane Perforation

The perforation is frequently central or subtotal and the annulus, infiltrated by calcium deposits, is well visualized. Frequently, submucous nodular deposits are encountered in the middle ear. Ossicular fixation or erosion due to devitalization as a result of loss of blood supply can also occur. The middle ear mucosa is very thin, with reduced vascularity. In some cases, tympanosclerotic plaques are seen extruding from the mucosa to present as white middle ear masses. See ▶ Fig. 7.48, ▶ Fig. 7.49, ▶ Fig. 7.50, ▶ Fig. 7.51, ▶ Fig. 7.52, ▶ Fig. 7.53, ▶ Fig. 7.54, ▶ Fig. 7.55, ▶ Fig. 7.56, ▶ Fig. 7.57, ▶ Fig. 7.58.

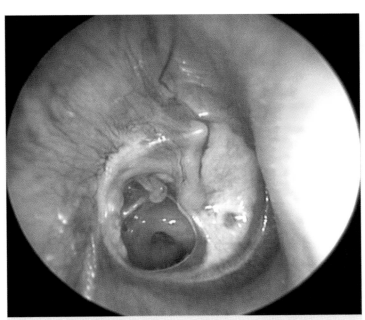

Fig. 7.48 Right ear. Perforation of the posteroinferior quadrant of the tympanic membrane, with myringosclerosis of the residual portions. The long process of the incus is eroded, resulting in conductive hearing loss.

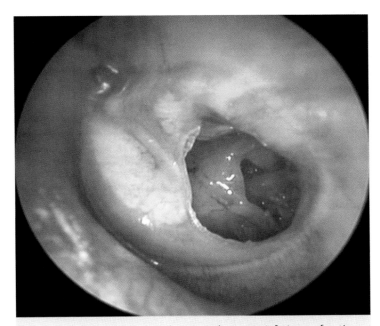

Fig. 7.49 Left ear. Tympanosclerosis with posteroinferior perforation. Two calcareous plaques are present (antero- and posteromalleolar). The incudostapedial joint and the round window are under view.

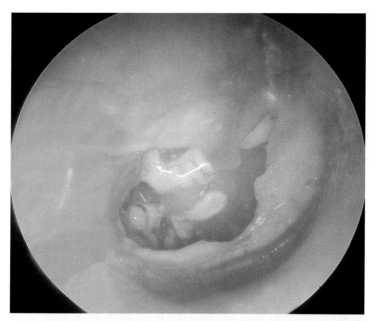

Fig. 7.50 Right ear. Tympanosclerosis associated with perforation. The tympanic membrane residues and the middle ear (promontory and hypotympanum) show the characteristic plaques. The malleus is blocked by tympanosclerosis.

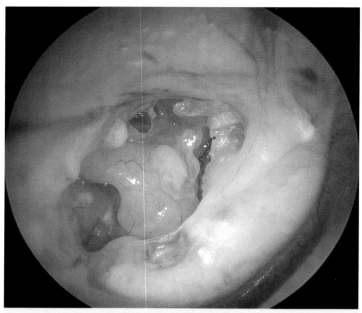

Fig. 7.51 Right ear. Tympanosclerosis with perforation. A large tympanosclerotic plaque is noted in the anterior residue of the tympanic membrane. The middle ear is also involved. The promontory, oval window, stapes footplate, and the round window can be appreciated.

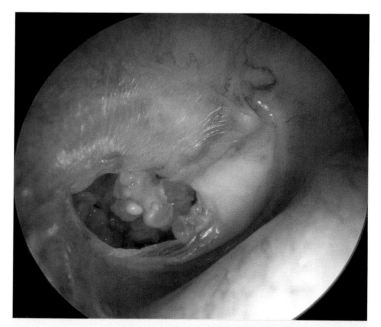

Fig. 7.52 Right ear. Perforations of the inferior quadrants with tympanosclerosis involving the residues of the tympanic membrane and the middle ear.

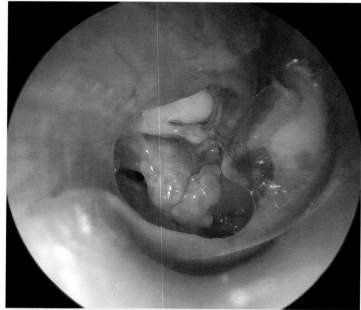

Fig. 7.53 Right ear. Tympanosclerosis with perforation. The tympanosclerotic process involves the anterior residues of the tympanic membrane and the mucosa of the promontory reaching to the posterior mesotympanum. At this level, ossification of the stapedius tendon is seen. The tympanic segment of the fallopian canal is covered by a sclerotic plaque. The long process of the incus is eroded.

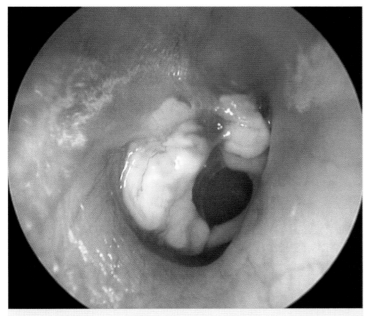

Fig. 7.54 Right ear. Thick tympanosclerosis with perforation of the anteroinferior quadrant. After recurrence of chronic otitis, the patient underwent computed tomography (CT) scan elsewhere for the suspect of cholesteatoma (see ▶ Fig. 7.55). CT scan alone is misleading in case of tympanosclerosis, because the radiological pattern could be similar to that of cholesteatoma. In cases like this, the patient should be revaluated with otoscopy after proper local therapy. If the discharge is persistent, a CT scan is recommended (see ▶ Fig. 7.56).

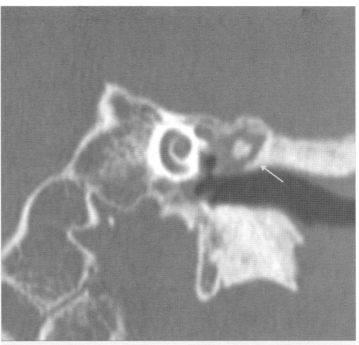

Fig. 7.55 CT scan of the previous case. Coronal view. The tympanosclerotic tissue has the same density of the soft tissue, as for cholesteatoma. Unlike attical cholesteatoma, scutum is not eroded in this case (*arrow*).

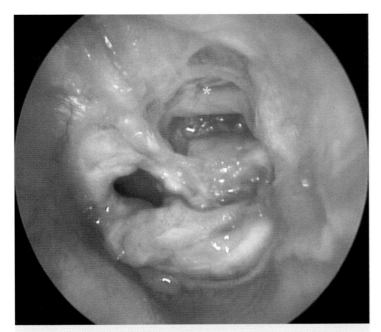

Fig. 7.56 Left ear. Tympanosclerosis with perforation of the tympanic membrane. There is a deep retraction of the posterosuperior quadrant with exposure of the second portion of the facial nerve (*asterisk*). The stapes and the long process of the incus are absent. The patient complained of persistent otorrhea, so he underwent a CT scan (▶ Fig. 7.57) that confirmed the presence of a cholesteatoma. An open tympanoplasty was performed.

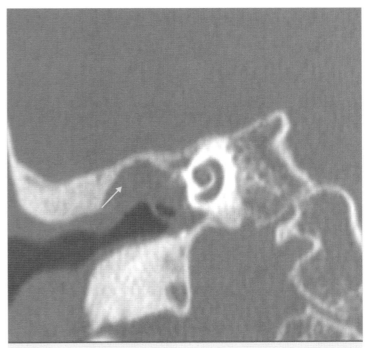

Fig. 7.57 Left ear. Tympanosclerosis associated with cholesteatoma. Unlike in ▶ Fig. 7.55, the scutum is eroded.

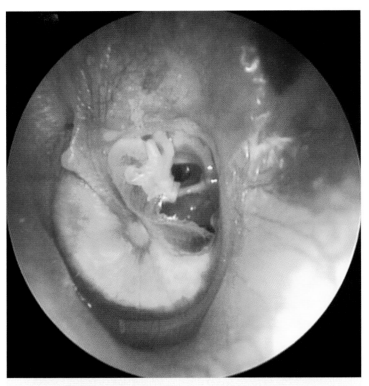

Fig. 7.58 Left ear. Tympanosclerosis associated with posterosuperior perforation. The perforation is marginal and irregular. Otorrhea is reported by the patient. In this case, CT scan is recommended to exclude the presence of a cholesteatoma.

7.8.2 Tympanosclerosis with Intact Tympanic Membrane

This is characterized by calcareous plaques (chalk patches) in the fibrous layer of the tympanic membrane. The antero- and poster-omalleolar regions are usually involved. The periannular region of the inferior quadrants is also affected, forming a horseshoe pattern. The pars tensa is rigid, thick, and loses is elasticity, assuming a whitish aspect. Atrophic and thinned areas can also occur. Infrequently, in very advanced cases, the tympanosclerotic plaques occupy all the middle ear spaces, attic, and aditus and completely block the ossicular chain. The tympanic membrane in these cases is very thick or even replaced by the plaques. See ▶ Fig. 7.59, ▶ Fig. 7.60, ▶ Fig. 7.61, ▶ Fig. 7.62, ▶ Fig. 7.63, ▶ Fig. 7.64, ▶ Fig. 7.65, ▶ Fig. 7.66.

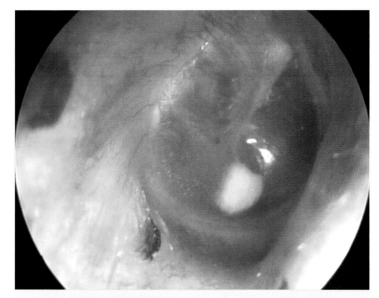

Fig. 7.59 Right ear. Small myringosclerotic plaque in the inferior quadrant. This is a typical outcome of previous otitis media with tympanic membrane perforation during childhood. Up to now, the patient does not complain hearing loss or other symptoms.

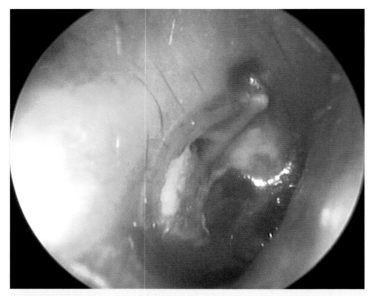

Fig. 7.60 Right ear. Tympanosclerosis with intact tympanic membrane. The anteroinferior quadrant of the tympanic membrane is atrophic. The left ear is similar (see ▶ Fig. 7.61). Bilateral conductive hearing loss is present, which is worst on the left side (see ▶ Fig. 7.62).

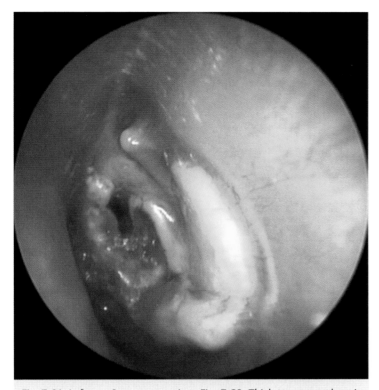

Fig. 7.61 Left ear. Same case as in ▶ Fig. 7.60. Thick tympanosclerosis of the tympanic membrane. A small atrophic remnant of the tympanic membrane is visible in the anterosuperior quadrant. The tubal orifice is visible in transparency. Considering hearing function (see ▶ Fig. 7.63), surgery is indicated. After removing tympanosclerotic plaques and involved ossicles, ossiculoplasty, with or without tympanic membrane reconstruction, should be performed. In case of stapes fixation, the surgery has to be staged.

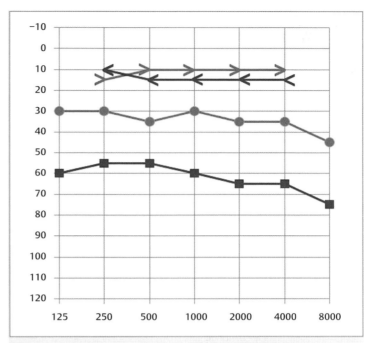

Fig. 7.62 Audiometry of the case in ▶ Fig. 7.60, ▶ Fig. 7.61. Bilateral mild to moderate conductive hearing loss (worse on the left side). Ossicular fixation should always be suspected in case of tympanosclerosis with intact tympanic membrane and air–bone gap.

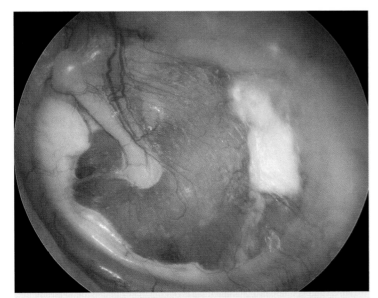

Fig. 7.63 Left ear. Tympanosclerosis and intact drum. The majority of the tympanic membrane is thinned due to atrophy of the fibrous layer. Two tympanosclerotic plaques are present near the anterior and posterior margins.

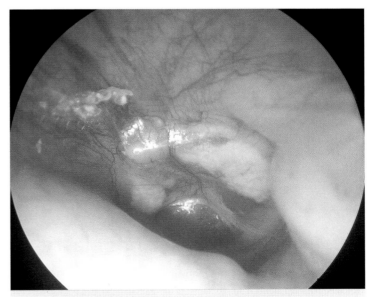

Fig. 7.64 Left ear. The intact tympanic membrane shows tympanosclerotic plaques lying both anterior and posterior to the malleus that alternate with areas of atrophy (in the inferior quadrants).

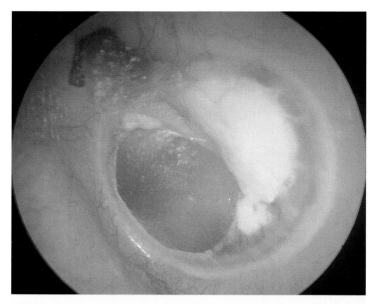

Fig. 7.65 Left ear. Tympanosclerosis with intact drum. A large plaque is visible in the posterior quadrants of the tympanic membrane. The anterior quadrants are thinned and atrophic, allowing visualization of the tubal orifice.

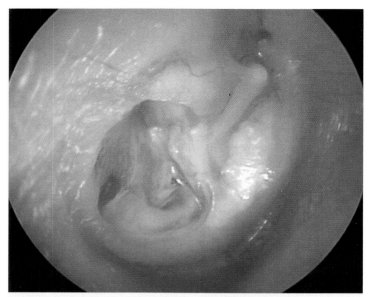

Fig. 7.66 Right ear. Tympanosclerosis with intact drum. A deep retraction pocket is visible in the posterior quadrants. The patients underwent myringoplasty and ossiculoplasty elsewhere with good audiological results (closure of the air–bone gap). After few years, the patient developed ipsilateral conductive hearing loss and underwent further ossiculoplasty due to stapes fixation. Despite the initial improvement of hearing function, the patient further developed hearing loss and stapes refixation was observed at the third surgery. A bone conduction hearing implant was finally applied.

Summary

Chronic otitis media associated with tympanosclerosis represents a more complex anatomopathological entity. In cases with intact tympanic membrane, surgery is indicated in the presence of a significant air–bone gap, signifying ossicular chain involvement. If erosion or fixation of the ossicles is found, ossiculoplasty is performed. Fixation of the stapes is an indication for stapedectomy.

In cases associated with tympanic membrane perforation, it is often possible to perform a single-stage reconstruction in which myringoplasty is performed with or without ossiculoplasty. A fixed stapes, however, is an indication for staging, where myringoplasty is performed first, followed by a second-stage stapedotomy after a few months. In all suspected cases, the patient should be informed preoperatively of the possibility of staging surgery.

In a small group of cases of chronic otitis media with tympanosclerosis, a good postoperative functional level can deteriorate with time due to refixation of the ossicular chain, with a consequent air–bone gap. In such cases, after achieving closure of the tympanic membrane, a hearing aid is recommended.

7.9 Principles of Myringoplasty

We prefer retroauricular incision in the majority of myringoplasties, as this approach gives better access to the entire tympanic membrane. In this approach, the tympanic membrane is repaired with an autologous temporalis fascia graft.

- Skin incision, harvest of temporalis fascia, and incision of the external auditory canal are conducted (▶ Fig. 7.67).

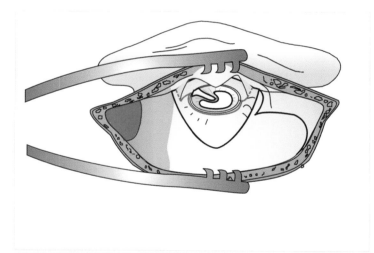

Fig. 7.67 Exposing the anterior wall by anterior extension of the lateral ends of the superior and inferior longitudinal incisions.

- To successfully reconstruct the tympanic membrane, a complete 360-degree view of the entire tympanic membrane is essential. If the anterior annulus is seen easily, the anterior meatal skin is left intact. Otherwise, the anterior meatal skin is transected laterally as a continuation of the superior and inferior longitudinal incisions that expose the anterior bony wall.
- Canalplasty is performed as described earlier (see Chapter 3).
- The annulus and meatal skin are inspected carefully. If these structures show any pathological involvement, such as granulation, everted mucosa, or scarring, the segment needs to be removed. The underlay technique is performed if any anterior residue of the tympanic membrane, at least the annulus, is

present after removing such pathological tissue. If not, the over-lay technique is indicated.

- Elevation of the anterior meatal skin, if necessary, should be conducted in a lateral to medial direction, so as not to disrupt the remaining epidermal layer.
- Do not detach the anterior meatal skin from medial (from the annulus) to lateral, as this maneuver may cause blunting of the anterior angle by insulting the tympanic annulus. It also has possibilities of cutting epidermization and leaving it in the tympanic cavity. Epidermis left inside the tympanic cavity and on the annulus may cause iatrogenic cholesteatoma and blunting of the anterior angle.
- Refreshing of the perforation edge and the undersurface of the tympanic membrane not only favors the attachment of the graft but also greatly reduces the risk of leaving entrapped skin inside, which may cause iatrogenic cholesteatoma (▶ Fig. 7.68). If everted mucosa is present on the lateral surface of the tympanic membrane, curetting it from the surface until the fibrous layer is reached, or total removal of that part, is also necessary for optimal epithelialization. If dense tympanosclerotic plaques are present in the tympanic membrane, removal of the plaque from the medial aspect without disrupting an epidermal layer or total removal of that part ensures an adequate vascularization of the graft and thus a higher success rate of closure (▶ Fig. 7.69).
- The posterior annulus is then elevated to allow access to the tympanic cavity (▶ Fig. 7.70, ▶ Fig. 7.71). If the perforation is large or located anteriorly, the tympanomeatal flap may be cut posteriorly (▶ Fig. 7.72), a maneuver that makes the posterior part of the flap appear like swing doors, thereby enhancing visualization of the tympanic cavity.
- The tympanic cavity is inspected carefully to check whether there is any pathology such as tympanosclerotic plaque and epidermis in the tympanic cavity (▶ Fig. 7.73). If present, it should be managed. The integrity of the ossicular chain is also evaluated at the same time by touching it gently with a blunt

dissector. Ossiculoplasty may be conducted in the same stage or in the second stage, depending on the pathological status.

- Bleeding should be completely controlled before starting reconstruction. Use a diamond burr on bone. Small pieces of Gelfoam, pressed down with Cottonoids, are placed on the tympanic cavity and held in position for a while. A bloodless surgical field allows precise estimation of middle ear structures followed by adequate arrangement of reconstruction materials.
- The tympanic orifice of the Eustachian tube is blocked with small pieces of Gelfoam soaked in physiological saline. According to our experience, this maneuver serves to prevent the graft from falling down toward the Eustachian tube and reduces the rate of failure.
- The tympanic cavity is packed with Gelfoam, soaked in physiological saline, to support the graft medially (▶ Fig. 7.74). Excessive packing of the tympanic cavity with Gelfoam from the beginning may push the graft laterally and prevent adequate reconstruction afterward.
- The temporalis fascia is dried completely as this helps precise maneuvers during reconstruction. While trimming the temporalis fascia, a small Cottonoid is placed over the Gelfoam to avoid blood falling down into the tympanic cavity. The graft is placed in the manner described later, depending on the pathological status. An example of underlay technique is shown (▶ Fig. 7.75).

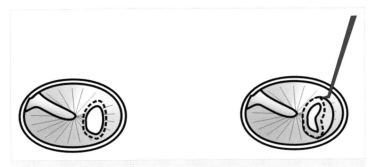

Fig. 7.68 Refreshing the edge of the perforation.

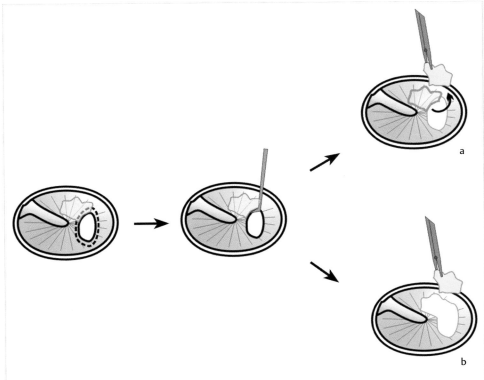

Fig. 7.69 A tympanosclerotic plaque can be removed from the medial aspect of the membrane without disturbing the epithelial layer (**a**) or by total removal of the part involved (**b**).

Transcanal

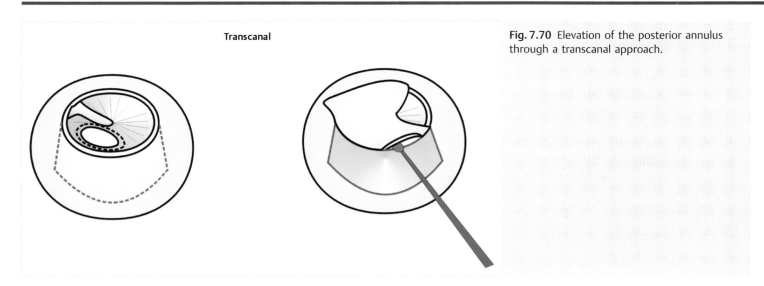

Fig. 7.70 Elevation of the posterior annulus through a transcanal approach.

Retroauricular

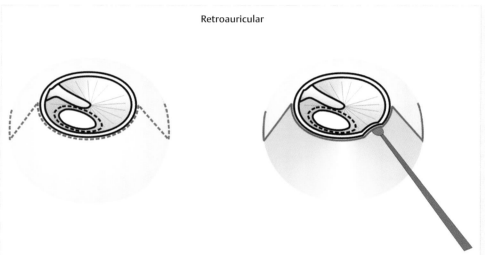

Fig. 7.71 Elevation of the posterior annulus through a retroauricular incision.

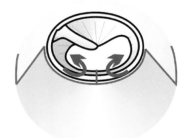

Fig. 7.72 The tympanomeatal flap cut posteriorly to enhance visualization of the tympanic cavity.

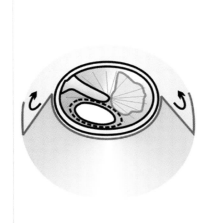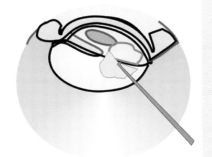

Fig. 7.73 The tympanic cavity is inspected for tympanosclerosis.

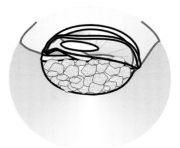

Fig. 7.74 Tympanic cavity filled with Gelfoam.

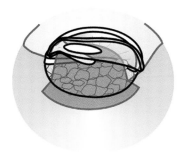

Fig. 7.75 Graft placed with underlay technique.

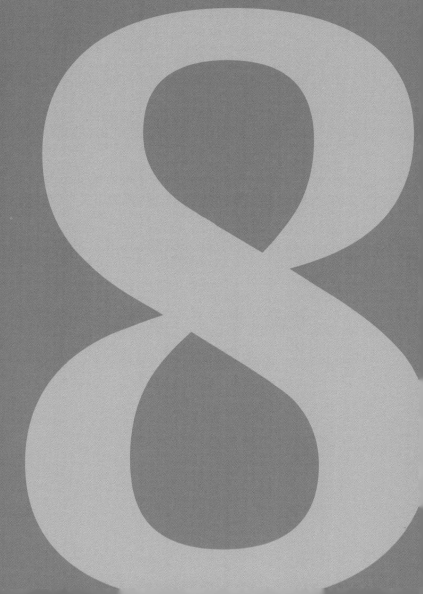

Chapter 8

Chronic Suppurative Otitis Media with Cholesteatoma

8 Chronic Suppurative Otitis Media with Cholesteatoma

Abstract

Cholesteatoma is an epidermal inclusion cyst localized in the middle ear. The "acquired type" can be caused by invasion of the skin of the external auditory canal into the middle ear through a marginal perforation. It can also originate from an epitympanic retraction pocket that becomes so deep that keratin debris can no longer be expelled, leading to its accumulation and subsequent cholesteatoma formation. Such retraction pockets can remain asymptomatic until they become infected, resulting in otorrhea and hearing loss. For this reason, we prefer to follow up these patients with otomicroscopy and endoscopy. In rare cases, the cholesteatoma can invade the labyrinth, cochlea, posterior and middle fossa durae, the internal auditory canal, and the petrous apex, forming a petrous bone cholesteatoma. Treatment of cholesteatoma is exclusively surgical and individualized (tympanoplasty).

Keywords: epitympanic cholesteatoma, mesotympanic cholesteatoma, closed tympanoplasty, open tympanoplasty, modified Bondy's technique

Cholesteatoma is an epidermal inclusion cyst localized in the middle ear, whose capsule and matrix are formed from stratified squamous epithelium. The desquamating debris includes pearly white lamellae of keratin that accumulate concentrically, forming the cholesteatoma mass.

The term cholesteatoma is actually a misnomer. It is derived from the Greek words "chole" or bile, "steatos" or fat, and "oma" or tumor. There is no relation between cholesteatoma and bile or fat. The suffix "oma" (tumor), however, is more appropriate because cholesteatoma can be considered an epidermal inclusion cyst.

Cholesteatoma can be divided into congenital (middle ear or petrous bone) and acquired (middle ear or petrous bone). Congenital cholesteatoma arises as a result of entrapped ectodermal cellular debris during embryonic development. When it involves the middle ear, it appears as a whitish retrotympanic mass that may be localized either anterior or posterior to the malleus (see Chapter 9). When it involves the petrous part of the temporal bone, it is termed congenital *petrous bone cholesteatoma* and in the majority of cases it is localized in the petrous apex (see Chapter 10). In this chapter, we will deal exclusively with cholesteatoma involving the middle ear. Petrous bone cholesteatoma is dealt with in a later chapter.

Acquired cholesteatoma of the middle ear can be caused by invasion of the skin of the external auditory canal into the middle ear through a marginal perforation. It can also originate from an epitympanic retraction pocket that becomes so deep that keratin debris can no longer be expelled, leading to its accumulation and subsequent cholesteatoma formation. Such retraction pockets can remain asymptomatic until they become infected, resulting in otorrhea and hearing loss. In other cases, the only symptom might be progressive hearing loss due to erosion of the ossicular chain by the developing cholesteatoma.

Because it is not always easy to establish a clear distinction between epitympanic or posterosuperior retraction pockets and cholesteatoma, we prefer to follow up these patients with otomicroscopy and endoscopy. In cases in which the retraction pocket becomes deep, giving rise to a cholesteatoma, a tympanoplasty is indicated. Because of the early stage of the disease, surgery can be done in a single stage. Fetid otorrhea and hearing loss are the main complaints in cholesteatoma. In addition, complicated cases can manifest with vertigo and/or facial nerve paralysis. Vertigo occurs as a result of labyrinthine fistula, which is most commonly located in the lateral semicircular canal. Facial paralysis can be caused by pressure of the cholesteatoma sac or neuritis.

In rare cases, the cholesteatoma can invade the labyrinth, cochlea, posterior and middle fossa durae, the internal auditory canal, and the petrous apex, forming a petrous bone cholesteatoma (see Chapter 10).

Treatment of cholesteatoma is exclusively surgical. Early in this century, radical mastoidectomy, a destructive procedure for the middle ear, was performed with the only goal being eradication of infection to save the ear and the life.

The concept of tympanoplasty was introduced in early 1950s. Tympanoplasty was aimed at eradication of infection as well as reconstruction of the tympano-ossicular system. Today, two types of tympanoplasty are employed: closed tympanoplasty, in which the posterior canal wall is preserved, and open tympanoplasty, in which the posterior canal wall is drilled. Both techniques, when performed appropriately and with the proper indications, can produce excellent results in terms of eradication of cholesteatoma and restoration of hearing. In children, the closed technique, performed in two stages, is preferred in the majority of cases due to children's highly cellular mastoids and in an attempt to preserve the anatomy of the ear as much as possible. In adults, particularly in epitympanic cholesteatoma with marked erosion of the scutum, in cases with sclerotic mastoids, or when middle ear atelectasis is present, an open tympanoplasty is performed (see also Chapter 14).

8.1 Epitympanic Retraction Pocket

See ▶ Fig. 8.1, ▶ Fig. 8.2, ▶ Fig. 8.3, ▶ Fig. 8.4, ▶ Fig. 8.5, ▶ Fig. 8.6, ▶ Fig. 8.7.

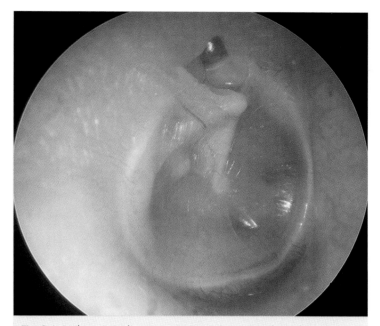

Fig. 8.1 Right ear. Early epitympanic retraction pocket. The tympanic membrane shows grade I atelectasis. Middle ear effusion with characteristic yellowish coloration of the drum is seen. In the anterosuperior quadrant, the tubal orifice is visible in transparency, whereas the long process of the incus is evident in the posterosuperior quadrant. In the area of the cone of light, an atrophic part of the tympanic membrane due to a precious myringotomy can be appreciated.

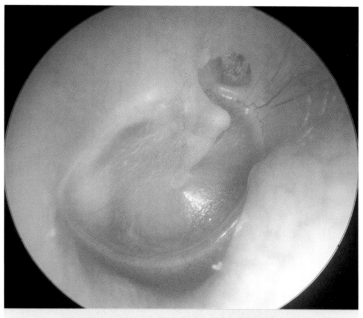

Fig. 8.2 Right ear. Epitympanic retraction pocket with the onset of tympanosclerosis of the pars tensa of the tympanic membrane.

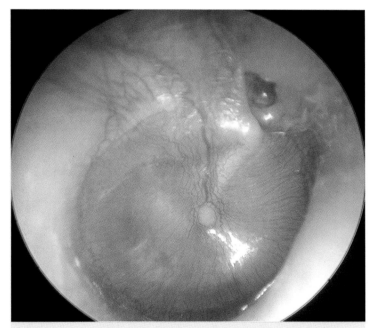

Fig. 8.3 Right ear. Similar case. The anterior quadrants of the pars tensa are retracted and thickened.

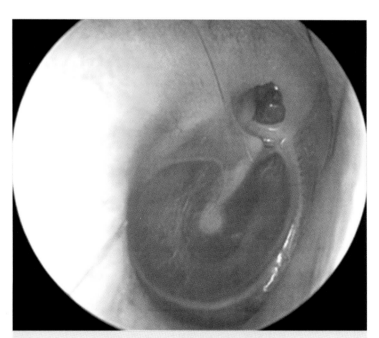

Fig. 8.4 Right ear. Epitympanic pocket. The neck of the malleus is visible.

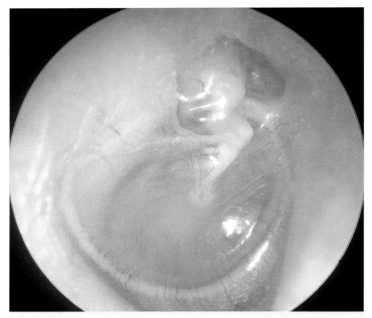

Fig. 8.5 Right ear. A large controllable epitympanic retraction pocket with erosion of the scutum. The head of the malleus is seen. Middle ear effusion gives the tympanic membrane the characteristic yellowish coloration. To prevent progression of the retraction pocket and formation of adhesions, myringotomy, ventilation tube insertion, and regular follow-up are indicated. These cases frequently represent the transition from a simple retraction pocket to an initial attic cholesteatoma. The distinction between the two is sometimes difficult. In suspected cases, a high-resolution computed tomography (CT) scan (with bone window) is beneficial for better evaluation of the extension of the retraction pocket. In cases where the condition remains stable with regular follow-up and where hearing is normal, no surgery is required. If the pocket extends deeper, giving rise to a frank cholesteatoma, surgery is indicated. If hearing is normal, an open tympanoplasty (modified Bondy's technique) is performed in a single stage.

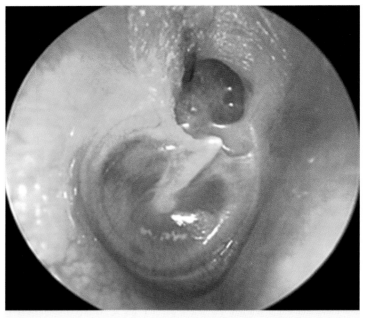

Fig. 8.6 Right ear. In this case, the retraction pocket is deeper than in ▶ Fig. 8.4. Even if the CT scan did not show a frank cholesteatoma, the patient referred occasional otorrhea. So, he underwent surgery (closed tympanoplasty with attic reconstruction with cartilage and bone pate). No cholesteatoma was found in the cavity.

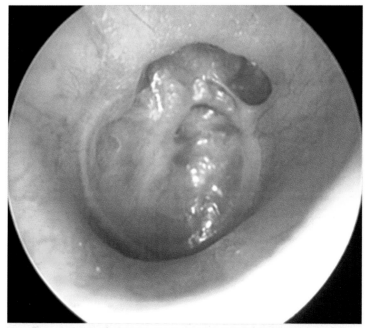

Fig. 8.7 Left ear. Deep epitympanic erosion extended to the posterior epitympanum. The neck of the malleus and the body of the incus are under view. The chorda tympani is also evident. The patient did not complained of otorrhea or hearing loss, but a strict follow-up should be assessed to avoid further development of a cholesteatoma.

8.2 Epitympanic Cholesteatoma

See ▶ Fig. 8.8, ▶ Fig. 8.9, ▶ Fig. 8.10, ▶ Fig. 8.11, ▶ Fig. 8.12, ▶ Fig. 8.13, ▶ Fig. 8.14, ▶ Fig. 8.15, ▶ Fig. 8.16, ▶ Fig. 8.17, ▶ Fig. 8.18, ▶ Fig. 8.19, ▶ Fig. 8.20, ▶ Fig. 8.21, ▶ Fig. 8.22, ▶ Fig. 8.23, ▶ Fig. 8.24, ▶ Fig. 8.25, ▶ Fig. 8.26, ▶ Fig. 8.27, ▶ Fig. 8.28, ▶ Fig. 8.29, ▶ Fig. 8.30, ▶ Fig. 8.31, ▶ Fig. 8.32, ▶ Fig. 8.33, ▶ Fig. 8.34, ▶ Fig. 8.35, ▶ Fig. 8.36, ▶ Fig. 8.37, ▶ Fig. 8.38.

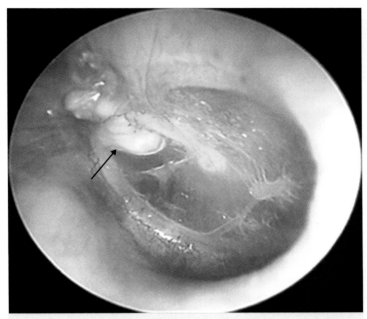

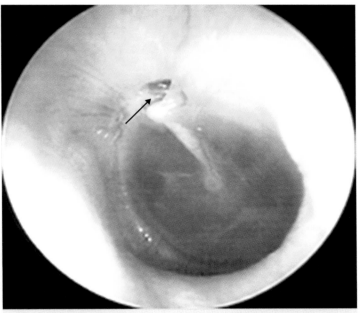

Fig. 8.8 Left ear. Epitympanic cholesteatoma in a 20-year-old man in the only hearing ear. The whitish cholesteatoma mass is visible anterior to the malleus (arrow). This is an example of how an epitympanic pocket can progressively led to a cholesteatoma. This patient underwent removal of a right petrous bone massive cholesteatoma (for definition and classification, see Chapter 10) through a transotic approach 5 years before. The left epitympanic retraction pocket (see ▶ Fig. 8.9) was followed up until the evidence of a cholesteatoma. The patient did not complain of any symptom on the left ear, and hearing function was normal. Considering the small size of the cholesteatoma, a left closed tympanoplasty was performed with preservation of the whole ossicular chain (see ▶ Fig. 8.12, ▶ Fig. 8.13, ▶ Fig. 8.14, ▶ Fig. 8.15, ▶ Fig. 8.16). A detailed description of the steps of open and closed tympanoplasties will be provided at the end of the chapter.

Fig. 8.9 Same case. Otoscopy performed 1 year before that on ▶ Fig. 8.8. A small controllable anteromalleolar epitympanic retraction pocket is visible (*arrow*). Considering that it is the only hearing ear, surgery is questionable at this stage, but a strictly follow-up is mandatory because early detection of a cholesteatoma is crucial for a correct management and outcome.

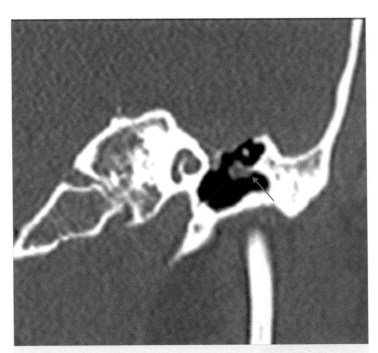

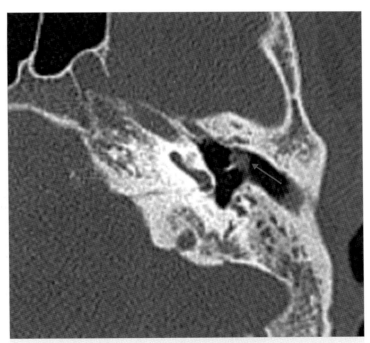

Fig. 8.10 CT scan, coronal view, of the same case. A small epitympanic cholesteatoma is visible (*arrow*).

Fig. 8.11 CT scan, axial view, of the same case.

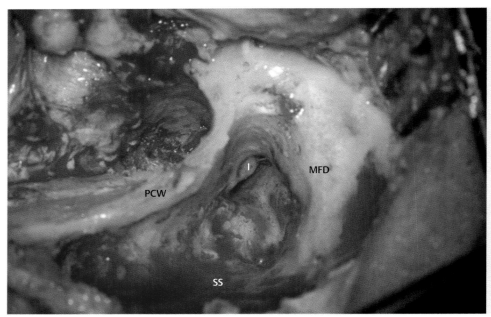

Fig. 8.12 Intraoperative picture of the same case. Canal wall-up mastoidectomy has been performed. The short process of the incus is visible. The mastoid is free from pathology. I, incus; MFD, middle fossa dura; PCW, posterior canal wall; SS, sigmoid sinus.

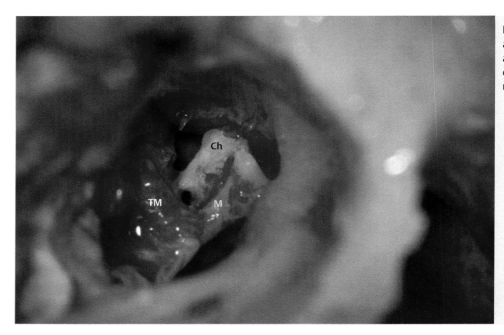

Fig. 8.13 The tympanic membrane is reflected anteroinferiorly and the cholesteatoma is visible anteromedially to the handle of the malleus. Ch, cholesteatoma; M, malleus; TM, tympanic membrane.

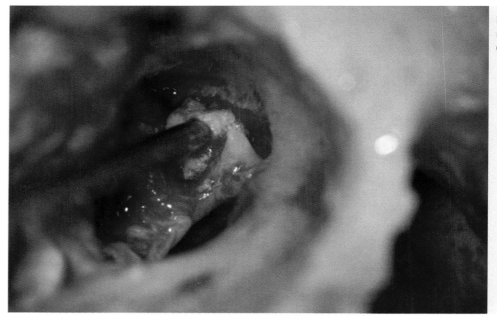

Fig. 8.14 The cholesteatoma is progressively removed with the help of the suction and Cottonoids (see ▶ Fig. 8.15).

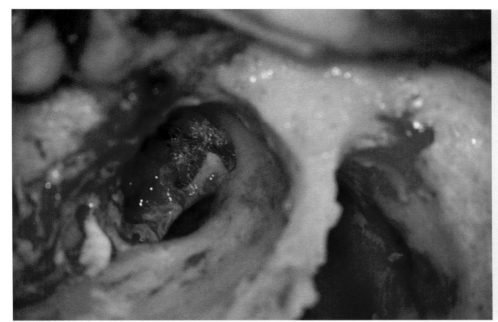

Fig. 8.15 Cottonoids are used to clean the medial surface of the handle of the malleus to avoid any residual pathology. In cases like this (cholesteatoma in the only hearing ear), it is of utmost importance to be radical in disease extirpation and careful to preserve structure and function of the middle ear.

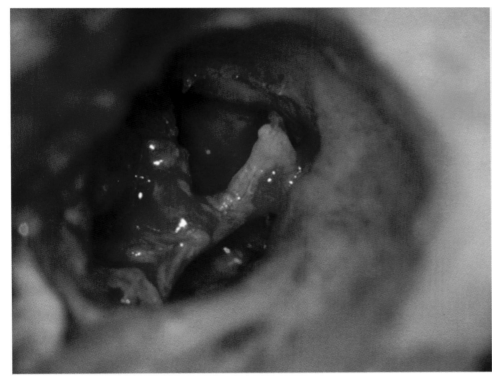

Fig. 8.16 View after disease clearance. The malleus and the middle ear cleft are free from the cholesteatoma. A 0- or 30-degree endoscope could be used to further check for any residual pathology. At the end of the procedure, the tympanic membrane is reflected and reconstructed/reinforced with a piece of fascia of the temporalis muscle, while the middle ear is filled with Gelfoam (see Chapter 7 for myringoplasty).

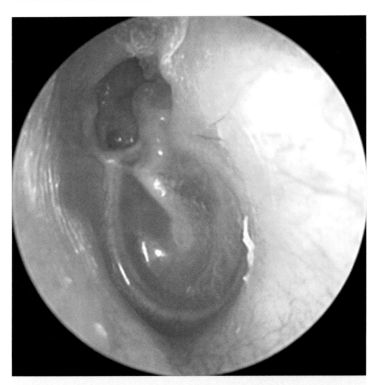

Fig. 8.17 Left ear. Epitympanic erosion with cholesteatoma. The head of the malleus and the supratubal recess are visible.

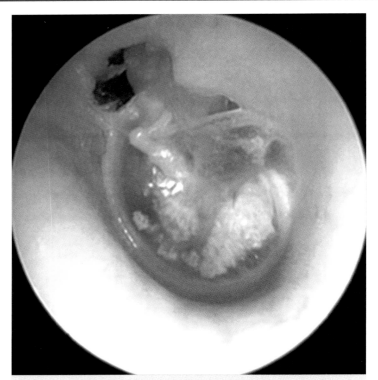

Fig. 8.18 Left ear. Epitympanic cholesteatoma. The head of the malleus and the body of the incus are visible. The inferior and posterior quadrants of the tympanic membrane are tympanosclerotic. The cholesteatoma was lateral to the ossicular chain (see ▶ Fig. 8.19). Hearing function was normal. A modified Bondy's technique tympanoplasty, was performed and no recurrence of cholesteatoma occurred during the follow-up.

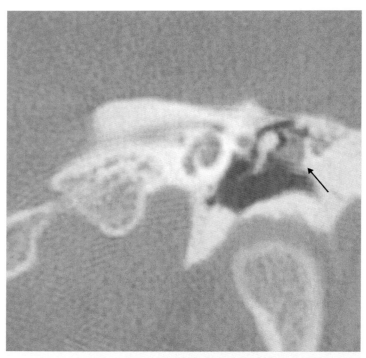

Fig. 8.19 CT of the previous case, coronal view. The cholesteatoma is located in the epitympanic area (arrow), lateral to the malleus. The middle ear is free.

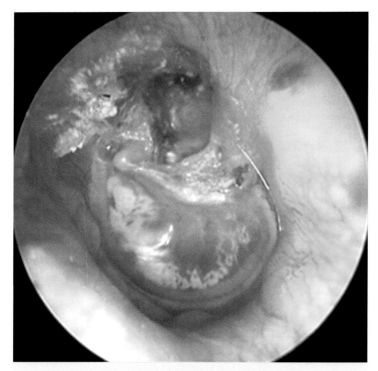

Fig. 8.20 Large epitympanic erosion with cholesteatoma. The head of the malleus and the body of the incus are eroded.

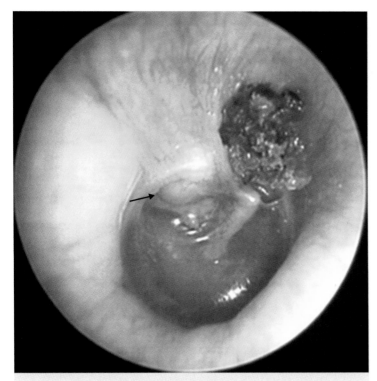

Fig. 8.21 Epitympanic cholesteatoma with erosion of the head of the malleus and the incus. The mass is in contact with the stapes (*arrow*), resulting in normal hearing. The rest of the tympanic membrane is slightly retracted (with myringostapedopexy) due to obstruction of the Eustachian tube. In cases like this, surgery could probably worsen the hearing function (with resulting conductive hearing loss), so the patient has to be informed for an eventual second-stage ossiculoplasty.

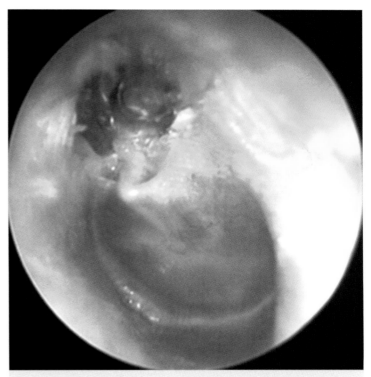

Fig. 8.22 Same patient as in ▶ Fig. 4.6, contralateral side. Large epitympanic erosion with cholesteatoma. Erosion of the head of the malleus is also visible. The CT scan (see ▶ Fig. 8.23, ▶ Fig. 8.24, ▶ Fig. 8.25) also showed involvement by the pathology at the level of the incudostapedial joint, antrum, and mastoid. Audiometry showed moderate conductive hearing loss. In this case, an open tympanoplasty is the treatment of choice. A second stage with ossiculoplasty could be eventually performed in case of poor hearing recovery or to exclude residual disease, after 10 to 12 months, via a transcanal approach.

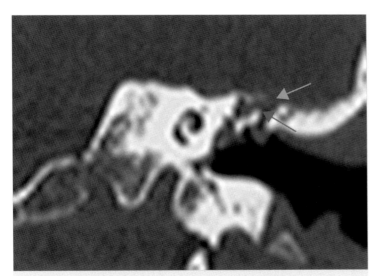

Fig. 8.23 CT scan, coronal view. Epitympanic cholesteatoma with erosion of the head of the malleus (*red arrow*) and thinning of the tegmen tympani (*green arrow*).

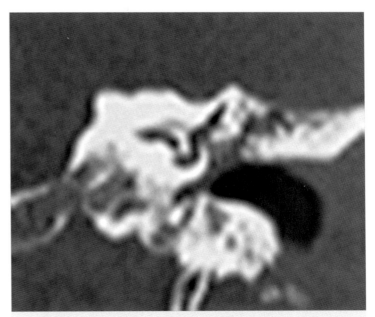

Fig. 8.24 CT scan, coronal view. The long process of the incus and stapes suprastructure seem involved and eroded by the cholesteatoma.

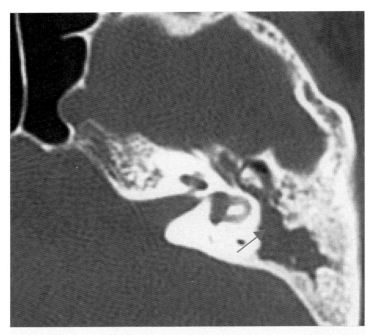

Fig. 8.25 CT scan, axial view. The cholesteatoma extends posteriorly toward the antrum and the mastoid (*arrow*).

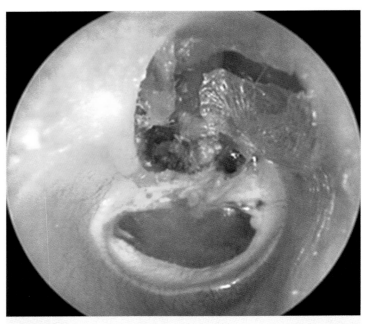

Fig. 8.26 Another case of epitympanic cholesteatoma. There is a deep erosion with involvement of the malleus and the incus.

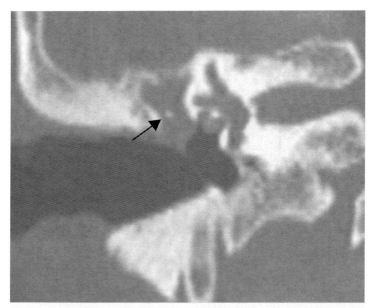

Fig. 8.27 CT scan, coronal view, of the same case. Epitympanic cholesteatoma with erosion of the long process of the incus (*arrow*).

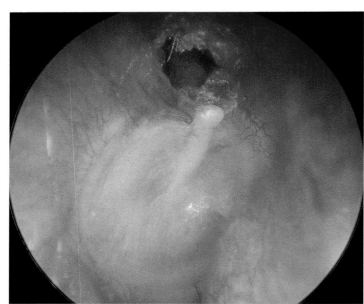

Fig. 8.28 Right ear. Epitympanic erosion with cholesteatoma. The tympanic membrane is completely tympanosclerotic. The patient did not complain of otorrhea (dry cholesteatoma).

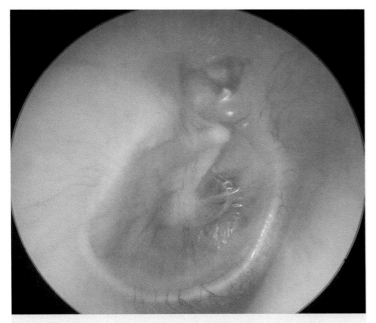

Fig. 8.29 Right ear of a 46-year-old patient suffering from bilateral cholesteatoma. An epitympanic erosion with cholesteatoma and middle ear effusion showing an air–fluid level can be seen. CT scan (▶ Fig. 8.31) demonstrates cholesteatoma extension into the mastoid. Intraoperatively, a fistula of the lateral semicircular canal was encountered, as well as erosion of the incus. A single-stage open tympanoplasty was performed with autologous incus interposition between the handle of the malleus and the head of the stapes. In patient with bilateral cholesteatoma, an open technique is preferred.

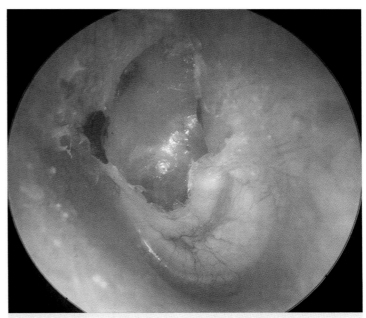

Fig. 8.30 Left ear of the same patient. Cholesteatoma with marked erosion of the scutum and epidermization of the attic and mesotympanum. The cholesteatoma debris was partially cleaned. The residual pars tensa shows tympanosclerosis. Intraoperatively, the ossicular chain was absent. The otoscopic view of the left ear is apparently more advanced than the right ear. This, however, was not the case intraoperatively since the marked epitympanic erosion shown here allowed self-cleaning of the cholesteatoma debris (see CT scan, ▶ Fig. 8.31). Because of the total destruction of the ossicular chain, a second stage was programmed for functional reconstruction.

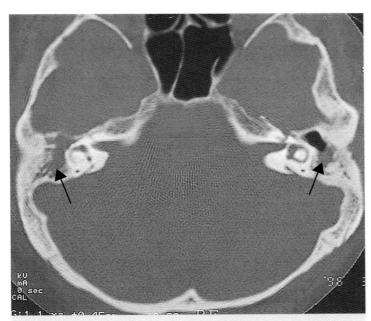

Fig. 8.31 CT of the previous case showing cholesteatoma extension in the mastoid in the right ear and self-cleaning of the cholesteatoma debris in the left ear (*arrows*).

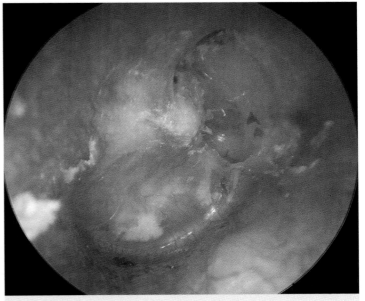

Fig. 8.32 Right ear. Large epitympanic erosion with cholesteatoma. This 18-year-old patient did not have otorrhea. Ipsilateral hearing was normal, whereas the contralateral side showed severe sensorineural hearing loss secondary to previous surgery of radical mastoidectomy. Given the intact ossicular chain, an open tympanoplasty (modified Bondy's technique) was performed. According to our strategy, cholesteatoma in the only hearing ear is one of the absolute indications for performing an open technique. The reason is that this technique, if properly performed, ensures complete eradication of the pathology and better long-term follow-up, thus minimizing the risk of recurrence. Further surgical interventions, with their potential risk even in the most experienced hand, are therefore avoided.

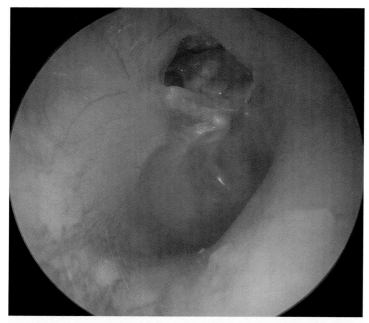

Fig. 8.33 Right ear. Large epitympanic erosion with cholesteatoma and polypoid tissue that covers the head of the malleus. The pars tensa is intact.

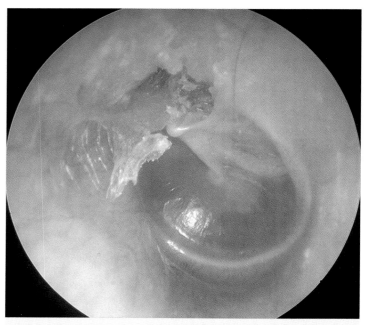

Fig. 8.34 Left ear. Epitympanic cholesteatoma. Extensive erosion of the scutum with excessive cholesteatomatous debris. The pars tensa shows grade I atelectasis with catarrhal middle ear effusion.

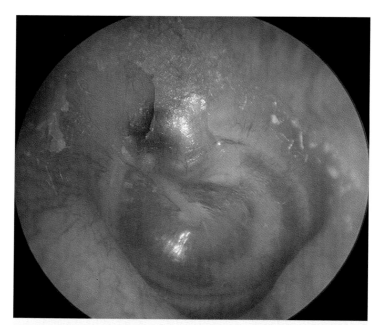

Fig. 8.35 Left ear. Cystic retrotympanic cholesteatoma situated posterior to the malleus. The tympanic membrane shows bulging at the level of the pars flaccida and slight retraction with tympano-sclerosis in the posterior quadrants.

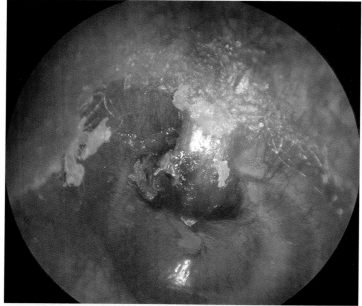

Fig. 8.36 Same case as in ▶ Fig. 8.35 during an acute inflammatory episode. Note the increase in size of the cholesteatomatous cyst.

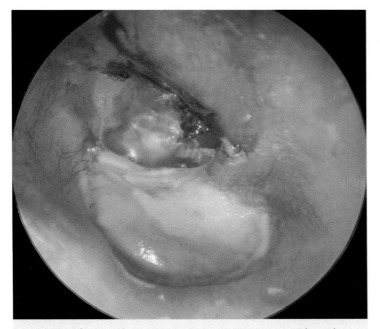

Fig. 8.37 Left ear. A large epitympanic erosion is seen with epidermization of the attic and posterior mesotympanum. The cholesteatoma, visible in transparency, causes bulging of the tympanic membrane in the posterior inferior quadrants. Resorption of the incus and head of the malleus is discernible.

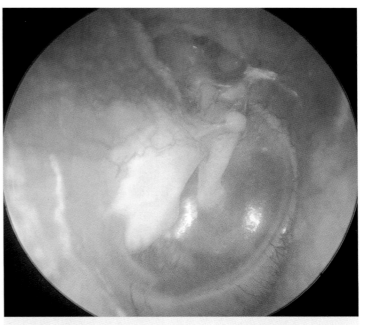

Fig. 8.38 Right ear. Epitympanic erosion with cholesteatoma. Extension of the cholesteatoma into the mesotympanum is seen through the bulging posterior quadrants of the tympanic membrane.

8.3 Mesotympanic Cholesteatoma

See ▶ Fig. 8.39, ▶ Fig. 8.40, ▶ Fig. 8.41, ▶ Fig. 8.42, ▶ Fig. 8.43, ▶ Fig. 8.44, ▶ Fig. 8.45, ▶ Fig. 8.46, ▶ Fig. 8.47, ▶ Fig. 8.48, ▶ Fig. 8.49, ▶ Fig. 8.50, ▶ Fig. 8.51, ▶ Fig. 8.52, ▶ Fig. 8.53, ▶ Fig. 8.54, ▶ Fig. 8.55, ▶ Fig. 8.56.

Summary

An epitympanic retraction pocket should be regularly checked with otomicroscopy. The 30-degree rigid endoscope allows visualization of the extent of the retraction pocket that can be difficult with the microscope. When progression of the epithelium into the epitympanum cannot be controlled, the presence of cholesteatoma is considered. In such cases, surgery should be performed. Whenever a minor epitympanic erosion is present, we adopt a closed technique with reconstruction of the attic using a cartilage and bone paste. This technique is valid particularly in children, in whom the mastoid is usually very pneumatized. Frequently, surgery is staged in these cases.

When a marked attic erosion is present, especially in adults, we perform an open technique to avoid cholesteatoma recurrence that can occur due to absorption of the material used for reconstruction of the attic defect. When preoperative hearing is normal in the presence of attic cholesteatoma with large bony erosion, we perform an open tympanoplasty in the form of a modified Bondy's technique. This technique allows single-stage eradication of the disease with conservation of the normal preoperative hearing.

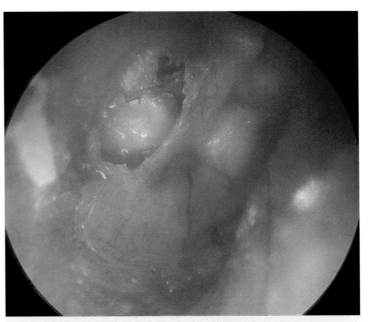

Fig. 8.39 Right ear. Mesotympanic cholesteatoma. The epithelial squamae can be seen through the retromalleolar perforation. Anterior to the malleus, the cholesteatoma mass causes bulging and whitish coloration of the tympanic membrane without perforating it. The entire middle ear is filled with cholesteatoma in this case.

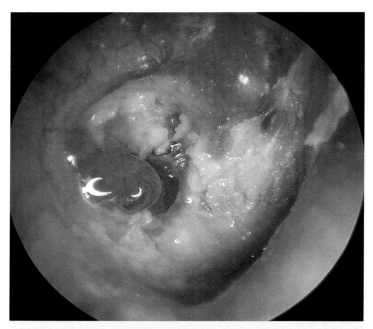

Fig. 8.40 Right ear. Posterior mesotympanic cholesteatoma associated with a polyp are seen at the level of the oval window. There is evidence of discharge.

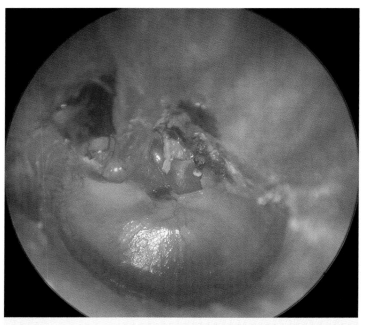

Fig. 8.41 Left ear. Small epitympanic erosion and mesotympanic retraction pocket with wax and cholesteatomatous squamae. Extension of the cholesteatomatous mass into the anteromalleolar region is seen through the retracted tympanic membrane.

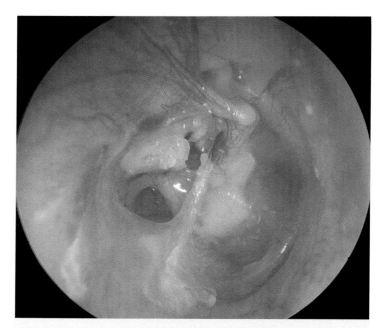

Fig. 8.42 Right ear. Posterior perforation with cholesteatoma in the posterior mesotympanum. The cholesteatomatous squamae cover the region of the oval window extending toward the attic and progress anterior to and under the handle of the malleus. The promontory and the round window are visible through the perforation.

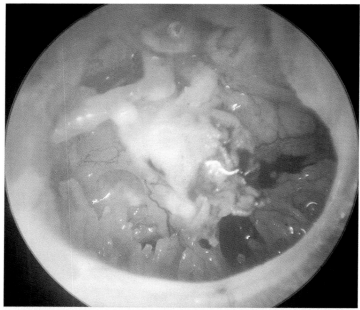

Fig. 8.43 Right ear. Total tympanic membrane perforation. The handle of the malleus is absent. The long process of the incus and part of the stapes are covered by cholesteatoma, which also involves the promontory. The round window, hypotympanic air cells, and tubal orifice are free from the pathology. In these cases, a staged closed tympanoplasty can be performed.

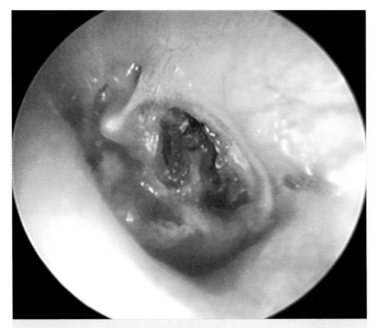

Fig. 8.44 Mesotympanic cholesteatoma. The long process of the incus is surrounded by cholesteatoma. The rest of the tympanic membrane is tympanosclerotic. In this case, a staged open tympanoplasty is the treatment of choice.

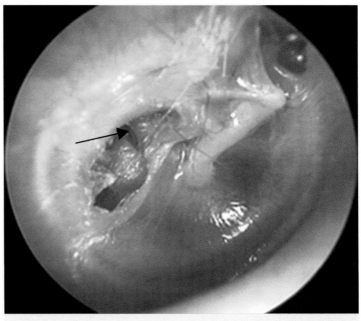

Fig. 8.45 Mesotympanic retraction pocket with cholesteatoma. An epitympanic retraction is also visible. The incudostapedial joint is completely epithelialized (*arrow*).

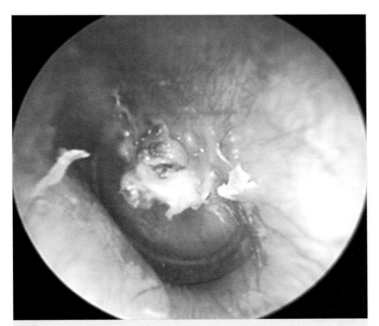

Fig. 8.46 Left ear. Mesotympanic cholesteatoma. The area of the incudostapedial joint is completely surrounded by cholesteatoma, resulting in erosion of both the long process of the incus and stapes suprastructure (see ▶ Fig. 8.47). The patient further underwent staged open tympanoplasty.

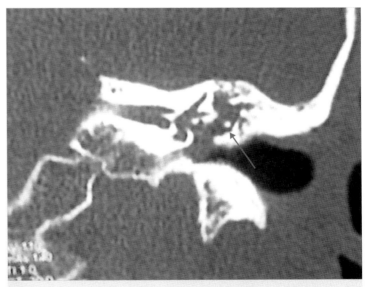

Fig. 8.47 CT scan, coronal view, of the same case. Cholesteatoma fills the middle ear cleft with erosion of the long process of the incus (*arrow*). The suprastructure of the stapes seems completely absent due to the cholesteatomatous process.

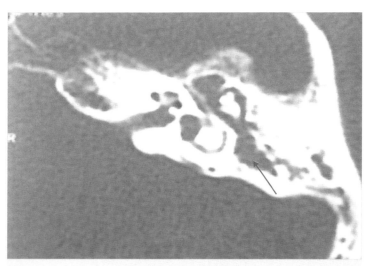

Fig. 8.48 CT scan, coronal view, of the same case. The cholesteatoma extends toward the antrum and the mastoid air cells (*arrow*).

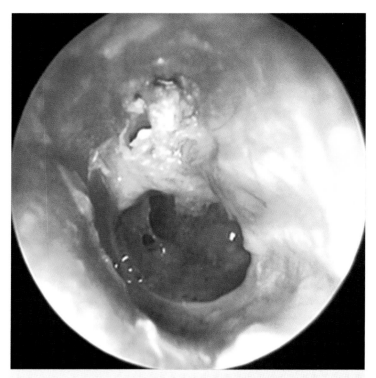

Fig. 8.49 Epi- and mesotympanic cholesteatoma. Both the malleus and the incus are completely involved by the pathology. The tympanic membrane shows a large perforation of the inferior quadrants. The mucosa of the middle ear is hypertrophic due to infection with fetid otorrhea.

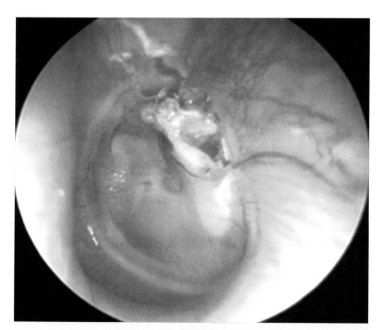

Fig. 8.50 Epi- and mesotympanic cholesteatoma. Even in this case, the long process of the incus is eroded by the pathology. The tympanic membrane shows tympanosclerosis.

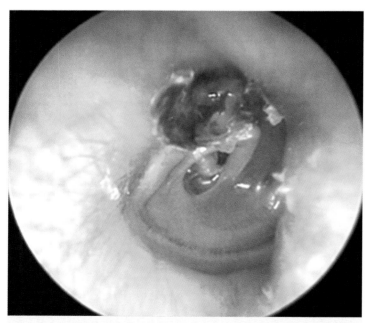

Fig. 8.51 Right ear. Epi- and mesotympanic cholesteatoma. There is a deep epitympanic erosion and a mesotympanic retraction pocket. The incudostapedial joint seems not disrupted, resulting in mild conductive hearing loss. However, in this case the involvement of the whole epitympanic area and the mastoid compartment led to a staged canal wall down (open) tympanoplasty.

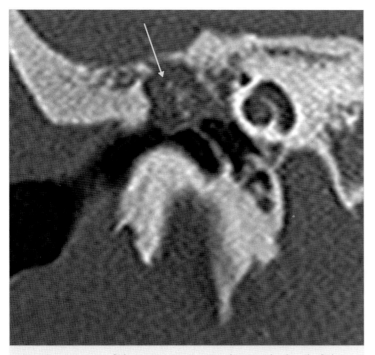

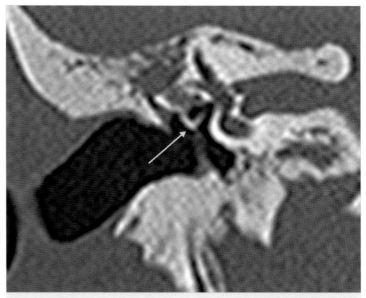

Fig. 8.53 CT scan of the same case, coronal view. The incudostapedial joint is not disrupted (*arrow*).

Fig. 8.52 CT scan of the same case, coronal view. The head of the malleus is eroded and engulfed by the disease (*arrow*).

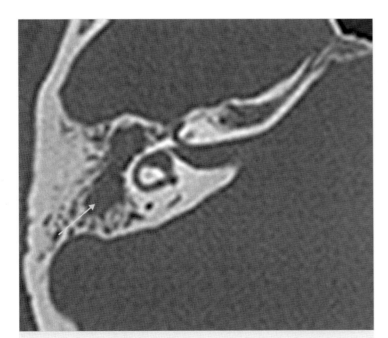

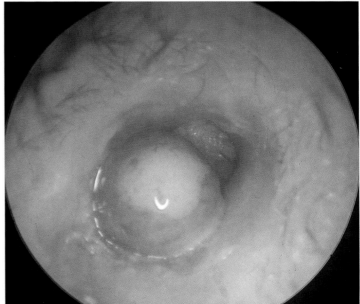

Fig. 8.54 CT scan of the same case, axial view. The cholesteatoma fills the mastoid cavity (*arrow*).

Fig. 8.55 Polyp in the external canal in a child presenting with continuous otorrhea and hearing loss. A CT scan (Fig. 8.56) shows the presence of a soft-tissue mass eroding the intercellular septa of the mastoid and the ossicular chain, suggestive of cholesteatoma. This was confirmed during surgery.

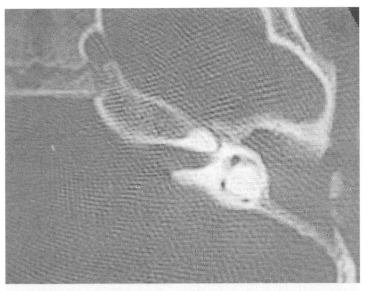

Fig. 8.56 CT scan, axial view. The entire mastoid is occupied by a soft-tissue mass. The intercellular septa of the mastoid and the ossicular chain are absent.

Summary

The presence of a posterior mesotympanic retraction pocket is usually associated with erosion of the ossicular chain. Surgery is indicated in these cases. The retraction pocket is completely removed after performing canalplasty of the posterior canal wall. In the same stage, the tympanic membrane is grafted, the posterosuperior quadrant of the tympanic membrane is reinforced, and middle ear aeration is restored using Silastic sheeting. One year later, if the tympanic membrane position remains normal (i.e., not retracted), the ossicular chain is reconstructed.

When an extensive erosion of the posterior wall is present, a modified radical mastoidectomy is indicated in the elderly, whereas a staged open tympanoplasty is performed in younger patients. The same strategy is also followed in patients presenting with bilateral cholesteatoma.

8.4 Cholesteatoma Associated with Atelectasis

See ▶ Fig. 8.57, ▶ Fig. 8.58, ▶ Fig. 8.59, ▶ Fig. 8.60, ▶ Fig. 8.61, ▶ Fig. 8.62.

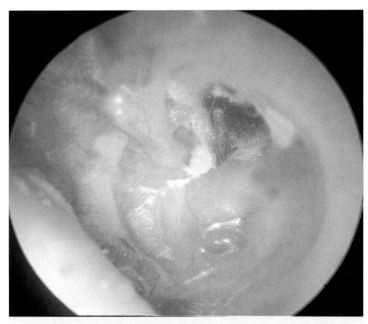

Fig. 8.57 Left ear. Grade IV tympanic membrane atelectasis with posterosuperior mesotympanic retraction pocket. A mixture of wax and cholesteatoma debris is seen. The middle ear mucosa is visible because of absence of the epithelial layer.

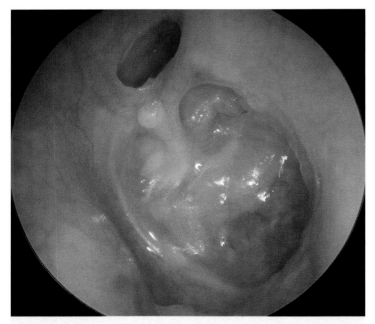

Fig. 8.58 Left ear. Epitympanic erosion through which a cholesteatoma is seen filling the attic and causing erosion of the head of the malleus. A grade IV atelectasis of the tympanic membrane (adhesive otitis) is seen, with formation of polypoidal granulation tissue in the middle ear. In the region posterior to the malleus, the cholesteatoma engulfs the ossicular chain.

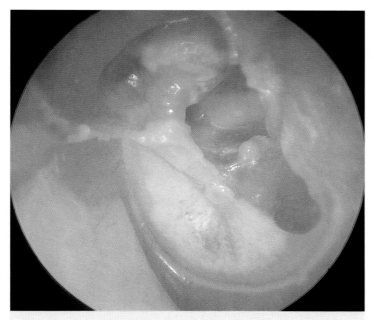

Fig. 8.59 Left ear. Epitympanic erosion with cholesteatoma associated with atelectasis of the tympanic membrane. The incus is absent. A natural myringostapedopexy has been created. The second portion of the facial nerve is seen superior to the stapes; inferiorly the round window is noted. The anterior part of the tympanic membrane is affected with tympanosclerosis. In these cases, as hearing loss is mild (< 30 dB), a modified radical mastoidectomy is indicated to maintain the normal preoperative hearing level obtained as a result of the spontaneous myringostapedopexy.

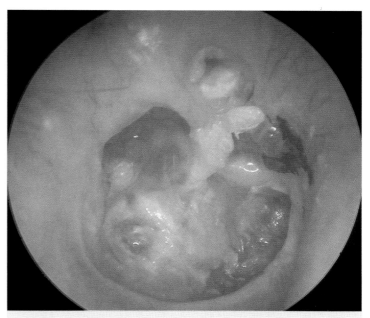

Fig. 8.60 Right ear. Epitympanic cholesteatoma associated with complete atelectasis of the tympanic membrane (see CT scan, ▶ Fig. 8.56).

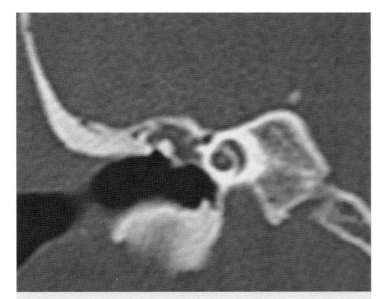

Fig. 8.61 CT scan of the previous case. An epitympanic cholesteatoma is found. Adhesions between the tympanic membrane and the promontory can be observed. This 45-year-old woman underwent a modified radical mastoidectomy with no interference in the middle ear.

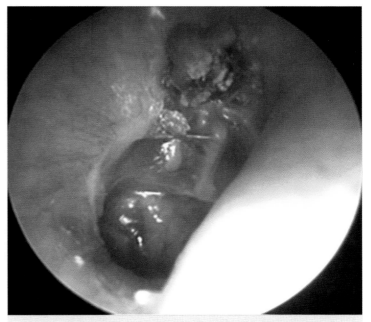

Fig. 8.62 Epitympanic cholesteatoma associated with complete retraction of the inferior quadrants of the tympanic membrane. There is atelectasis on the round window. The anterior quadrants are not completely visible due to anterior hump of the external auditory canal. An open tympanoplasty with proper canalplasty is indicated in this case. Eventually, a ventilation tube can be inserted in the same stage.

Summary

In adult patients with extended epitympanic erosion or with bilateral cholesteatoma, we prefer to perform an open technique. In all cases of spontaneous tympanostapedopexy with normal preoperative hearing or elderly patients with normal contralateral hearing, we prefer to leave the atelectatic tympanic membrane untouched after having verified the absence of any middle ear cholesteatoma. In the presence of mesotympanic cholesteatoma, staging is indicated. In the first operation, a closed tympanoplasty is performed with reconstruction of the tympanic membrane, and a Silastic sheet is positioned in the middle ear. Silastic favors regeneration of the middle ear mucosa and prevents the formation of adhesions. In the second stage, performed 6 to 8 months later, the middle ear is checked for the presence of any residual cholesteatoma. The ossicular chain is then reconstructed using, preferably, an autologous incus. In children, we always try to perform a staged closed tympanoplasty. If a recurrent cholesteatoma (epitympanic retraction pocket) is encountered in the second stage, we do not hesitate to switch to an open technique.

8.5 Cholesteatoma Associated with Complications

See ▶ Fig. 8.63, ▶ Fig. 8.64, ▶ Fig. 8.65, ▶ Fig. 8.66, ▶ Fig. 8.67, ▶ Fig. 8.68, ▶ Fig. 8.69, ▶ Fig. 8.70, ▶ Fig. 8.71, ▶ Fig. 8.72.

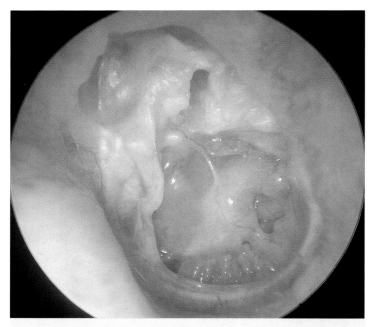

Fig. 8.63 Left ear. Large epitympanic with pars tensa perforation. Cholesteatomatous squamae are present in the attic and mesotympanic area. The handle of the malleus is present. The tympanic annulus is intact. A preoperative CT scan showed the suspicion of a fistula of the lateral semicircular canal, which was encountered during surgery. In such cases, because of the presence of marked epitympanic erosion and of the fistula, an open tympanoplasty is indicated.

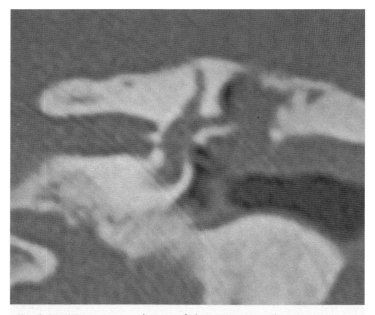

Fig. 8.64 CT scan, coronal view, of the same case. The CT scan, performed 3 months before surgery, showed middle ear pathology compatible with cholesteatoma and suspected fistula of the lateral semicircular canal. The ear was discharging and the patient referred vertigo, while inner ear function was preserved.

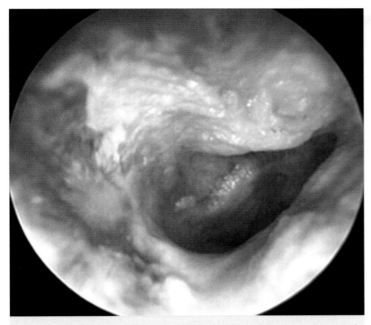

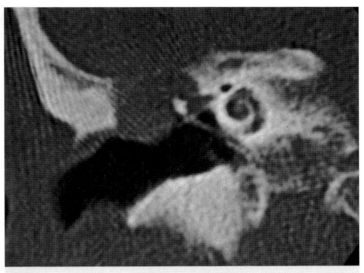

Fig. 8.66 CT scan, coronal view, of the same case. Large bony defect of the tegmen tympani with soft tissue protruding into the middle ear.

Fig. 8.65 Right ear. Bulging of the whole epitympanic area suspected for epitympanic cholesteatoma with meningoencephalic herniation. The CT scan (▶ Fig. 8.66) showed a large bony defect of the tegmen with soft tissue in the middle ear. Intraoperatively, cerebral tissue herniation surrounded by cholesteatoma was found in the middle ear and mastoid. A subtotal petrosectomy was performed.

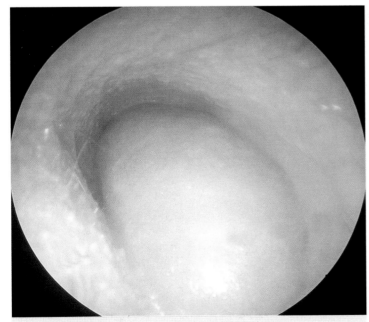

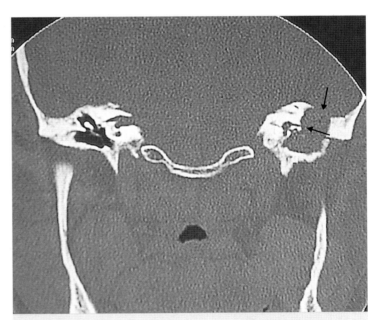

Fig. 8.67 Left ear. Large polyp obstructing the external auditory canal. The patient complained of fetid otorrhea, hearing loss, and vertigo. A high-resolution CT scan of the temporal bone was ordered (▶ Fig. 8.68). A CT scan of the temporal bone should always ordered in patients with chronic suppurative otitis media suffering from vertigo and/or instability.

Fig. 8.68 CT scan of the previous case. A huge cholesteatoma causing a fistula of the lateral semicircular canal and erosion of the tegmen can be seen (*arrows*).

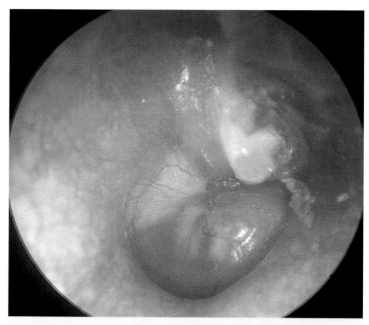

Fig. 8.69 Right ear. Epi- and mesotympanic cholesteatoma. The cholesteatoma debris protruded through the epitympanic erosion. In the posterosuperior quadrant, the cholesteatoma sac can be seen in transparency, causing bulging of the tympanic membrane. The skin surrounding the attic erosion is hyperemic. The pars tensa is intact. The patient complained of frequent episodes of vertigo. A CT scan (see ▶ Fig. 8.70) demonstrated the presence of a fistula of the lateral semicircular canal.

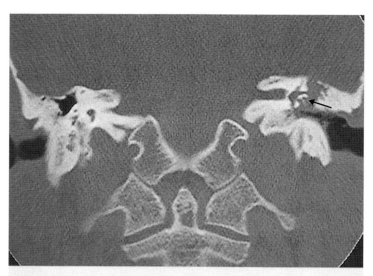

Fig. 8.70 CT scan of the previous case. The interruption of the lateral semicircular canal caused by the cholesteatoma is apparent (*arrow*).

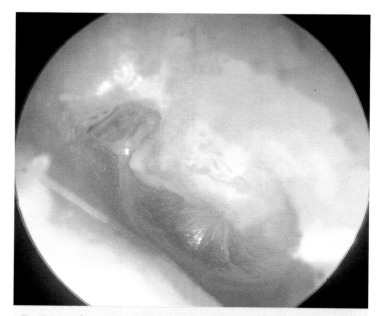

Fig. 8.71 Left ear. Small epitympanic retraction pocket in a patient presenting with hearing loss, tinnitus, and recurrent episodes of otitis media with effusion. The contralateral ear had been operated on elsewhere using an open tympanoplasty that resulted in total hearing loss and facial nerve paralysis. A CT scan of the temporal bone revealed the presence of an epitympanic cholesteatoma that caused a fistula of the superior semicircular canal and erosion of the tegmen (see ▶ Fig. 8.72). The patient underwent open tympanoplasty. Being the only hearing ear, the cholesteatoma matrix was left over the fistula, whereas the tegmental erosion was repaired using cartilage to avoid a meningoencephalic herniation (see Chapter 12).

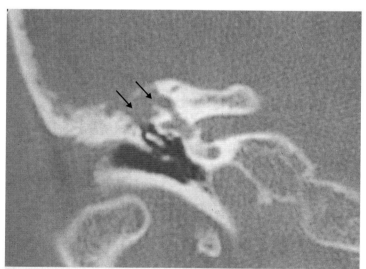

Fig. 8.72 CT scan of the previous case. Cholesteatoma caused a fistula of the superior semicircular canal and erosion of the tegmen (*arrows*).

Summary

At present, with the diagnostic methods at hand and increased medical care, it is very rare to find a cholesteatoma with intracranial complications (e.g., meningitis, brain abscess, lateral sinus thrombophlebitis). However, cases of cholesteatoma with massive bone destruction, labyrinthine fistulas, severe sensorineural hearing loss resulting in deaf ear, and facial nerve paralysis are not infrequently encountered. In general, it is not necessary to order a CT scan to diagnose a cholesteatoma. However, in the presence of headache, vertigo, facial nerve paralysis, severe sensorineural hearing loss, or sudden deafness, a high-resolution CT scan of the temporal bone becomes highly important. Axial and coronal cuts without contrast are required. When intracranial complications are suspected, contrast injection and MRI are also needed.

A labyrinthine fistula is found in less than 10% of cases. The lateral semicircular canal, being the most superficial, is the most commonly involved. Treatment of a labyrinthine fistula depends on the type (bony or membranous) and size of the fistula.

A tegmental erosion can be repaired using cartilage and bone paste.

Facial nerve paralysis is either due to infection of the exposed nerve or secondary to compression by the cholesteatoma. In the majority of cases, removing the cholesteatoma and clearing the infection are sufficient for the paralysis to resolve. It is very rare to find fibrosis or thinning of the nerve. In these cases, facial nerve reconstruction varies from rerouting and end-to-end anastomosis to nerve grafting, according to the degree of injury and length of the injured segment.

8.6 Surgical Treatment of Cholesteatoma: Individualized Technique

Various techniques for cholesteatoma surgery have been developed, practiced, criticized, and favored by different otologists. The current dilemma regarding the choice of technique reflects differences of option between various schools of thinking in otology. However, both the open and closed techniques have now been individualized, and the choice of procedure can be made in accordance with certain indications to optimize the results.

Until the mid-1980, we were very strong proponents of closed cavity techniques. However, we now use open procedures in a large number of cholesteatoma cases and plan the operation in an individualized manner, on a case-by-case basis.

A modified Bondy's mastoidectomy is indicated in epitympanic cholesteatoma when the patient has good hearing and an intact ossicular chain and pars tensa, thus allowing one-stage mastoid cavity exteriorization with removal of the cholesteatoma while preserving the preoperative hearing levels.

We use both the open and closed techniques in patients with a labyrinthine fistula. The cholesteatoma matrix is generally left over the fistula site in open cavity cases, while in closed cavity cases, the matrix is removed with small fistulas, and a second-look operation is performed after 6 months. We prefer an open technique in patients who have a labyrinthine fistula in the only hearing ear, in those with small mastoids, and in other situation in which an open technique is indicated.

We generally prefer the closed techniques in patients with extensively pneumatized mastoids and in children, as we prefer not to create a cavity to prevent the possible later limitations of activity that may result.

However, we do not hesitate to carry out a switch to open cavities in these patients, either during second-stage surgery or whenever there is recurrent disease. Difficulties have been encountered with regard to cavity care and water tolerance in some cases, but the incidence of this is very low in our hands. We attribute this to the effective reduction of the cavity size achieved using the surgical technique we have adopted.

Care is taken to remove all the overhanging margins, to amputate the mastoid tip when an extensively pneumatized mastoid is present, and to create a round cavity; all of these procedures help the prolapse of the adjacent tissues into the cavity, thereby genuinely reducing the size of the cavity.

8.6.1 Canal Wall Up (Closed) Tympanoplasty

Indications

- Cholesteatoma in children and in patients with highly pneumatized mastoids.
- Minor epitympanic erosion.
- Mesotympanic cholesteatoma.
- Cochlear implants.
- Facial nerve decompression.
- Some cases of class B tympanojugular paragangliomas.

In chronic otitis media without cholesteatoma, tympanoplasty without mastoidectomy gives the same result as that with mastoidectomy regarding rate of graft failure and postoperative hearing status. We perform mastoidectomy only in patients with cholesteatoma in the mastoid cavity.

Whenever minor epitympanic erosion is present, we adopt a closed technique with reconstruction of the attic using cartilage and bone paste.

There is no single procedure to treat all cases of cholesteatoma. The surgeon should be flexible and prepared to choose a surgical technique suitable for the particular patient. In general, we use canal wall down (CWD; open) tympanoplasty in most cases of cholesteatoma, as the canal wall up (CWU; closed) technique results in higher residual and recurrent rates compared with the CWD technique. Surgical intervention for cholesteatoma using CWU tympanoplasty should be completed by the second-stage operation, as the objective of the surgery is not only to reconstruct the sound transmission system but also to eradicate any residual cholesteatoma. Currently, we use the closed technique only in selected cases.

In patients with highly pneumatized mastoid, CWU tympanoplasty is also indicated to avoid having a very large cavity. In children, we try to perform a staged CWU tympanoplasty because of their highly cellular mastoids and in an attempt to preserve the anatomy of the ear as much as possible. However, even in such cases, if there is large epitympanic erosion or surgery reveals intensive involvement of the middle ear by cholesteatoma, we use the CWD technique. CWD tympanoplasty is also chosen for the only hearing ear. In the presence of mesotympanic cholesteatoma, especially in young patients, closed tympanoplasty may be indicated. In the first operation, a CWU tympanoplasty is performed with reconstruction of the tympanic membrane, and a Silastic sheet is placed through a posterior tympanotomy toward the Eustachian tube to cover both the tympanic cavity and the mastoid. Silastic favors regeneration of the middle ear mucosa and prevents the formation of adhesions. However, if the posterior wall interferes with the view of the cholesteatoma matrix, for example, by extension toward the Eustachian tube, open tympanoplasty is adopted, especially in old patients.

If the surgeon is not sure whether removal of the posterior canal wall is suitable, every surgical step is performed as CWU tympanoplasty.

Once it turns out that CWD tympanoplasty is indicated, conversion of the technique by removing the posterior wall is not a major effort. Time spent in canalplasty and tympanotomies is worthwhile for the patient.

In the second stage, usually performed 8 to 12 months later, the middle ear is checked for eradication of any residual cholesteatoma. The approach for the second stage is transmeatal, transcanal, or transmastoid, depending on the localization of the cholesteatoma and the approach used in primary surgery. If a recurrent cholesteatoma or absorption of the posterior canal wall is encountered in the second stage, we transform the technique into CWD without hesitation.

Postoperatively, regular otoscopic follow-up, for at least 10 years, is essential to identify the formation of a retraction pocket or recurrent cholesteatoma. If these occur, there should be no hesitation in switching to a CWD tympanoplasty, as we believe that they indicate a persistent underlying pathology, even after the earlier CWU tympanoplasty.

Surgical Technique

The technique used for mastoidectomy in closed tympanoplasty should be the same as for open tympanoplasty. The only difference from the open technique is preservation of posterior canal wall, which may impede the view of the tympanic membrane. Adequate saucerization of the mastoid cavity, with complete drilling of the sinodural angle and bony overhang on the cavity edges should be performed before posterior epitympanotomy and posterior tympanotomy. The saucerized cavity maximizes the surgical view and surgical visualization of the tympanic membrane. The canal wall should therefore not be thinned at the outset.

A meatal skin flap is elevated medially, and the meatal bone is calibrated if necessary. To obtain better control of any pathology and to facilitate reconstruction, it is important to be able to visualize the entire annulus without moving the microscope.

The attic is opened from behind, with the superior wall of the external auditory canal being left intact. The direction of the drilling should be from medial to lateral. The posterior atticotomy should have sufficient anterior extension to allow the whole attic to be visualized.

The utmost care should be taken not to touch the ossicular chain with the burr. If there is any risk, the incudostapedial joint should be disarticulated first. In this case, reconstruction of the ossicular chain may be performed either at the end of the procedure or during the second-stage operation, depending on the pathology. Care should be taken not to fenestrate the superior wall of the external auditory canal. If this occurs, reconstruction with cartilage and bone paste is performed.

A retraction pocket with a small epitympanic erosion can be dissected and pushed back to the external auditory canal from the posterior cavity using a small Cottonoid. If there is attic cholesteatoma, the head of the malleus is cut and the cog is removed with either a burr or a curette to open the anterior attic recess.

In cases of retraction pocket and attic cholesteatoma, it is important in the closed technique to drill the invisible edge of the lateral attic wall, or to scratch it with a curette, to avoid leaving skin in the middle ear. However, one should avoid creating a large atticotomy, to avoid recurrence.

The posterior wall of the external auditory canal is thinned out. The final step is preferably performed using a large diamond burr. It is important not to make the posterior wall of the external auditory canal too thin. Inadvertent opening and postoperative atrophy of the bony canal wall can lead to recurrent cholesteatoma, even a considerable time after surgery in cases of tubal insufficiency.

To avoid injury to the facial nerve, the third portion of the nerve is identified using a large cutting burr, parallel to the course of the nerve, and with continuous suction and ample irrigation. The nerve is only skeletonized, never exposed. Care should be taken not to open the ampulla of the lateral semicircular canal, which is located just medial to the facial nerve. The chorda tympani is also identified.

Using a diamond burr or a curette, the facial recess between the facial nerve and the chorda tympani is opened. The chordal crest can be seen in this step. A small buttress of bone is left intact posterior to the short process of the incus, to protect the ossicular chain from the burr.

The posterior tympanotomy allows control of the incudostapedial joint and the oval and round windows. It can be opened inferiorly to allow control of the hypotympanum, by cutting the chorda tympani.

To ventilate the epitympanum via the supratubal recess, the overhanging cog is removed with a curette after the malleus head has been mobilized.

Medium to thick Silastic sheeting—shaped to cover the medial wall of the middle ear, including the tubal orifice, the epitympanum, the opened facial recess, and the mastoid—is inserted from the posterior cavity in cases of cholesteatoma, atelectatic ear, and extensive defect of mucosa in the medial wall. The Silastic sheeting helps avoid adhesions between the graft and the denuded tympanic wall and promotes good mucosal regeneration.

The Eustachian tube is blocked with small pieces of Gelfoam, and the tympanic cavity is filled with the same material. Any defect in the tympanic membrane is reconstructed with the temporalis fascia.

At the end of the procedure, the external auditory canal is packed with small pieces of Gelfoam.

This surgical technique is shown in ▶ Fig. 8.73, ▶ Fig. 8.74, ▶ Fig. 8.75, ▶ Fig. 8.76, ▶ Fig. 8.77, ▶ Fig. 8.78, ▶ Fig. 8.79, ▶ Fig. 8.80, ▶ Fig. 8.81, ▶ Fig. 8.82, ▶ Fig. 8.83, ▶ Fig. 8.84, ▶ Fig. 8.85, ▶ Fig. 8.86.

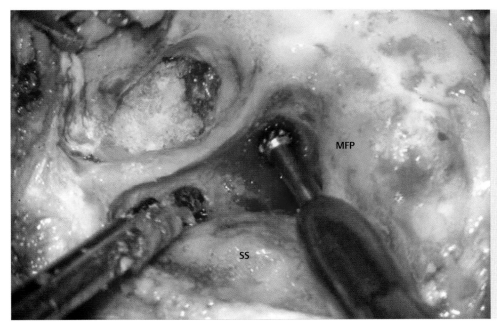

Fig. 8.73 Left ear, a case of epitympanic cholesteatoma. Canal wall up tympanoplasty is performed. The middle fossa plate and the sigmoid sinus are skeletonized. MFP, middle fossa plate; SS, sigmoid sinus.

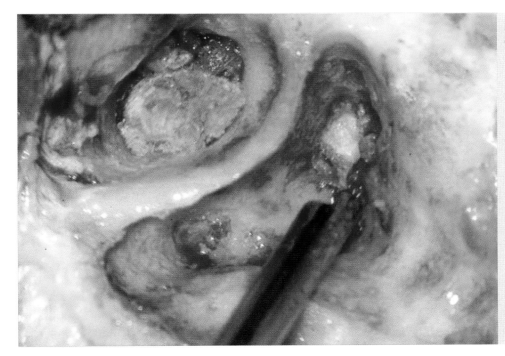

Fig. 8.74 Opening of the antrum visualizes the cholesteatoma filling the antrum.

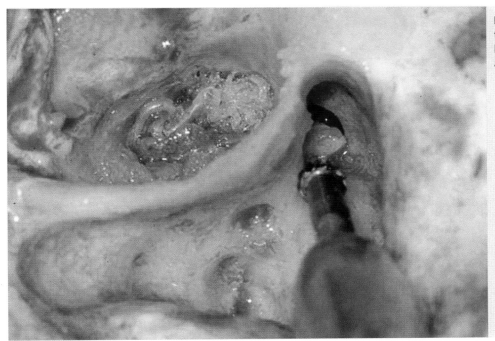

Fig. 8.75 Drilling has been advanced anteriorly to open the attic from the mastoid. Care should be taken not to make the canal wall too thin so as to avoid fenestration.

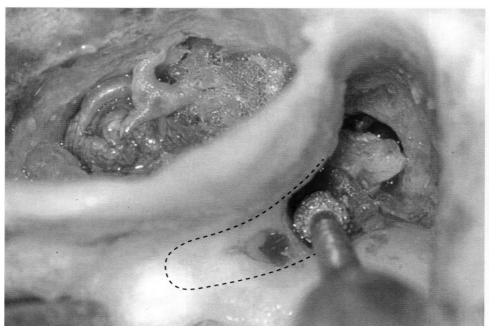

Fig. 8.76 With a diamond burr, the fossa incus is extended inferiorly to perform posterior tympanotomy. Since the incus is already eroded in this case, the procedure does not threaten the ossicular chain. The area to be drilled is indicated by the dotted line. The tympanotomy can be extended more inferiorly by sacrificing the chorda tympani nerve when it is necessary to manage hypotympanum from the mastoid.

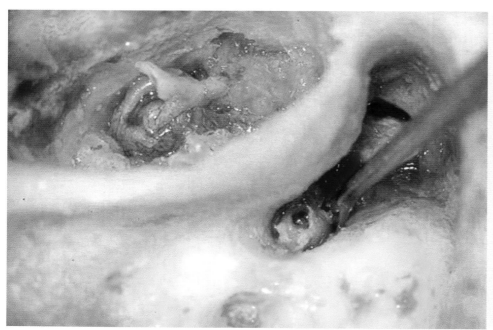

Fig. 8.77 Cholesteatoma is seen filling the facial recess.

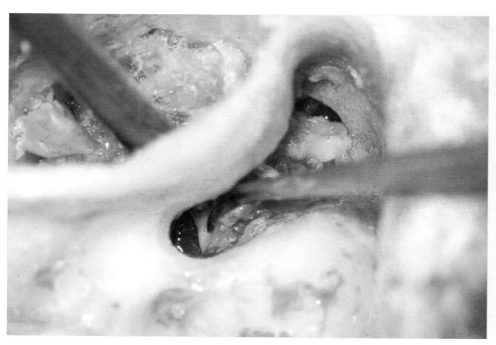

Fig. 8.78 A combined approach is performed to dissect cholesteatoma matrix from the area of the stapes. A suction tube is introduced into the area through the canal, and the dissector through the posterior tympanotomy to obtain a better view of the area. Meticulous care should be taken to remove pathology around the stapes.

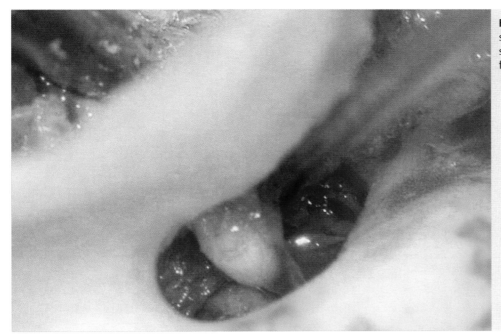

Fig. 8.79 The matrix is dissected from the superstructure of the stapes. The dissection should be performed along the long axis of the footplate.

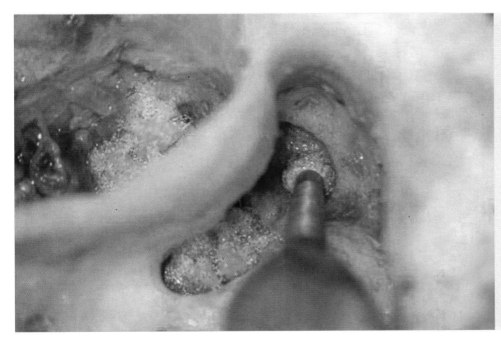

Fig. 8.80 The malleus has been removed to allow removal of cholesteatoma matrix from the supratubal recess. The cog separating the recess from the posterior attic is removed with a diamond burr.

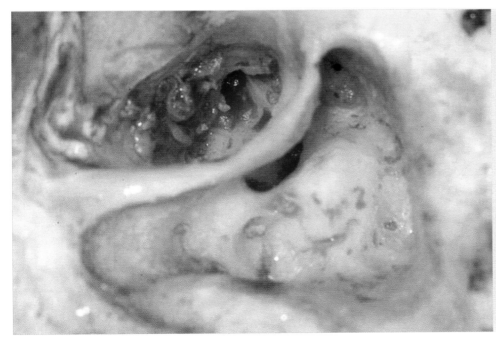

Fig. 8.81 The cholesteatoma is eradicated from the middle ear. Note that the middle fossa plate and the sigmoid sinus are well skeletonized, and the sinodural angle is opened.

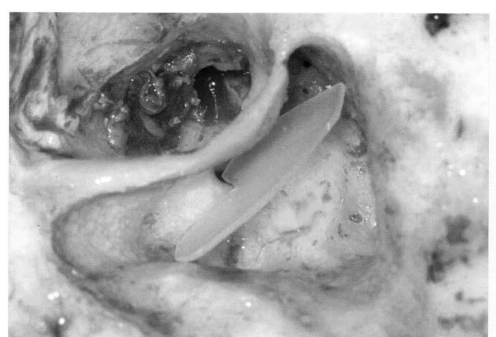

Fig. 8.82 A piece of Silastic sheeting is used to prevent postoperative adhesion of the tympanic membrane.

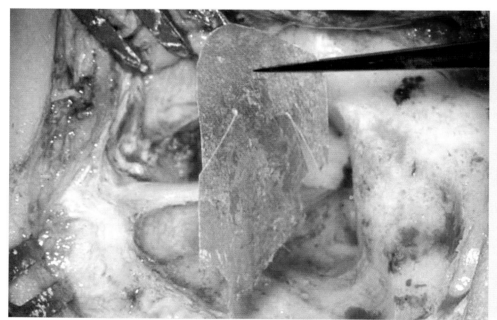

Fig. 8.83 A piece of temporalis fascia is prepared to reconstruct the tympanic membrane. Two small cuts are made in the fascia. One tongue goes under the bony annulus inferiorly, and the other goes under the lateral wall of the attic to facilitate intimate attachment.

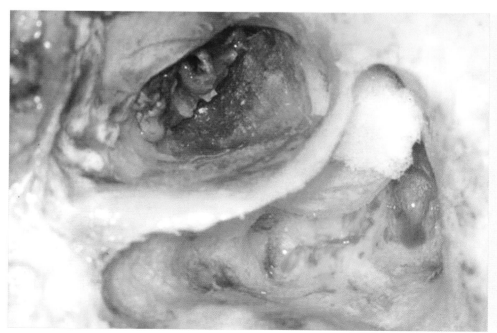

Fig. 8.84 The temporalis fascia is grafted underlay.

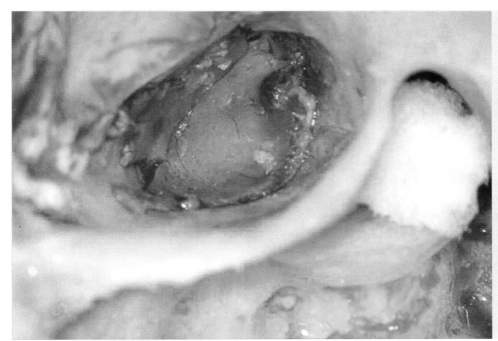

Fig. 8.85 The tympanomeatal flap is replaced over the fascia.

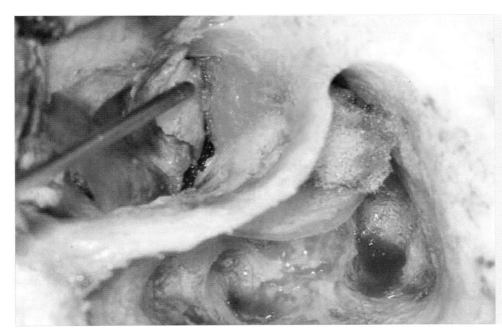

Fig. 8.86 The erosion of the attic is closed with sandwich technique, with two pieces of cartilage and bone paste in between.

8.6.2 Canal Wall Down (Closed) Tympanoplasty

Indications

- Cholesteatoma in cases of:
  - Contracted mastoid.
  - Large epitympanic erosions.
  - Recurrence after the closed tympanoplasty.
  - Bilateral cholesteatoma.
  - Cleft palate and Down's syndrome.
  - Only hearing ear.
  - Large labyrinthine fistula.
  - Severe sensorineural hearing loss.
- Some benign tumors involving the middle ear.
- Some malignancy in the external auditory canal.

When marked attic erosion is present in cholesteatoma, especially in adults, we perform a CWD (open) technique to avoid cholesteatoma recurring. This can occur because of absorption of the material used for reconstruction of the attic defect. In cases with sclerotic mastoids, or when middle ear atelectasis is present, a CWD tympanoplasty is also performed. The number of CWD techniques performed in our center is gradually increasing. As described, we now use the CWU (closed) technique in only limited numbers of cases (fewer than 10%) because of its higher risk of recurrence and residual cholesteatoma.

Today, we apply CWD techniques mainly in cholesteatoma surgery. In our experience, a well-performed CWD operation has a better chance of preventing a second operation and results in minimal reduction of both hearing and quality of life. In CWD tympanoplasty, execution of correct technique is the key to successful surgery. In this technique, since the posterior wall of the external auditory canal is removed, the mastoid and the external auditory canal became a common communicating cavity exposed to the outside after surgery. To avoid postoperative complications, it is very important to create an ideal cavity during the first operation by following correct procedures, such as sufficient saucerization of the cavity and appropriate meatoplasty.

Saucerization of the entire cavity and removal of any overhanging edges not only increases the working space but also allows soft tissue to fill in the bony defect. This makes the cavity smaller without the use of other material for obliteration. We always perform meatoplasty in CWD operations, as this technique allows reduction of raw surfaces and also results in a relatively small and shallow cavity, by enlarging its opening. An adequate meatoplasty is an essential prerequisite for consistent success in CWD tympanoplasties. If all procedures are properly performed, the cavity appears small, shallow, rounded in shape, dry, and well epithelialized.

On the other hand, a badly produced cavity may appear wet and irregular, and the periphery may be difficult to reach. The cavity may be lined with granulation tissue covered by accumulated debris. We have found that technical mistakes commonly seen in the failed cavity are a very narrow meatus and insufficient bone removal, such as a high facial ridge, an overhanging edge, and a prominent mastoid tip. Each of these factors impedes self-cleansing of cerumen and debris from the cavity, resulting in an inflammatory reaction. In addition, the risk of residual and recurrent cholesteatoma is higher in such a cavity.

Those patients who have recurrent cholesteatoma tend to have either poor physiological function of the Eustachian tube or the most difficult-to-manage disease state. Revision surgery preserving the canal wall is likely to cause the patient and family extra expense for additional surgery. Therefore, once cholesteatoma has recurred, we have no hesitation in converting the procedure to CWD technique by removing the posterior canal wall.

Surgical Technique

Local anesthesia (2% lidocaine and 1:100,000 epinephrine) is used in 95% of cases. General anesthesia is required in the remainder, when the patients are young or apprehensive. Using a postauricular skin incision, temporalis fascia is harvested for graft material.

The bone over the tegmen is thinned out to identify the middle fossa dura through the bone. Disease over the dura, if present, is gently removed. If there is any doubt about residual matrix on the dura, it is coagulated using bipolar cautery, as previously described by Sanna et al (1993a). The air cells behind the sigmoid sinus are removed, and the sinodural angle is opened widely.

Usually, the antrum requires wide opening. The posterior canal wall is removed. The perilabyrinthine and the mastoid tip cells are also removed. A prominent, well-pneumatized mastoid tip should be removed to reduce the volume of the mastoid cavity. Drilling starts from the level of the stylomastoid foramen and continues posteriorly, in a rotatory fashion parallel to the digastric ridge, until the tip is undermined. It is important to create a fracture line lateral to the stylomastoid foramen to avoid any traction on the facial nerve in the following process. The

remaining bony shell is mobilized and pulled out in a rotatory fashion with a bone rongeur, and detached from the muscle using electrocautery. This amputation of the mastoid tip not only reduces the cavity volume, but also prevents a "sink trap" effect that may cause postoperative accumulation of skin debris.

The facial nerve should be distinguished from the disease. The two consistent structures for identifying the facial nerve are the cochleariform process and the digastric ridge. The digastric ridge is identified and then followed to the stylomastoid foramen.

The ossicles are usually absent or eroded.

The anterior buttress and the bony spur superior to the cochleariform process are removed along with the anterior attic cells. The zygomatic air cells are exteriorized, thereby removing all the air cells in the epitympanic space and the supratubal recess. The skin of the anterior and inferior bony ear canal is reflected toward the annulus and protected with aluminum foil. The ear canal is enlarged, with care being taken not to uncover the capsule of the temporomandibular joint. The tympanic membrane is then inspected, as usually there is some residual anterior and inferior tympanic membrane present.

The posterior buttress and the facial ridge are lowered to the floor of the external ear canal or the facial nerve itself. The disease is then cleared from the facial recess, sinus tympani, and hypotympanum. At the end of the procedure, the cavity edges are smooth, rounded, and well saucerized. The appearance of white cortical bone signifies total exteriorization of all accessible air cells. Sometimes, a retroauricular, anteroinferiorly based, soft-tissue flap is used to obliterate the area of the mastoid tip.

One of the most important steps in creating a trouble-free cavity is obtaining a wide meatus, to provide an adequate surface-to-volume ratio for aeration, epithelial stability, and good postoperative visualization of the cavity. The conchal incision is made in an anterior to posterior direction, with the help of a nasal speculum. The conchal cartilage is further exposed by dissecting the skin from it. The cartilage on each side of the incision is excised in a triangular fashion. The skin flaps are sutured together with the subcutaneous tissue, so as to lie on the posterosuperior and posteroinferior aspects of the mastoid cavity. These skin flaps cover the remaining edge of the conchal cartilage, thereby preventing the possibility of perichondritis.

In cases in which staged procedures are necessary, medium thickness Silastic is placed on the promontory, with a long extension into the Eustachian tube orifice.

Temporalis fascia is placed on the Gelfoam bed medial to the annulus, spreading over to cover the facial ridge, epitympanum, and mastoid cavity. The residual tympanic membrane and canal skin are placed over it. The cavity and the ear canal are then filled with Gelfoam. The postauricular incision is sutured in layers, and a mastoid bandage is applied.

This surgical technique is shown in ► Fig. 8.87, ► Fig. 8.88, ► Fig. 8.89, ► Fig. 8.90, ► Fig. 8.91, ► Fig. 8.92, ► Fig. 8.93, ► Fig. 8.94, ► Fig. 8.95, ► Fig. 8.96, ► Fig. 8.97, ► Fig. 8.98, ► Fig. 8.99, ► Fig. 8.100, ► Fig. 8.101, ► Fig. 8.102, ► Fig. 8.103, ► Fig. 8.104.

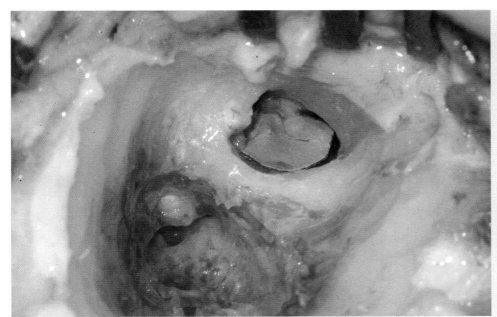

Fig. 8.87 Canal wall down mastoidectomy is performed. The posterior end of cholesteatoma reaching the antrum is beginning to be seen. The tympanomeatal flap is detached from the bony meatus and protected with aluminum sheeting for canalplasty.

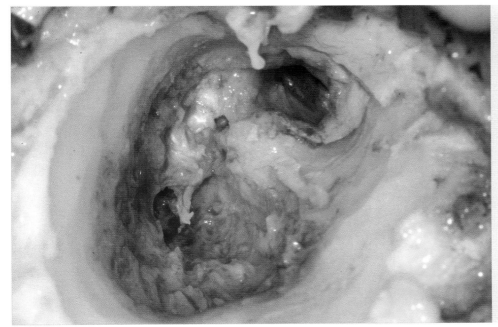

Fig. 8.88 The canalplasty is completed, and the scutum is removed with a curette after thinning the bony bridge lateral to the chain. The cholesteatoma in the attic is visualized.

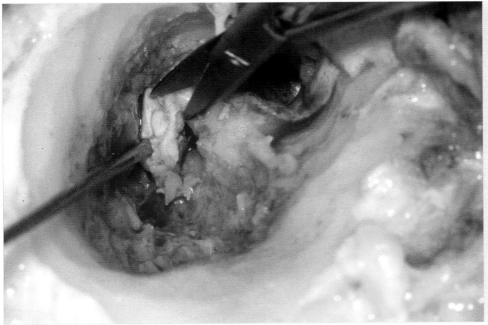

Fig. 8.89 Debulking and piecemeal removal of cholesteatoma is of importance to visualize structures around the matrix and to make room for dissection.

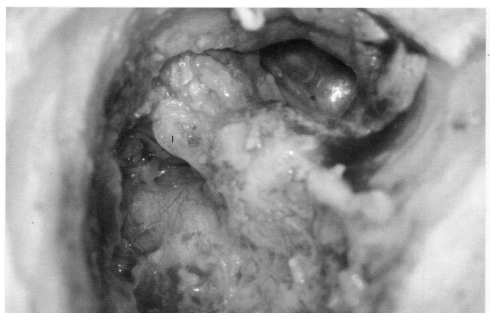

Fig. 8.90 The facial ridge is further lowered to the level of the tympanic membrane to obtain a good rounded cavity. The tympanomeatal flap should be protected by aluminum sheeting during drilling.

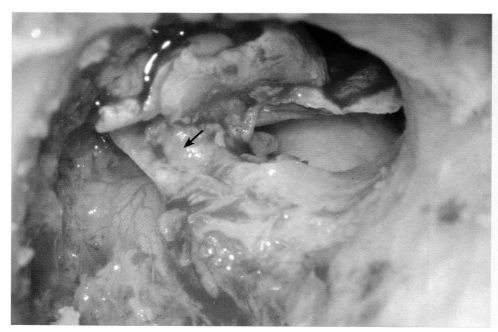

Fig. 8.91 The fibrous annulus is detached to verify absence of cholesteatoma from the tympanic cavity. The long process of the incus is seen (*arrow*).

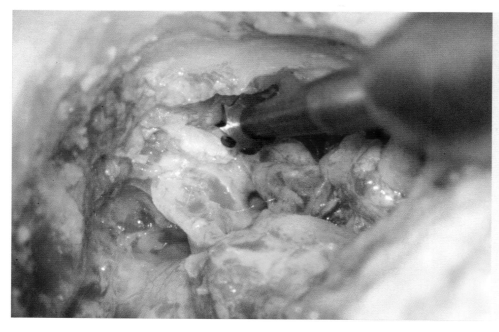

Fig. 8.92 Bony overhangs are removed with a cutting burr to expose the cholesteatoma extending anteriorly. To avoid contact with the ossicular chain, the drill should be moved either from the area near the chain to elsewhere or parallel to the chain.

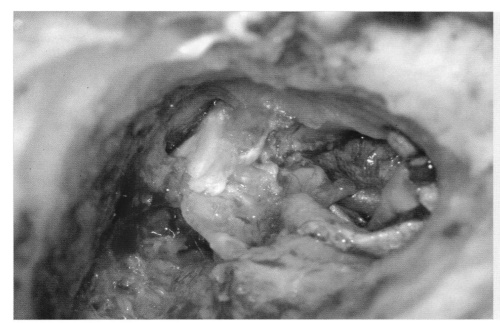

Fig. 8.93 Bony overhangs are removed with a cutting burr to expose the cholesteatoma extending anteriorly. To avoid contact with the ossicular chain, the drill should be moved either from the area near the chain to elsewhere or parallel to the chain.

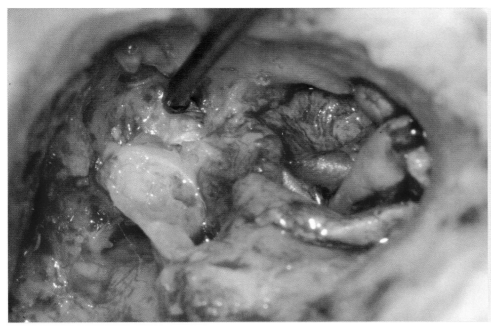

Fig. 8.94 Debulking of the cholesteatoma reveals considerable invagination of the matrix anteriorly to the malleus. Since access to this area is blocked by the ossicular chain, removal of the malleus and the incus is indicated.

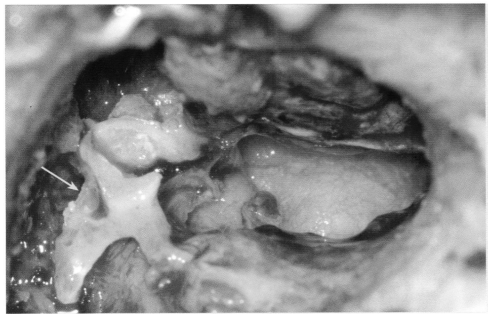

Fig. 8.95 The incudomallear joint is disarticulated, and the incus is taken out. The erosion in the lateral face of the body of the incus is seen (*arrow*).

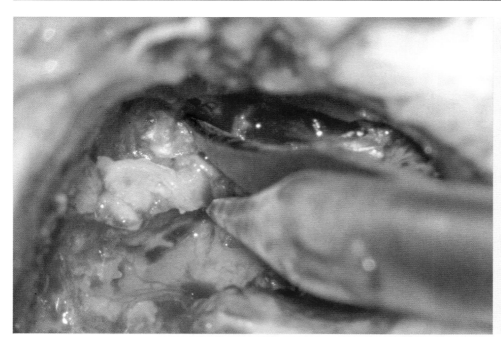

Fig. 8.96 The head of the malleus blocking access to the supratubal recess is removed.

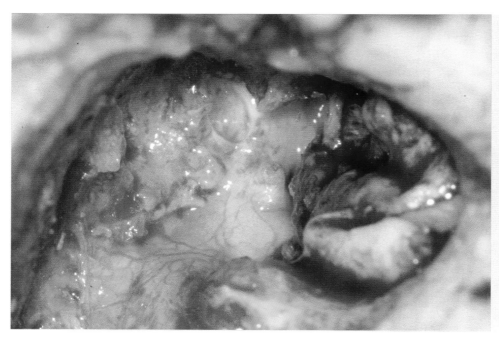

Fig. 8.97 The cholesteatoma is eradicated from the middle ear. The transection of the tendon followed by inferior reflection of the tympanic membrane has sufficiently enlarged the approach to the supratubal recess.

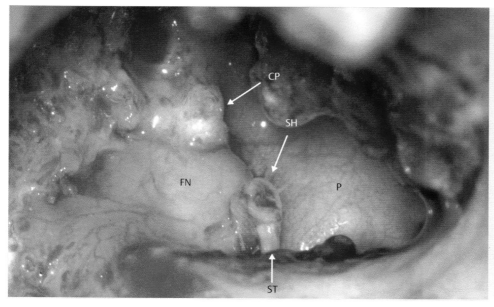

Fig. 8.98 The anatomy around the stapes is shown. Note the prominent bulging of the facial nerve reaching to the stapes. CP, cochleariform process; FN, facial nerve; P, promontory; SH, head of stapes; ST, tendon of stapes.

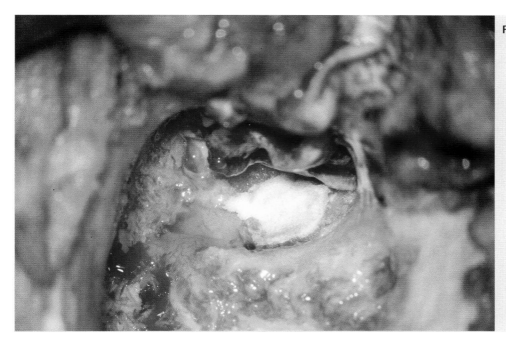

Fig. 8.99 The cavity is packed with Gelfoam.

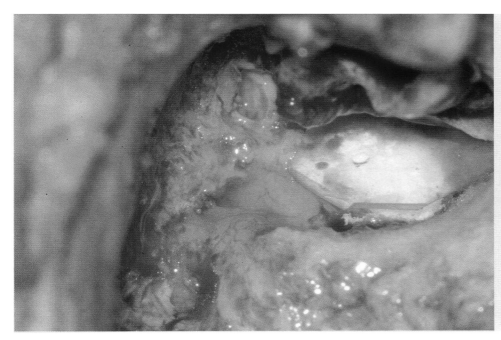

Fig. 8.100 Silastic sheeting is used to avoid postoperative adhesion of the tympanic membrane to the structures in the medial wall.

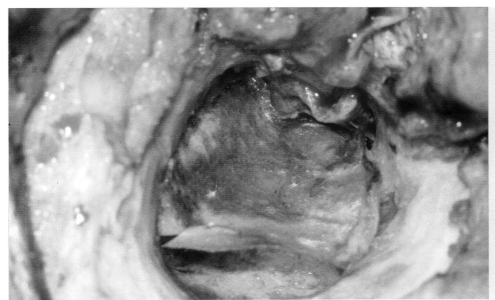

Fig. 8.101 A large piece of temporalis fascia is grafted underlay.

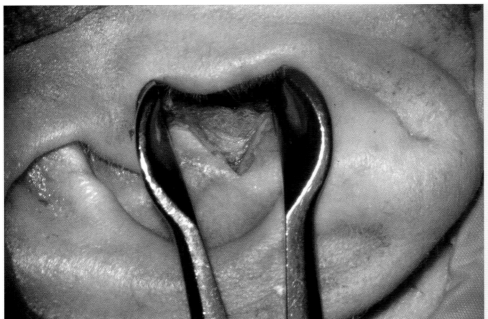

Fig. 8.102 Meatoplasty. A piece of gauze is put over the cavity to prevent blood running into the cavity. A skin cut is made with a Beaver blade including underlying the conchal cartilage. The cut runs almost parallel to the crus of the helix, toward the antihelix. Under the cut, folded gauze that prevents blood from running into the cavity is seen.

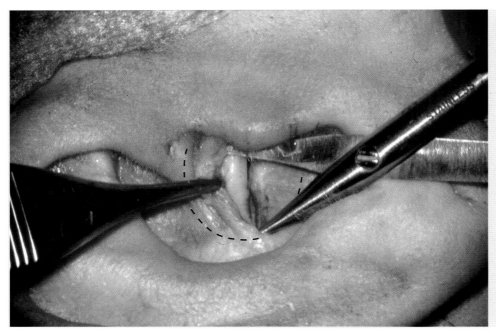

Fig. 8.103 The conchal cartilage is dissected from subcutaneous tissue with scissors to expose a sufficient area. Because the cartilage is fragile, it is wise to hold the skin during this procedure. The cartilage to be removed is indicated by the dashed line.

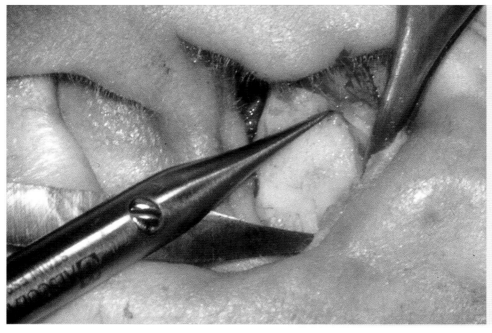

Fig. 8.104 A sufficiently large piece of cartilage is resected at the superior and inferior edges. Finally, the skin flaps are sutured to appropriate positions superiorly and inferiorly to open the meatus widely and to cover the edge of the conchal cartilage. When adequately sutured, the meatus keeps its shape by itself.

8.6.3 Modified Bondy's Technique

Indications

- Epitympanic cholesteatoma in a normal or good hearing ear with an intact tympanic membrane, ossicular chain, and tympanic cavity.
- Epitympanic cholesteatoma in the better or only hearing ear with slightly injured ossicular chain.
- Some cases of bilateral postinflammatory canal stenosis.

In modified Bondy's technique, the posterior canal wall is removed, but the articulations between the ossicles are not touched.

The prerequisite conditions for using this technique are an intact ossicular chain and the tympanic membrane with cholesteatoma located laterally to the chain, usually epitympanic cholesteatoma. A contracted mastoid is preferred. Significant benefits of this technique are constant retention of preoperative hearing, due to the preservation of ossicular articulations, low recurrence, and low rate of residues compared with closed technique, and that it is a one-stage operation that does not necessitate a second intervention.

The risk of this procedure is sensorineural hearing loss at the high frequencies due to acoustic trauma, especially when drilling around the chain, as the ossicular chain remains intact throughout the surgery. Drilling around the chain should be conducted correctly and meticulously. With appropriate selection of cases, there are no further disadvantages compared with other open mastoidectomy procedures.

Surgical Technique

A mastoidectomy is completed using one of two techniques described earlier. Sufficient lowering of the facial ridge to the level of the tympanic annulus is of tremendous importance.

The drill should be moved parallel to the nerve during this procedure. A highly pneumatized mastoid tip should be amputated as described previously. Extensive pneumatizations in the cavity are filled with cartilage or bone paste.

If canalplasty is required, the anterior meatal skin is cut and folded medially. The inferior canal wall is widened to give a round cavity. The tympanomeatal flap should be protected with a thin aluminum sheet during the drilling. The facial bridge is removed with a curette, taking special care not to injure the chain. Burrs may be used, but because the ossicular chain remains intact, this might carry more risks. The anterior and the posterior buttresses are also removed in the same way. The anterior epitympanum should be fully opened. The facial ridge is further lowered. Cholesteatoma is removed from the attic and the mastoid. The posterosuperior annulus is partially detached from the tympanic sulcus, and the tympanic cavity is carefully inspected to ensure absence of cholesteatoma. Pathological tissue, such as scar and granulation tissue, if any, is dissected with meticulous care from the ossicular chain. Minor invagination of cholesteatoma matrix behind the body of the incus and the head of the malleus is carefully dissected from the chain.

Meatoplasty is performed to obtain sufficiently large access to the cavity postoperatively. The conchal cartilage is harvested for the subsequent reconstruction.

A piece of cartilage is placed in the attic, medially to the body of the incus and the head of the malleus. This cartilage prevents retraction of the reconstructed tympanic membrane behind the ossicles. Bone paste should not be used in this area to avoid fixation of the ossicular chain. The Eustachian tube and the tympanic cavity are packed with Gelfoam.

A longitudinal cut is made in the temporalis fascia. One tongue is placed medial to the body of the incus and the head of the malleus, extending anteriorly under the anterosuperior quadrant of the tympanic membrane. The other tongue is inserted lateral to the long process of the incus and medial to the handle of the malleus making the fascia underlay. In some cases, a thin piece of cartilage may be inserted over the long process of the incus to avoid retraction of the posterosuperior quadrant.

As large an exposed bony surface as possible is covered with the posterior extension of the fascia. Another piece of fascia may be placed to cover exposed bone and materials used for obliteration. The tympanomeatal flap is replaced on the temporal fascia.

If the ossicular chain is substantially involved in the cholesteatoma and its dissection is difficult, it is necessary to remove the body of the incus with or without the head of the malleus. This converts the technique to open tympanoplasty. The chain may be reconstructed in the same stage.

This surgical technique is shown in ▶ Fig. 8.105, ▶ Fig. 8.106, ▶ Fig. 8.107, ▶ Fig. 8.108, ▶ Fig. 8.109, ▶ Fig. 8.110, ▶ Fig. 8.111, ▶ Fig. 8.112. Also see ▶ Table 8.1 and ▶ Table 8.2.

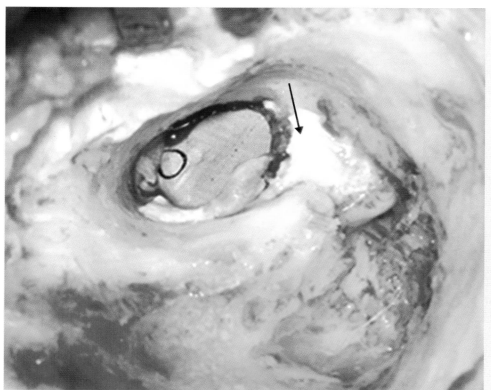

Fig. 8.105 Left ear. Epitympanic cholesteatoma with normal hearing and apparently intact ossicular chain. The former surgical steps are the same of that of a CWD technique. The cholesteatoma is visible lateral to the incus (*arrow*).

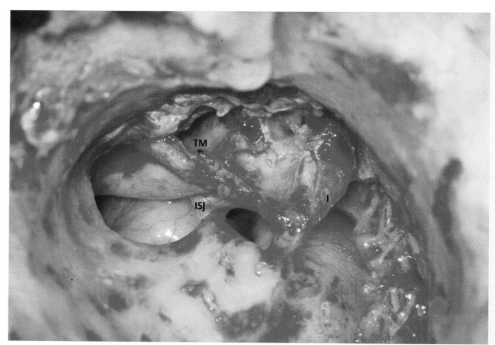

Fig. 8.106 After removal of the cholesteatoma, the intact ossicular chain is exposed. I, incus; ISJ, incudostapedial joint; TM, tympanic membrane.

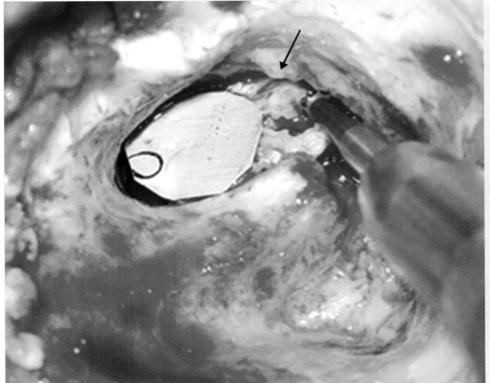

Fig. 8.107 The bony overhang in the attic from the middle fossa plate (*arrow*) is performed with cutting burr to expose the epitympanum. Care should be taken not to touch the ossicular chain, since articulations between the ossicles remain intact in modified Bondy's technique.

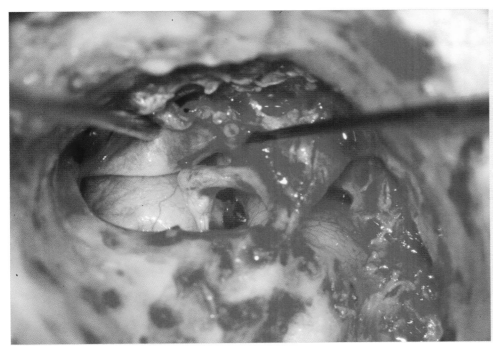

Fig. 8.108 The ossicular chain is further cleaned and checked to avoid any residual disease.

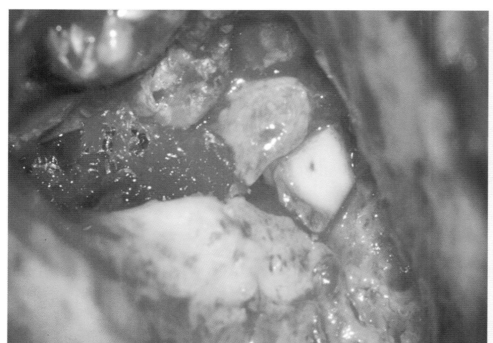

Fig. 8.109 A piece of cartilage is placed in the attic, medially to the body of the incus and the head of the malleus to prevent retraction.

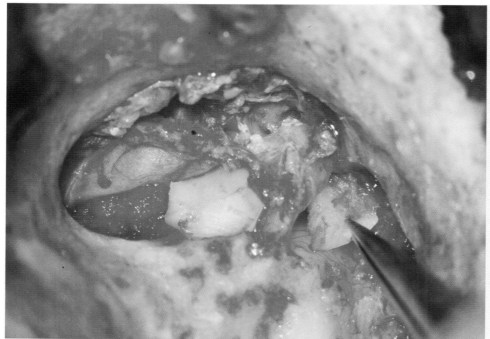

Fig. 8.110 Another piece of conchal cartilage is placed in the attic.

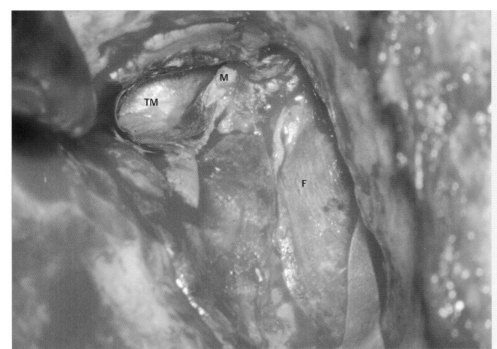

Fig. 8.111 Reconstruction is completed with a piece of temporalis fascia placed over the cartilage and the ossicular chain. F, fascia; M, malleus; TM, tympanic membrane.

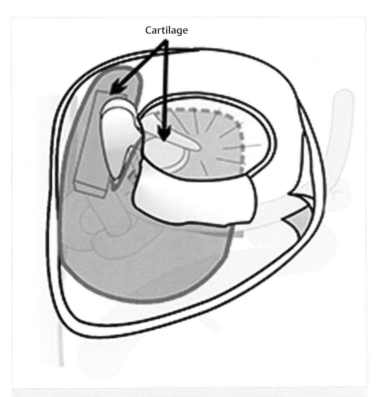

Fig. 8.112 Reconstruction in a modified Bondy's technique tympanoplasty.

Table 8.1 Hearing outcomes in 303 patients operated at the Gruppo Otologico with modified Bondy's technique tympanoplasty for epitympanic cholesteatoma (1983–2014)

Hearing outcomes	Preoperative	Postoperative	
		First year	Fifth year
PTA AC	30 ± 11.8 dB (range 10–66 dB)	30.8 ± 12.25 dB (range 10–80 dB)	30.8 ± 12.3 dB (range 10–80 dB)
PTA BC	16.3 ± 7.5 dB (range 0–45 dB)	16.6 ± 7.5 dB (range 5–51 dB)	16.7 ± 7.6 dB (range 5–51 dB)
PTA ABG	13.6 ± 7 dB (range 0–25 dB)	14.1 ± 7.2 dB (range 0–48 dB)	14 ± 7.5 dB (range 0–48 dB)

Note: Patients had at least 5 years of follow-up. The pure tone averages (PTA) were noted for air conduction (AC) and bone conduction (BC) recorded before and after surgery as the mean of 500, 100, 2,000, and 4,000 Hz. Air–bone gap (ABG) was calculated using the AC and BC values determined at the same time.

Table 8.2 Postoperative sequelae after modified Bondy's procedure in this series (303 cases with 5 years of follow-up, 1983–2014)

Postoperative sequelae	Patients (%)
Recidivism	
• Residual cholesteatoma (lateral to the reconstructed tympanic membrane)	8.1
• Residual cholesteatoma (medial to the reconstructed tympanic membrane)	0
• Recurrent cholesteatoma	0
Effusion	5
Retraction pocket	3.1
Discharging ear	1.5
Perforation	1.5
Meatal stenosis	1.2

Chapter 9

Congenital Cholesteatoma of the Middle Ear

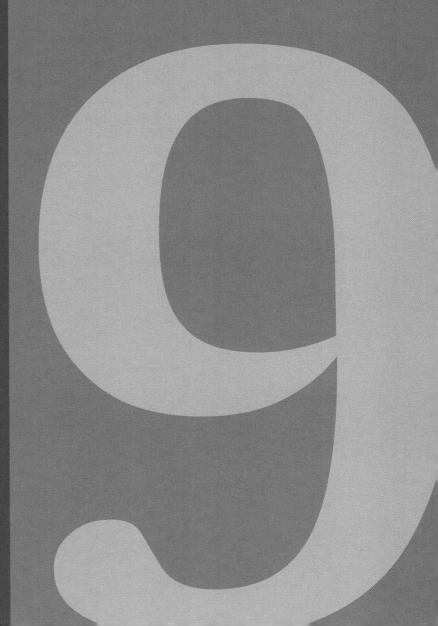

9 Congenital Cholesteatoma of the Middle Ear

Abstract

Congenital cholesteatoma is defined as an epidermoid cyst that develops behind an intact tympanic membrane in a patient with no history of otorrhea, trauma, or previous ear surgery. Thus, otoscopy is characterized by a whitish bulging of the posterior or anterior quadrants. The treatment of this condition is surgical (tympanoplasty).

Keywords: congenital cholesteatoma, Michaels' structure, tympanoplasty

Congenital cholesteatoma is defined as an epidermoid cyst that develops behind an intact tympanic membrane in a patient with no history of otorrhea, trauma, or previous ear surgery. Michaels studied fetal temporal bones and demonstrated the presence of an epidermoid structure between 10 and 33 weeks of gestation. This structure tends to involute spontaneously until it completely disappears. Michaels hypothesized that the persistence of this structure could act as anlage and lead to congenital cholesteatoma. The fact that the most classic location of congenital cholesteatoma, namely, in the anterosuperior part of the tympanum, corresponds to the site of the fetal Michaels' structure supports this theory. In our cases, however, and contrary to the few studies reported in literature (Cohen 1987, Derlacki and Clemis 1965, Friedberg 1994, Levenson et al 1989), the most common site of congenital cholesteatoma was the posterior mesotympanum (see ► Table 9.1). As no existing theory can truly explain the origin of congenital cholesteatoma in the posterior location, a strong conjecture can be made that these lesions might represent a different entity from those of the anterior location and may originate from epithelial cell rest that are trapped in the posterior mesotympanum during the development of the temporal bone. Diagnosis is occasional in the asymptomatic patient, or the patient may complain of hearing loss due to erosion of the ossicular chain or of recurrent attacks of secretory otitis media due to occlusion of the tubal orifice by the cholesteatomatous mass. A high degree of suspicion and thorough examination are essential in detecting the presence of these lesions. Refer to ► Fig. 9.1, ► Fig. 9.2, ► Fig. 9.3, ► Fig. 9.4, ► Fig. 9.5, ► Fig. 9.6, ► Fig. 9.7, ► Fig. 9.8, ► Fig. 9.9, ► Fig. 9.10, ► Fig. 9.11, ► Fig. 9.12, ► Fig. 9.13, ► Fig. 9.14, ► Fig. 9.15, ► Fig. 9.16, ► Fig. 9.17, ► Fig. 9.18, ► Fig. 9.19, ► Fig. 9.20, ► Fig. 9.21, ► Fig. 9.22, ► Fig. 9.23, ► Fig. 9.24.

Congenital cholesteatoma could slowly and silently progress, involving the mastoid space or causing tympanic membrane perforation, especially in cases without symptoms. In such cases, classification between acquired and congenital cholesteatoma is more difficult.

Even more rarely, facial nerve palsy or sensorineural hearing loss could suddenly occur as a result of progression of a congenital cholesteatoma of the middle ear into a petrous bone cholesteatoma (see Chapter 10).

Table 9.1 Classification of congenital cholesteatoma of the middle ear and rate at our Institution

Type	Location	Percent
Type A	Mesotympanic	52.27
Type A1	Premalleolar	5.55
Type A2	Retromalleolar	46.72
Type B	Epitympanic	6.83
Type A/B	Mixed	40.90

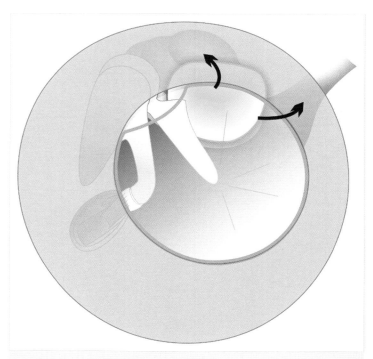

Fig. 9.1 Type A1 congenital cholesteatoma.

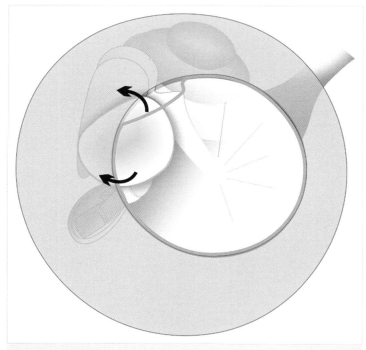

Fig. 9.2 Type A2 congenital cholesteatoma.

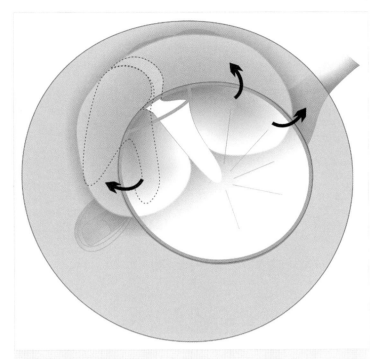

Fig. 9.3 Type B congenital cholesteatoma.

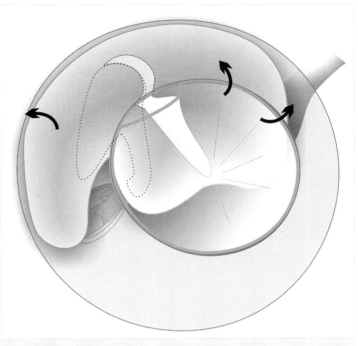

Fig. 9.4 Type A/B congenital cholesteatoma.

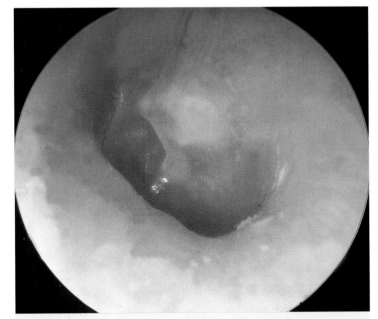

Fig. 9.5 Left ear. Congenital cholesteatoma (type A2) seen as a white retrotympanic mass causing bulging of the posterosuperior quadrant of the tympanic membrane. Neither drum perforation nor bony erosion is detected. In this case, the cholesteatoma caused erosion of the long process of the incus with resultant conductive hearing loss.

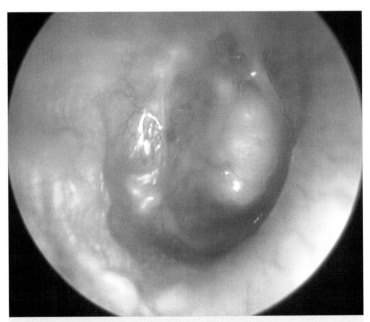

Fig. 9.6 Right ear. Type A1 congenital cholesteatoma. The cholesteatoma is located in the area of the Eustachian tube, causing middle ear dysventilation and tympanic membrane retraction. Audiometry showed mild conductive hearing loss.

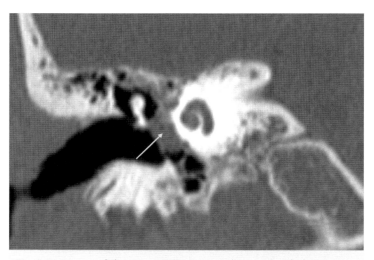

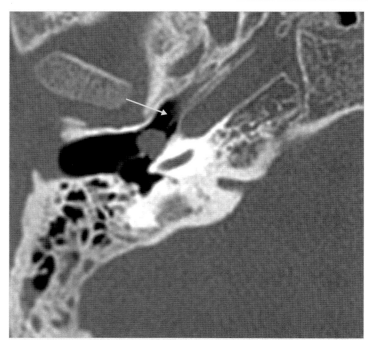

Fig. 9.7 CT scan of the same patient, coronal view. The cholesteatoma pearl is clearly visible medial to the malleus (*arrow*).

Fig. 9.8 CT scan of the same patient, axial view. The cholesteatoma is in contact with the promontorium and tends to block the Eustachian tube (*arrow*).

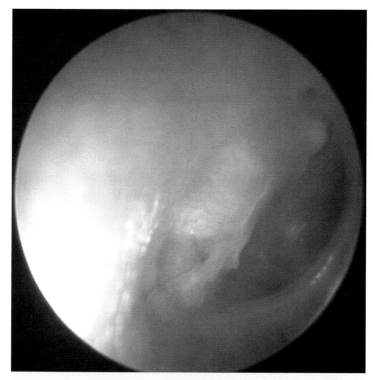

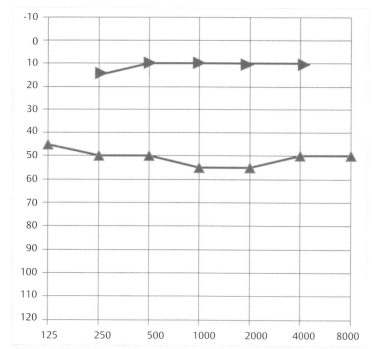

Fig. 9.10 Audiometry of the previous case showing right conductive hearing loss.

Fig. 9.9 Congenital cholesteatoma in an 18-year-old female patient with the onset of right hearing loss since 2 months. No history of chronic otitis was reported. A white mass is clearly visible in the mesotympanic area. A CT scan showed the presence of a cholesteatoma involving both the epitympanic and the mesotympanic areas (type A/B). Audiometry showed moderate right conductive hearing loss (see ▶ Fig. 9.10).

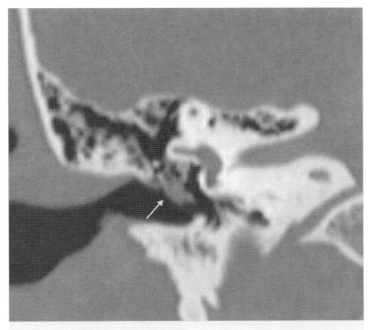

Fig. 9.11 CT scan of the same case, coronal view. The cholesteatoma mass erodes the long process of the incus and the stapes suprastructure (*arrow*).

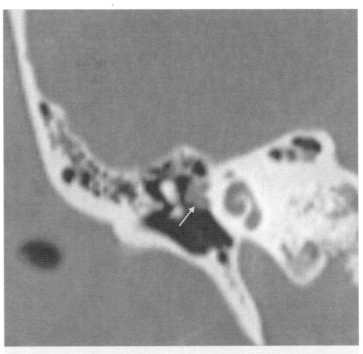

Fig. 9.12 CT scan of the same case, coronal view. The cholesteatoma mass extends to the anterior epitympanic area, medial to the malleus (*arrow*).

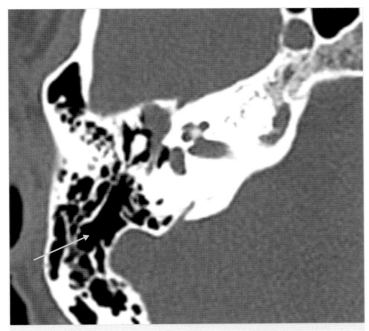

Fig. 9.13 CT scan of the same case, axial view. The cholesteatoma involves both the epitympanic and slightly the mesotympanic area. The mastoid is free from the disease (*arrow*).

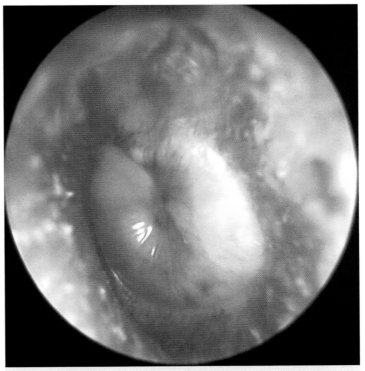

Fig. 9.14 Another case of congenital cholesteatoma (type A/B) evolved slowly in a 40-year-old female patient with no history of otitis. The patient referred to our center for the worsening of a left subjective hearing loss. She had never had ENT consultations before ours. CT scan showed massive involvement of the mastoid and erosion of the incudostapedial joint. Audiometry showed severe conductive hearing loss. A staged canal wall down (open) tympanoplasty was performed.

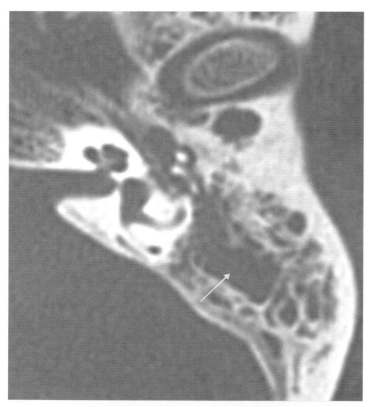

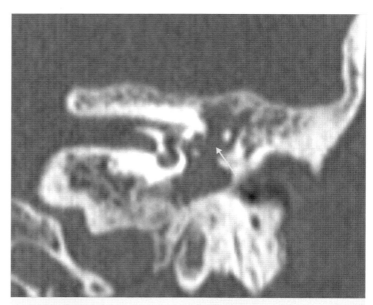

Fig. 9.15 CT scan of the same patient, axial view. The cholesteatoma involves the middle ear cleft and the mastoid air cells (*arrow*).

Fig. 9.16 CT scan of the same patient, coronal view. The cholesteatoma caused erosion of the incudostapedial joint arrow, resulting in hearing loss.

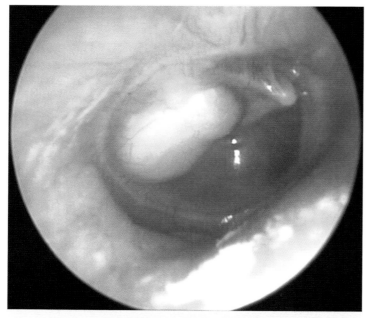

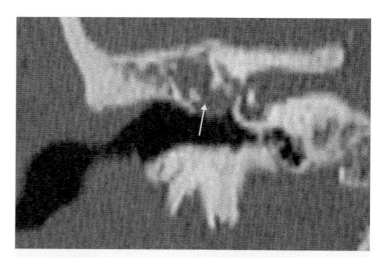

Fig. 9.18 CT scan, coronal view, of the same case. The cholesteatoma (*arrow*) involves the posterior epitympanum and the mesotympanic area. The hypotympanum seems free from the disease.

Fig. 9.17 Case of congenital cholesteatoma (type A2) evolved slowly in a 36-year-old male patient with no history of otitis. In this case, the patient complained of fullness and hearing loss. CT scan showed mesotympanic cholesteatoma with involvement of the posterior epitympanic area and the mastoid (see ▶ Fig. 9.18, ▶ Fig. 9.19). Audiometry showed slight conductive hearing loss (10–15 dB air–bone gap). A staged canal wall up tympanoplasty has been planned.

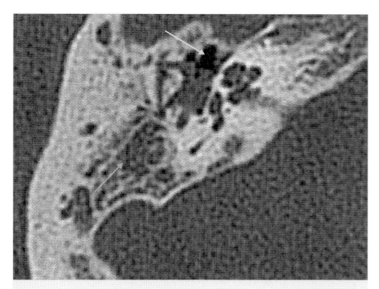

Fig. 9.19 CT scan, axial view, of the same case. The anterior epitympanum is free from the disease (*yellow arrow*), while the mastoid (poorly pneumatized) seems involved (*green arrow*).

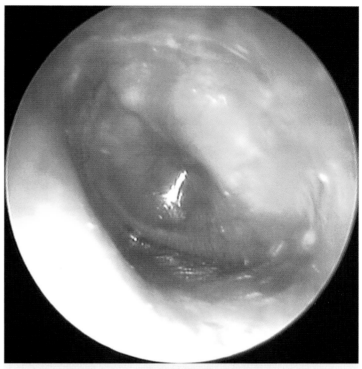

Fig. 9.20 Congenital cholesteatoma in a 7-year-old boy presenting with left hearing loss. The otoscopy shows a classic whitish retrotympanic mass. The CT scan (see ▶ Fig. 9.21, ▶ Fig. 9.22) confirmed the presence of a mesotympanic retromalleolar cholesteatoma (type A2). A staged canal wall up (closed) tympanoplasty was performed.

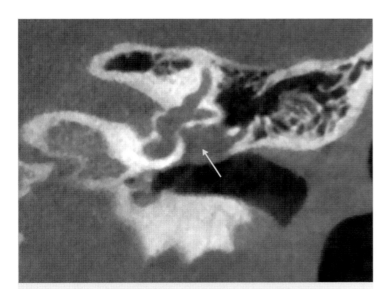

Fig. 9.21 Cone-beam CT scan, coronal view, of the same case. The cholesteatoma involves the mesotympanic area, eroding the incudostapedial joint (*arrow*).

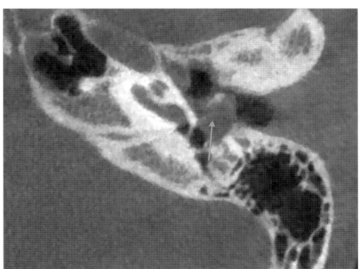

Fig. 9.22 Cone-beam CT scan, axial view, of the same case. The cholesteatoma mass is visible in the mesotympanum, engulfing the incudostapedial joint.

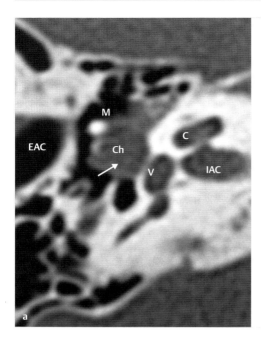

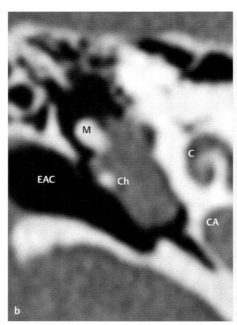

Fig. 9.23 (a,b) A case similar to that of
► Fig. 9.20. Congenital cholesteatoma in an 11-year-old child. On otoscopic examination, a whitish mass is seen in the tympanic cavity with transparency. The CT examination demonstrated that cholesteatoma (arrow) is localized mainly in the tympanic cavity, with small extension toward the attic. The incus is eroded, and continuity of the ossicular chain is impaired. C, cochlea; CA, carotid artery; Ch, cholesteatoma; EAC, external auditory canal; IAC, internal auditory canal; M, malleus; V, vestibule.

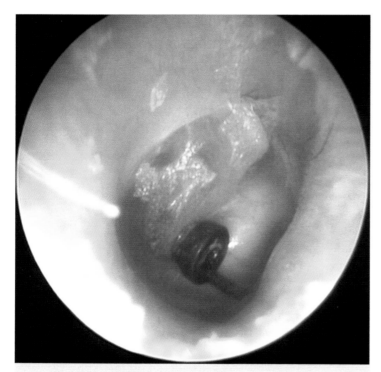

Fig. 9.24 Right ear. This 12-year-old male patient referred to our institution after insertion of a ventilation tube elsewhere for slight conductive hearing loss. The otoscopy reveals a clear congenital cholesteatoma in the area of the Eustachian tube (type A1). Surgical removal of the cholesteatoma has been planned.

Summary

Congenital cholesteatoma of the middle ear is an infrequent pathology during infancy and childhood. It presents behind an intact tympanic membrane, either anterior or posterior to the handle of the malleus.

Anterosuperior cholesteatoma can be removed through an extended tympanotomy that permits the preservation of the tympanic membrane and ossicular chain integrity. Posterior cholesteatoma, however, requires a staged closed tympanoplasty. The second stage serves to check for any residual cholesteatoma. The ossicular chain, which is generally eroded in the posterior type, can be reconstructed at this stage.

Chapter 10

Petrous Bone Cholesteatoma

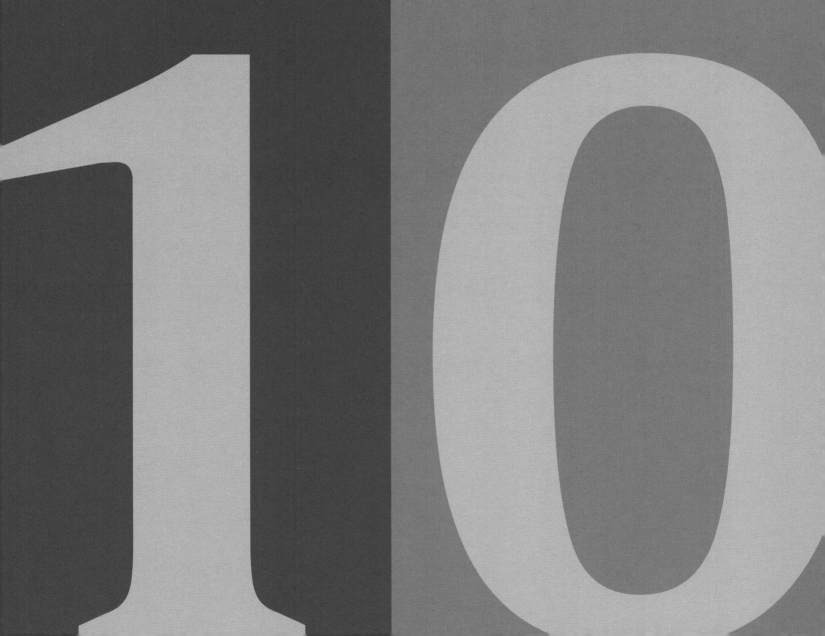

10 Petrous Bone Cholesteatoma

Abstract

Petrous bone cholesteatomas (PBCs) are slow-growing expansile epidermoid lesions arising in the petrous portion of the temporal bone. In such cases, the first symptoms are facial nerve paralysis, vertigo, and deaf ear due to invasion of the facial nerve and labyrinth. Otoscopy may be irrelevant or only demonstrates pars flaccida perforation or an open mastoid cavity with evidence of suppurative discharge. Radiological examinations (computed tomography and magnetic resonance imaging scans) are fundamental to evaluate the extension of the lesion and to determine the surgical management. The classification proposed by Sanna divides PBCs into five groups based on the relationship of the disease to the labyrinthine block (supralabyrinthine, infralabyrinthine, infralabyrinthine-apical, massive, apical types). This radiological classification allows standardization in reporting and a clear planning of the surgical approach, which has to be suitable for a safer management of the facial nerve, dura, internal carotid artery, sigmoid sinus, and jugular bulb.

Keywords: petrous bone cholesteatoma, facial nerve, Sanna classification, transotic approach, transcochlear approach

Petrous bone cholesteatomas (PBCs) are slow-growing expansile epidermoid lesions arising in the petrous portion of the temporal bone with an incidence of 4 to 9% of all petrous pyramid lesions. These could be congenital, acquired, or iatrogenic. Congenital PBCs are most plausibly explained by the persistence of fetal epidermoid formation in the petrous bone or the middle ear from which it expands to the petrous bone. In such cases, the first symptoms are facial nerve paralysis, vertigo, and deaf ear due to invasion of the facial nerve and labyrinth. The acquired variety is due to the migration of squamous epithelium into the petrous bone secondary to a perforation in the tympanic membrane. The iatrogenic variety is due to the implantation of cholesteatoma after an otologic surgery. Fetid otorrhea, progressive facial palsy, vertigo, and hearing loss of any type (conductive, sensorineural, mixed) are usually encountered in these patients.

Otoscopy may be irrelevant or only demonstrates pars flaccida perforation or an open mastoid cavity with evidence of suppurative discharge. A computed tomography (CT) scan and magnetic resonance imaging (MRI) are fundamental to evaluate the extension of the lesion and to determine the surgical management.

The rarity of these lesions, slow and silent growth pattern, their complex location in the skull base, proximity to vital neurovascular structures (facial nerve, internal carotid artery, sigmoid sinus, jugular bulb, lower cranial nerves, dura), and tendency to recur make PBCs very challenging to diagnose and treat. PBCs have shown to be locally aggressive by involving the petrous bone and the areas surrounding it, such as the clivus, nasopharynx, sphenoid sinus, and the infratemporal fossa, and even extending intradurally. Also, the close proximity of the disease to the labyrinth and the facial nerve puts to risk both hearing and facial nerve function, which is reflected in the high incidence of facial nerve palsy (34.6–100%) seen in the important series reported in literature.

Surgery remains the mainstay of treatment of PBCs. The choice of surgical approach has evolved from radical petromastoid exenteration with marsupialization of the cavity to closed and obliterative techniques following complete eradication Advancements in neuroradiology and microscopic lateral skull base surgery have made it possible today to completely extirpate these lesions safely with minimal recurrences and perioperative morbidity. The primary objective in surgical approaches for PBCs is to ensure total disease eradication along with complete control and safety of the surrounding important neurovascular structures. The development of the transotic and transcochlear approaches, combined with various other skull base approaches, has helped achieve both these objectives and is considered the mainstay of surgery for PBCs.

The classification proposed by Sanna divides PBCs into five groups based on the relationship of the disease to the labyrinthine block. This radiological classification allows standardization in reporting and a clear planning of the surgical approach (▶ Table 10.1, ▶ Table 10.2). Also see ▶ Fig. 10.1, ▶ Fig. 10.2, ▶ Fig. 10.3, ▶ Fig. 10.4, ▶ Fig. 10.5, ▶ Fig. 10.6, ▶ Fig. 10.7, ▶ Fig. 10.8, ▶ Fig. 10.9, ▶ Fig. 10.10, ▶ Fig. 10.11, ▶ Fig. 10.12, ▶ Fig. 10.13, ▶ Fig. 10.14, ▶ Fig. 10.15, ▶ Fig. 10.16, ▶ Fig. 10.17, ▶ Fig. 10.18, ▶ Fig. 10.19, ▶ Fig. 10.20, ▶ Fig. 10.21, ▶ Fig. 10.22, ▶ Fig. 10.23, ▶ Fig. 10.24, ▶ Fig. 10.25, ▶ Fig. 10.26, ▶ Fig. 10.27, ▶ Fig. 10.28, ▶ Fig. 10.29, ▶ Fig. 10.30, ▶ Fig. 10.31, ▶ Fig. 10.32, ▶ Fig. 10.33, ▶ Fig. 10.34, ▶ Fig. 10.35, ▶ Fig. 10.36, ▶ Fig. 10.37, ▶ Fig. 10.38, ▶ Fig. 10.39, ▶ Fig. 10.40, ▶ Fig. 10.41, ▶ Fig. 10.42, ▶ Fig. 10.43, ▶ Fig. 10.44.

Table 10.1 Updated Sanna classification of petrous bone cholesteatomas

Updated Sanna Classification of Petrous Bone Cholesteatomas (2016)		
Class	**Cholesteatoma location**	**Relations, extension, and features**
Class I: Supralabyrinthine 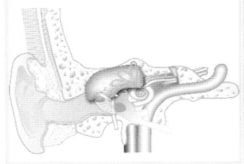	Centered on the geniculate ganglion area of the FN and the anterior epitympanum 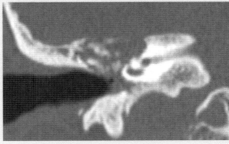	Superior: Tegmen or dura Inferior: Semicircular canals, apical turns of the cochlea Medial: Limited extension beyond the otic capsule into the petrous apex Lateral: Antrum, epitympanum and further into middle ear Anterior: Horizontal part of the pICA Posterior: Posterior bony labyrinth Features: Usually associated with fistula of the semicircular canals, erosion of tegmen, involvement of the FN
Class II: Infralabyrinthine 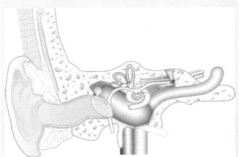	Centered on the infracochlear, infralabyrinthine, and hypotympanic cells 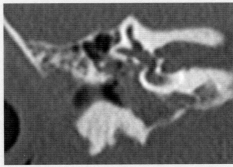	Superior: Basal turn of the cochlea, vestibule Inferior: Jugular bulb, lower cranial nerves, occipital condyle Medial: Limited extension beyond the otic capsule into the petrous apex Lateral: Hypotympanum and further into middle ear, retrofacial cells Anterior: Vertical and horizontal part of pICA Posterior: Posterior semicircular canal, IAC Features: Fistula of the semicircular canals, erosion of the cochlea, jugular bulb, carotid canal, involvement of the lower cranial nerves
Class III: Infralabyrinthine-Apical 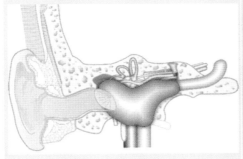	Involves infralabyrinthine cell tracts extending medially into the petrous apex 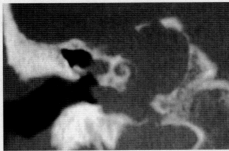	Superior: Basal turn of the cochlea, vestibule Inferior: Jugular bulb, lower cranial nerves, occipital condyle Medial: Extension into the petrous apex, lower clivus, along the greater wing of sphenoid into the foramen spinosum, foramen ovale; may extend up to sphenoid sinus Lateral: Hypotympanum and further into middle ear, retrofacial cells Anterior: Vertical and horizontal part of pICA Posterior: IAC, dura of the posterior cranial fossa (posterolaterally) Features: Fistula of the semicircular canals, erosion of the cochlea, jugular bulb, involvement of the lower cranial nerves, extensive destruction of the carotid canal, involvement of the internal auditory canal
Class IV: Massive 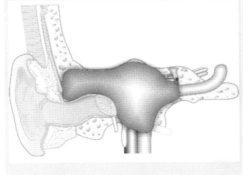	Centered on the otic capsule 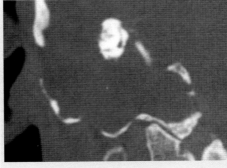	Superior: Dura of the middle fossa, may extend intradurally Inferior: Hypotympanic cells, infralabyrinthine cells, jugular bulb, lower cranial nerves Medial: Extension into the petrous apex, along the greater wing of sphenoid into the foramen spinosum, foramen ovale; may extend up to sphenoid sinus Lateral: Middle ear, antrum, retrofacial cells Anterior: Vertical and horizontal part of pICA Posterior: IAC, dura of the posterior cranial fossa, may extend intradurally Features: Various degrees of destruction of the otic capsule, involvement of FN

(continued)

▶

Table 10.1 Updated Sanna classification of petrous bone cholesteatomas (*continued*)

Updated Sanna Classification of Petrous Bone Cholesteatomas (2016)		
Class	**Cholesteatoma location**	**Relations, extension, and features**
Class V: Apical 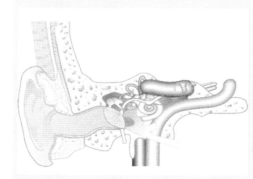	Centered on the petrous apex 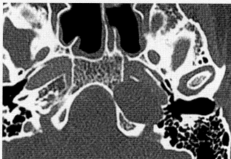	Superior: Dura of the middle fossa, Meckel's cave, may extend intradurally Inferior: Hypotympanic cells, infralabyrinthine cells, jugular bulb, lower cranial nerves, infratemporal fossa Medial: Extension into the spheno-petro-clival junction, midclivus, along the greater wing of sphenoid into the foramen spinosum, foramen ovale; may extend up to sphenoid sinus Lateral: Otic capsule Anterior: Horizontal part of pICA and foramen lacerum Posterior: IAC, dura of the posterior cranial fossa, may extend intradurally Features: Otic capsule may be eroded medially, erosion of horizontal petrous carotid, clivus and intradural extensions into middle fossa or posterior fossa; extensions also possible into sphenoid, nasopharynx, or infratemporal fossa

Table 10.2 Updated Sanna subclassification of petrous bone cholesteatomas

Updated Subclassification of Petrous Bone Cholesteatomas (2016)	
Subclasses	**Relations and features**
Clivus (C) 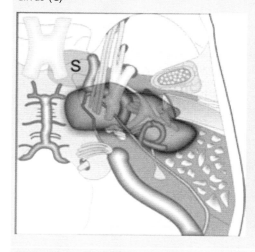	Superior and mid clival extensions are seen from massive, infralabyrinthine-apical and apical PBC whereas the lower clival involvement is a feature of infralabyrinthine-apical PBC 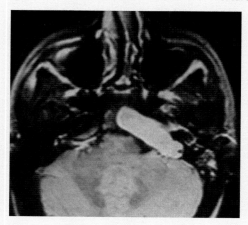
Sphenoid sinus (S) 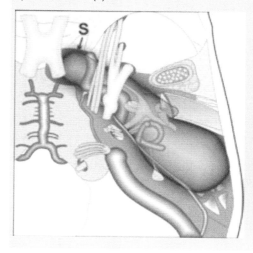	Sphenoid sinus involvement is seen from anteromedial extensions of massive, infralabyrinthine-apical and apical PBC; it is a rare extension 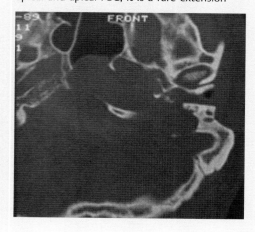

Table 10.2 Updated Sanna subclassification of petrous bone cholesteatomas (*continued*)

Updated Subclassification of Petrous Bone Cholesteatomas (2016)	
Subclasses	**Relations and features**
Nasopharynx (N) 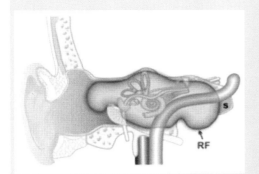	It is the rarest extension of the PBC; it is an extension of infralabyrinthine-apical or massive PBC, which may extend through the clivus beneath the sphenoid sinus into the nasopharynx 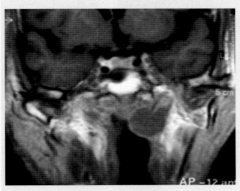
Intradural (I) 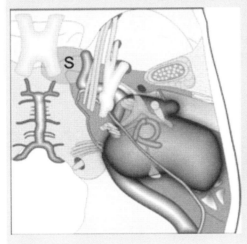	Intradural extensions may arise from the massive, infralabyrinthine-apical and apical PBCs usually into the posterior cranial fossa and rarely into the middle cranial fossa 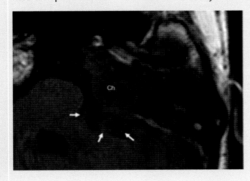

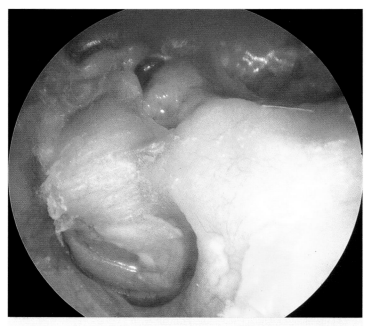

Fig. 10.1 Left acquired or iatrogenic supralabyrinthine petrous bone cholesteatoma in a radical cavity. A whitish retrotympanic mass is seen at the level of the second portion of the facial nerve. The patient presented with progressive facial nerve paralysis and total hearing loss. A correct diagnosis depends not only on otoscopy but also on the symptomatology (facial paralysis, anacusis) and a high-resolution CT scan.

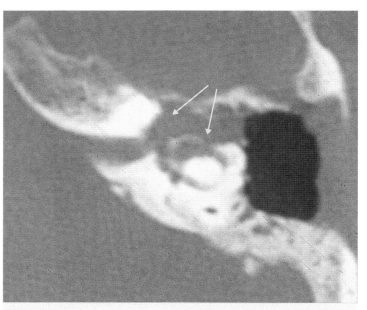

Fig. 10.2 CT scan of the case presented in ▶ Fig. 10.1, axial section. Involvement of the lateral semicircular canal and the vestibule (*arrows*) is well visualized. The cholesteatoma invades the cochlea anteriorly, while medially it reaches the fundus of the internal auditory canal. The posterior semicircular canal is not invaded.

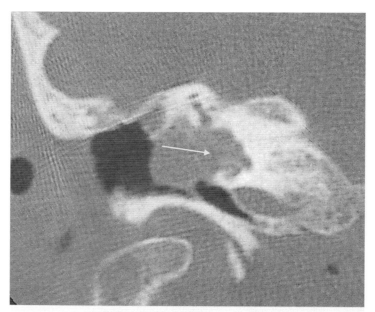

Fig. 10.3 CT scan of the case presented in ▶ Fig. 10.1, coronal section. The medial extension of the cholesteatoma can be appreciated (*arrow*).

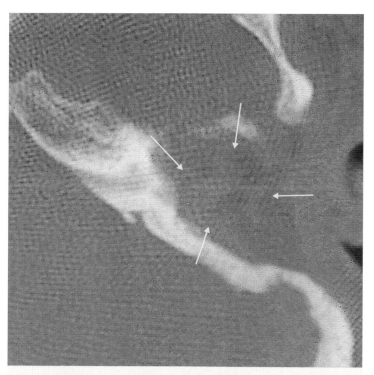

Fig. 10.4 Postoperative CT scan. A transcochlear approach was performed and the operative cavity was obliterated with abdominal fat (*arrows*).

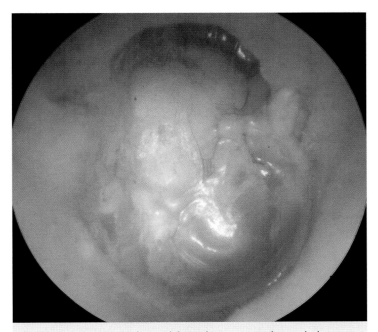

Fig. 10.5 Right acquired supralabyrinthine petrous bone cholesteatoma. A whitish mass is present in the mastoid cavity of an open tympanoplasty. The mass occupies the whole epitympanum and extends interiorly behind the tympanic membrane. The patient presented with ipsilateral facial paralysis and conductive hearing loss.

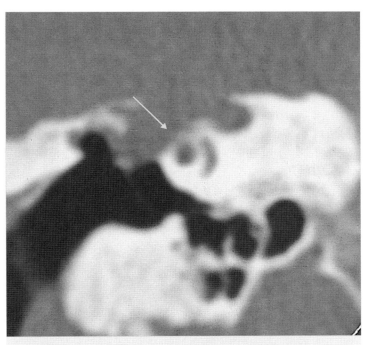

Fig. 10.6 CT scan of the case presented in ▶ Fig. 10.5. The cholesteatoma invades the cochlea (arrow). Total removal of the pathology was accomplished using a transcochlear approach with obliteration of the operative defect using abdominal fat. The external auditory canal was closed as cul de sac. The facial nerve was infiltrated at the level of the geniculate ganglion and was repaired using a sural nerve graft.

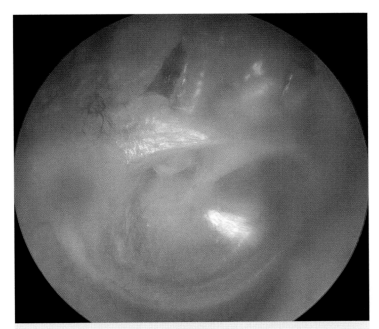

Fig. 10.7 Another example of right acquired supralabyrinthine petrous bone cholesteatoma. The patient presented with right facial nerve paralysis. Otoscopy reveals a right epitympanic erosion.

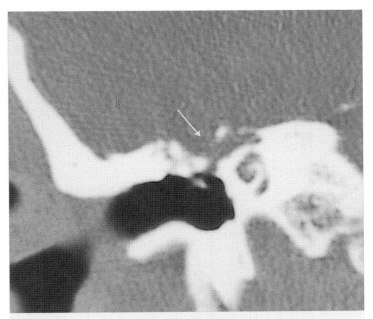

Fig. 10.8 CT scan of the case presented in ▶ Fig. 10.7, coronal view. Typical location and erosion of acquired small supralabyrinthine petrous bone cholesteatoma (arrow).

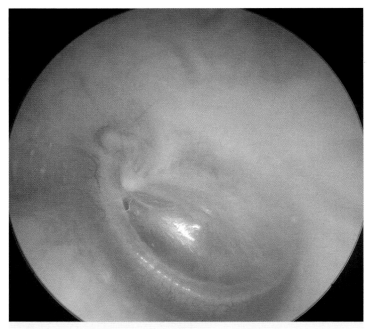

Fig. 10.9 Left congenital supralabyrinthine petrous bone cholesteatoma with extension toward the apex.Otoscopy is negative. The patient complained of progressive facial nerve paralysis of 5 years' duration as well as conductive hearing loss (▶ Fig. 10.10, ▶ Fig. 10.11).

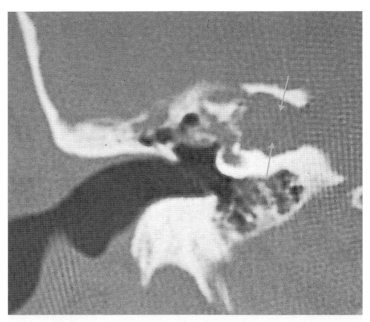

Fig. 10.10 CT scan of the case presented in ▶ Fig. 10.9. Coronal view showing extension of the cholesteatoma into the internal auditory canal (*arrows*).

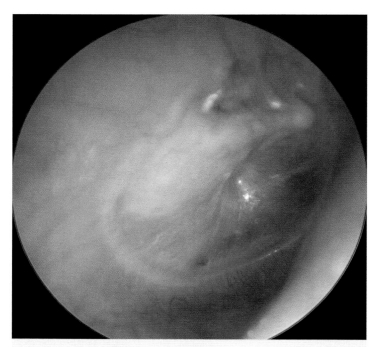

Fig. 10.11 Right congenital infralabyrinthine apical petrous bone cholesteatoma in a 30-year-old female patient. In the posterosuperior quadrant, a white retrotympanic view is observed. The patient had complained of right anacusis since childhood and instability of 1-year duration. The facial nerve was normal.

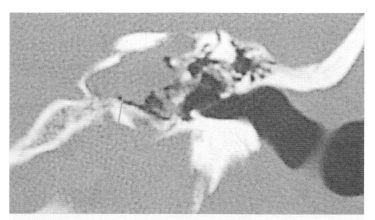

Fig. 10.12 CT scan of the case presented in ▶ Fig. 10.11. Coronal view demonstrating the involvement of the infralabyrinthine apical compartment by the cholesteatoma (*arrow*).

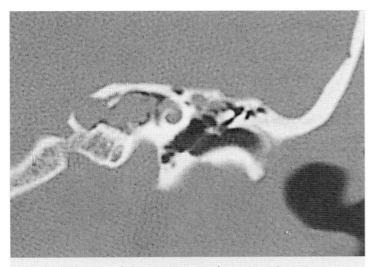

Fig. 10.13 CT scan of the case presented in ▶ Fig. 10.11. A more anterior coronal view at the level of the cochlea.

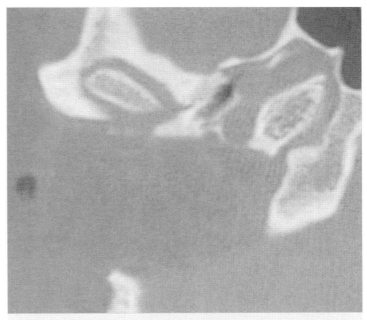

Fig. 10.14 Postoperative CT scan showing total removal of the cholesteatoma through the transcochlear approach and obliteration of the operative cavity using abdominal fat.

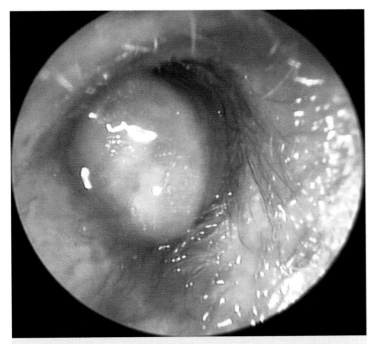

Fig. 10.15 Polyp in the external auditory canal in a patient who had undergone a myringoplasty. The patient presented with otorrhea and sensorineural hearing loss.

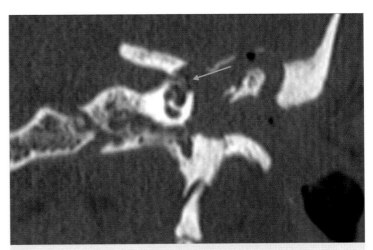

Fig. 10.16 CT scan of the case on ▶ Fig. 10.15, coronal view. A cholesteatoma involving the basal turn of the cochlea is visible (*arrow*).

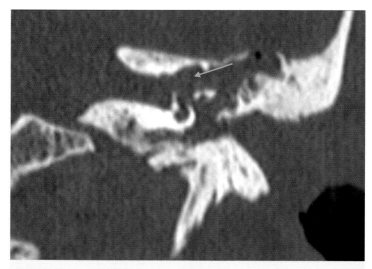

Fig. 10.17 CT scan of the same case, coronal view. The PBC (massive type) involves the labyrinth (*arrow*).

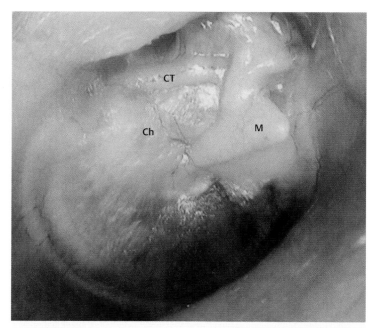

Fig. 10.18 Right ear. This 60-year-old male patient presented with anacusis and facial nerve palsy. The otoscopy showed a dry clean retraction in the attic. Presence of whitish matter behind the tympanic membrane was the only clue for the presence of cholesteatoma. The CT scan (see ► Fig. 10.19, ► Fig. 10.20) revealed the presence of a supralabyrinthine PBC extended to the petrous apex. A modified transcochlear type A approach was performed. Ch, cholesteatoma; CT, chorda tympanic nerve; M, malleus.

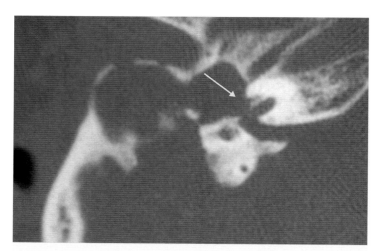

Fig. 10.19 CT scan of the same case, axial view. The cholesteatoma causes erosion of the cochlea and involvement of the facial nerve (*arrow*).

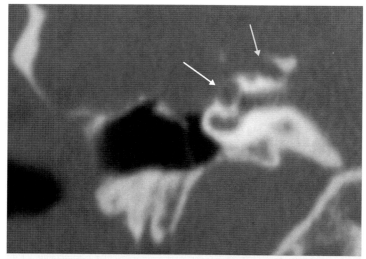

Fig. 10.20 CT scan of the same case, coronal view, shows severe erosion of the otic capsule (*white arrow*) and extensive extension of the cholesteatoma medially to the labyrinth, toward the internal auditory canal (*yellow arrow*).

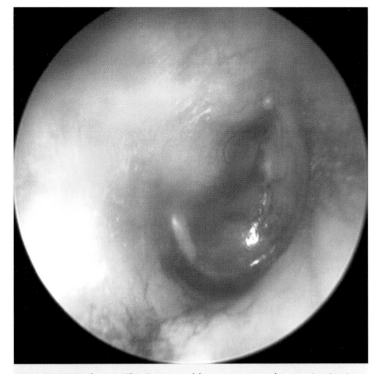

Fig. 10.21 Right ear. This 24-year-old man presented to our institution after two tympanoplasties for cholesteatoma. He complained of persistent otorrhea, severe hearing loss (mixed type), and vertigo. CT scan revealed the presence of a supralabyrinthine PBC with involvement of the semicircular canals. A transotic approach with preservation of the cochlea was performed. Facial nerve was grade I House–Brackmann scale after surgery.

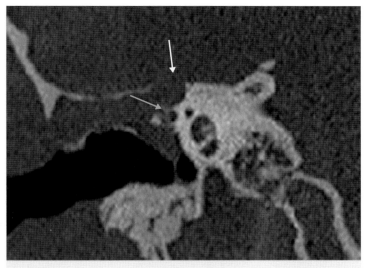

Fig. 10.22 CT scan, coronal view. The cholesteatoma involves the supralabyrinthine compartment, causing erosion of the middle fossa dura plate (*white arrow*). The cochlea is not invaded by the disease, while the second portion of the facial nerve is in close contact with the pathology (*green arrow*). However, facial nerve function is normal.

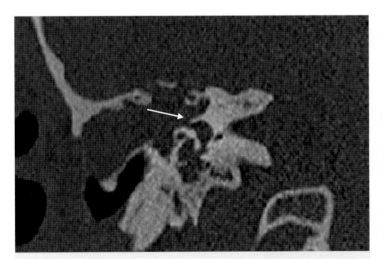

Fig. 10.23 CT scan, coronal view. The cholesteatoma involves the lateral semicircular canal (*arrow*).

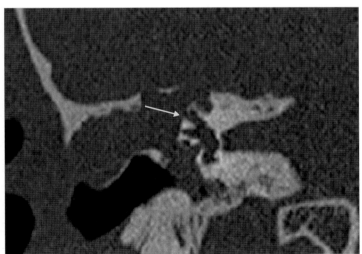

Fig. 10.24 CT scan, coronal view. The cholesteatoma involves the superior semicircular canal (*arrow*).

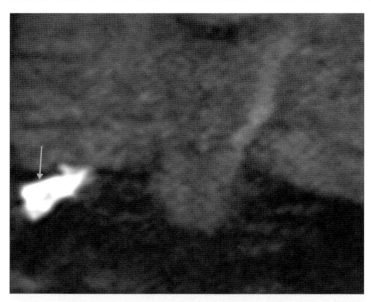

Fig. 10.25 MRI scan, diffusion-weighted image (DWI), coronal view. The cholesteatoma is typically hyperintense in this sequence (*arrow*). The DWI technique is particularly important in the follow-up, because it allows the detection even of small (> 2 mm) residual/recurrent disease.

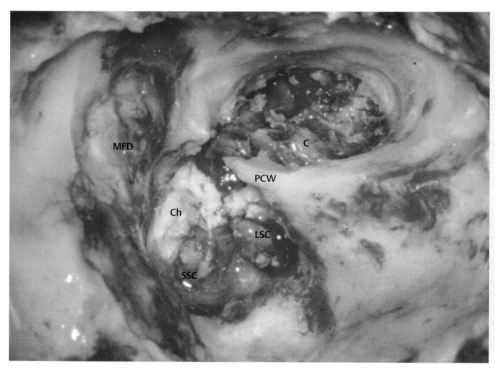

Fig. 10.26 Intraoperative picture of the same case. Blind sac closure of the external auditory canal, removal of the tympanic membrane and the ossicles, and mastoidectomy have been performed. The cholesteatoma (Ch) involves both the lateral (LSC) and the superior semicircular canal (SSC). C, cochlea; MFD, middle fossa dura; PCW, posterior canal wall.

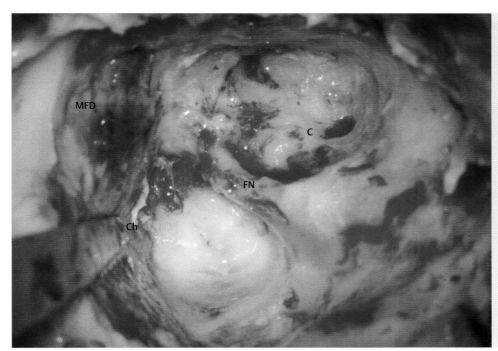

Fig. 10.27 Surgical view after labyrinthectomy. There is still some cholesteatoma matrix on the middle fossa dura, which is gently elevated with a retractor. The third portion of the facial nerve is completely skeletonized. After having removed all the cholesteatoma, the cavity is obliterated with abdominal fat. C, cochlea; Ch, cholesteatoma; FN, facial nerve; MFD, middle fossa dura.

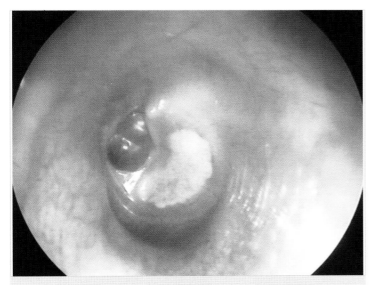

Fig. 10.28 Left ear. Otoscopy showed myringosclerosis of the posterior quadrants and a retraction pocket on the anterior quadrant. The patient complained of left progressive hearing loss evolved in anacusis and facial nerve paralysis for the last 2 years. A CT scan revealed the presence of a PBC on both sides: massive type on the left side (see ▶ Fig. 10.29, ▶ Fig. 10.30) and supralabyrinthine type on the right side (▶ Fig. 10.32). Surgery on this side was performed through a transcochlear approach.

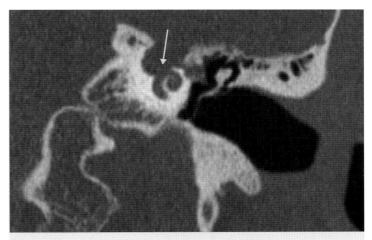

Fig. 10.29 CT scan of the same case, coronal view. The cholesteatoma has eroded the basal turn of the cochlea (*arrow*).

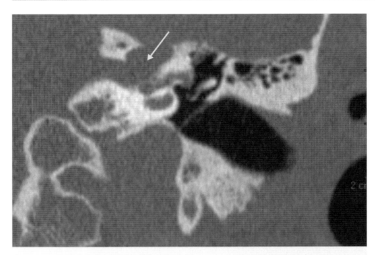

Fig. 10.30 CT scan of the same case, coronal view. The cholesteatoma has engulfed the labyrinth, going medial toward the roof of the internal auditory canal (*arrow*).

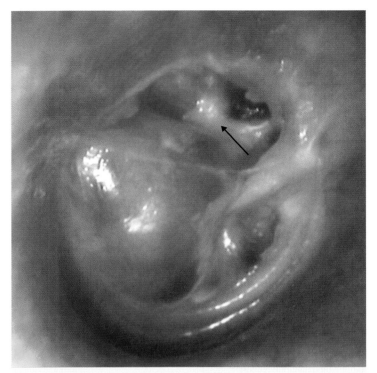

Fig. 10.31 Right ear, same case. The posterior half of the tympanic membrane is scarred, and touched to the promontory. The posterosuperior quadrant goes deep toward the attic, touching the superstructure of the stapes (*arrow*). Hearing function is normal, even though the cholesteatoma has determined a fistula of the lateral semicircular canal (see ► Fig. 10.32). A transmastoid + middle fossa approach was chosen with the purpose of preserving right hearing function.

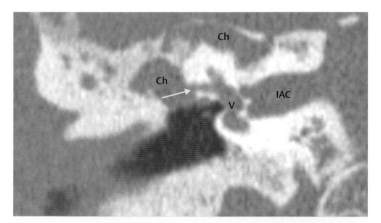

Fig. 10.32 CT scan of the same case, coronal view. A fistula in the lateral semicircular canal is clearly seen (*arrow*). The cholesteatoma infiltrates medially along the middle fossa plate to reach the petrous apex. Ch, cholesteatoma; IAC, internal auditory canal; V, vestibule.

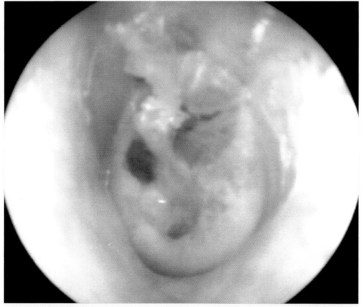

Fig. 10.33 Left ear. Otoscopy shows diffuse myringosclerosis of the tympanic membrane with an anterosuperior retraction pocket. This patient underwent two myringoplasties elsewhere. The patient complained of left anacusis and facial nerve palsy (both lasting for 5 years). Lower cranial nerves paralysis has developed since 2 months before our consultation. CT and MRI scans revealed the presence of a massive PBC that extended intracranially and toward the clivus and sphenoid sinus. A single-stage modified transcochlear approach was performed for the removal of the disease.

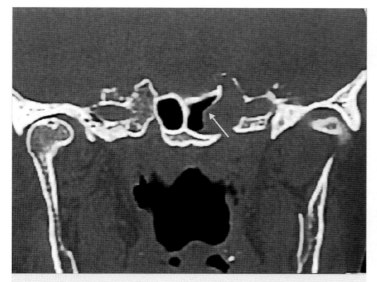

Fig. 10.34 CT scan of the same case, coronal view. The cholesteatoma invades the sphenoid sinus (*arrow*).

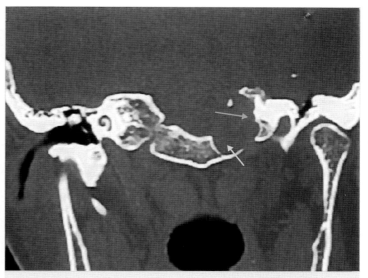

Fig. 10.35 CT scan of the same case, coronal view. The cholesteatoma erodes the clivus (*yellow arrow*). The cochlea is not recognizable due to massive engulfment by the disease (*green arrow*).

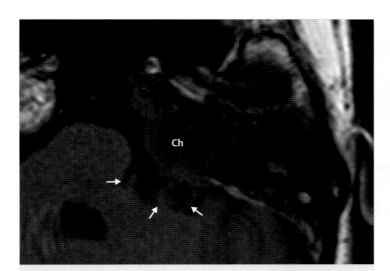

Fig. 10.36 MRI of the same case (T1W), axial view. The cholesteatoma causes compression of the brain stem protruding from the petrous apex (*arrows*). Ch, cholesteatoma.

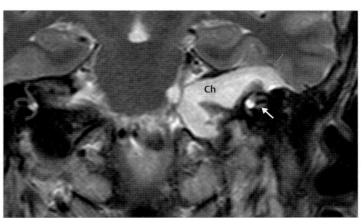

Fig. 10.37 MRI of the same case (T2W), coronal view, which shows a large petrous apex lesion elevating the middle fossa dura to compress the temporal lobe (*red arrow*). The vestibule and the semicircular canal can be identified (*white arrow*). Ch, cholesteatoma.

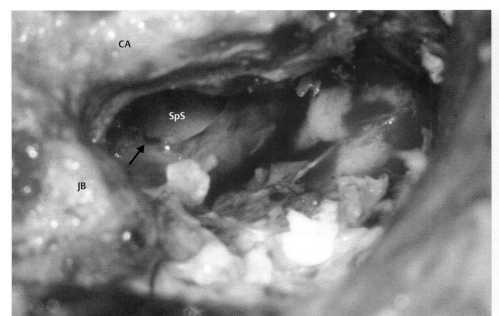

Fig. 10.38 Intraoperative picture. The cholesteatoma has been nearly completely removed from the area of the sphenoid sinus. The opening of sphenoid sinus is seen in the petroclival area medially to the carotid artery (*arrow*). CA, carotid artery; JB, jugular bulb; SpS, sphenoid sinus.

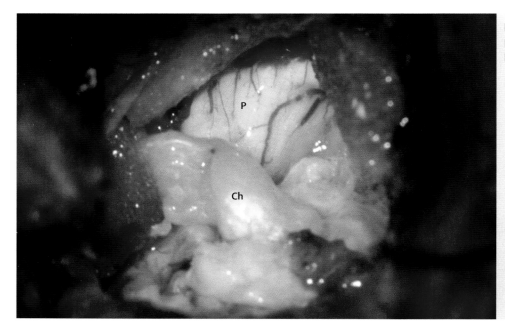

Fig. 10.39 Intraoperative picture. The intradural portion of the cholesteatoma attached to the pons is shown. Ch, cholesteatoma; P, pons.

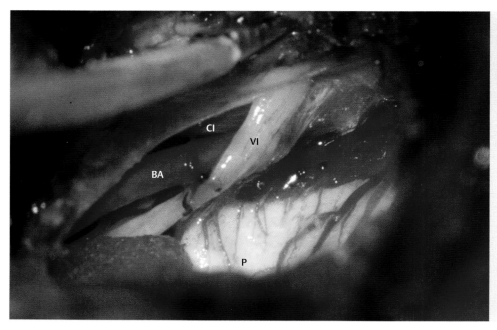

Fig. 10.40 Intraoperative picture. The majority of cholesteatoma is removed from the cerebellopontine angle. BA, basilar artery; Cl, clivus; P, pons; VI, abducens nerve.

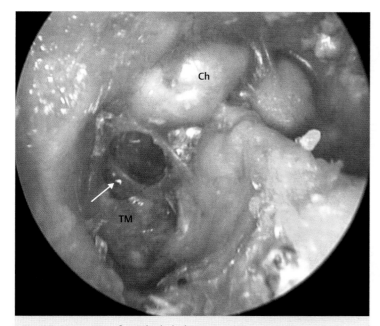

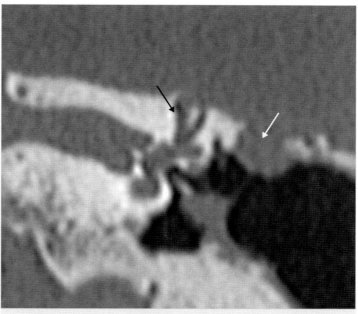

Fig. 10.41 A case of residual cholesteatoma in an open cavity is shown. The patient underwent cholesteatoma surgery with canal wall down technique elsewhere. Residual cholesteatoma (Ch) is seen at the tegmen of the cavity, just superiorly to the tympanic membrane. A deep dimple (*arrow*) is seen in the superior part of the tympanic membrane (TM), and the facial ridge remains very high.

Fig. 10.42 CT scan of the same case, coronal view, shows the presence of soft tissue eroding the tegmen of the antrum (*white arrow*). The cholesteatoma infiltrates medially to the superior semicircular canal eroding the ampulla (*black arrow*).

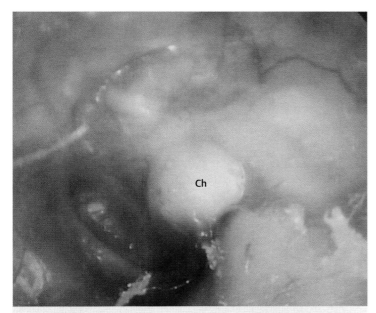

Fig. 10.43 A case similar to that of ▶ Fig. 10.41. Residual cholesteatoma in a canal wall down tympanoplasty. Otoscopy shows a whitish mass in the canal wall cavity located beneath the posterosuperior quadrant of the tympanic membrane. Ch, cholesteatoma.

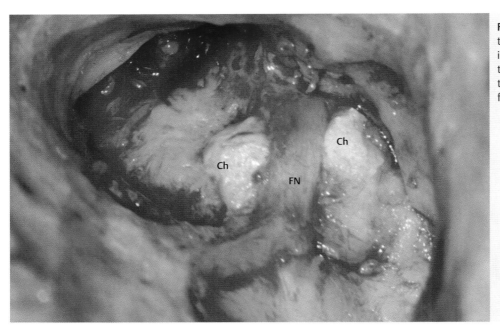

Fig. 10.44 Intraoperative picture. The cholesteatoma is medial to the facial nerve and involves both the cochlea and the labyrinth. A transotic approach was performed, thus leaving the facial nerve in situ. Ch, cholesteatoma; FN, facial nerve.

10.1 Surgical Management

The classification of PBC is of paramount importance as it gives information regarding the anatomical position and the extent of the disease. The subclassification proposed by us aims at preoperatively diagnosing the extension of PBC beyond the temporal bone (clivus, sphenoid sinus rhinopharynx, intradural space). This helps to plan the surgical approach, which is important to clear the disease from these areas. The choice of surgical approach has evolved from radical petromastoid exenteration with marsupialization of the cavity to closed and obliterative techniques following complete eradication. Decision-making is the crucial aspect of surgical management. It depends on several factors, the most significant of which are the extent of the disease and preoperative facial nerve function. The approach is chosen depending on the type of PBC and its extent, which should be determined according to the CT scan and MRI findings.

The main factors to be taken into consideration while treating these lesions are as follows: (1) complete eradication of the disease, (2) preservation of facial nerve function, (3) prevention of cerebrospinal fluid (CSF) leak and meningitis, (4) cavity obliteration, and (5) hearing preservation whenever feasible.

In supralabyrinthine PBC, if hearing is normal without any evidence of a fistula in the basal turn of the cochlea, we prefer a middle fossa approach which may be combined with a transmastoid approach depending on the extension of the disease. In the presence of sensorineural hearing loss or CT evidence of a fistula in the basal turn of the cochlea, we prefer a radical approach (subtotal petrosectomy/enlarged translabyrinthine approach/transotic approach) with cavity obliteration. In infralabyrinthine PBC, bone conduction can be preserved with subtotal petrosectomy and blind sac closure of the external auditory canal with cavity obliteration. Hearing preservation is usually not possible in infralabyrinthine-apical and massive PBC; hence, we use a transotic approach or a modified transcochlear approach type A depending on preoperative facial nerve function. Modified transcochlear approaches provide excellent access to the petrous apex, clivus, sphenoid sinus, rhinopharynx, and intradural space depending on the type used. The posterior rerouting of the facial nerve carries the disadvantage of postoperative facial paresis. Therefore, we prefer a transotic approach when facial nerve function is normal. Whenever the cholesteatoma involves the apical portion of the temporal bone or when it extends further to the clivus, sphenoid sinus, or rhinopharynx, an infratemporal fossa approach type B or modified transcochlear approach type A is incorporated into the transotic approach depending on the preoperative status of the facial nerve.

10.1.1 The Transotic and Modified Transcochlear Approaches

The original transcochlear approach described by House and Hitselberger (1976) includes identification of the internal auditory canal, posterior rerouting of the facial nerve, and removal of the cochlea and petrous apex with preservation of the middle ear and external auditory canal.

Fisch (1978) described the transotic approach in which he removed the external auditory canal and middle ear but keeps the facial nerve in situ.

Our modified transcochlear approach, on the other hand, combines the removal of the external auditory canal and middle ear with the posterior rerouting of the facial nerve, thus removing the major impediment to anterior extension of the approach. This allows better control of the vertical and horizontal intrapetrous internal carotid artery and facilitates the total removal of the petrous apex. The extensive anterior bone removal provides an excellent control of the ventral surface of the brainstem without cerebellar and brainstem retraction. We have further classified this approach into four types according to the extension. Type A represents the basic approach; types B, C, and D denote the anterior, superior, and inferior extensions, respectively.

The transotic and modified transcochlear approaches have been shown in ► Fig. 10.45 and ► Fig. 10.46.

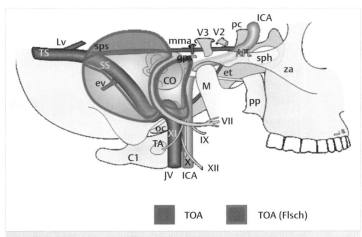

Fig. 10.45 A schematic drawing showing the outlines of the transotic approach. C1, first cervical vertebra; CO, cochlea; ET, Eustachian tube; EV, emissary vein; FN, facial nerve; IAC, internal auditory canal; ICA, internal carotid artery; IX, glossopharyngeal nerve; JV, jugular vein; Lv, Labbé's vein; M, mandible; MMA, middle meningeal artery; OC, occipital condyle; pc, posterior clinoid; pp, pterygoid process; SS, sigmoid sinus; SPH, sphenoid; TA, transverse process of the atlas; TS, transverse sinus; V2, second branch of the trigeminal nerve; V3, third branch of the trigeminal nerve; VII, facial nerve; XII: Hypoglossal nerve, XI, accessory nerve; ZA, zygomatic process.

Fig. 10.46 A schematic drawing showing the outlines of the modified transcochlear approach type A. About three-fourths of the vertical internal carotid artery (ICA-V) are under control in contrast to only one-fourth of the horizontal internal carotid artery (ICA-H) using this approach.

Indications of the Transotic Approach

- Some cases of cerebellopontine angle tumors with anterior extension and preoperative normal facial nerve function (i.e., epidermoids).
- PBCs.
- Some cases of petrous bone tumors with preoperative normal facial nerve function.

Indications of the Modified Transcochlear Approach (Type A—Basic Type)

- *Extradural lesions*: extensive petrous bone apex lesions with preoperative facial nerve and inner ear compromise, that is:
  - PBC of the massive infralabyrinthine apical and supralabyrinthine types.
  - Recurrent acoustic neurinoma with petrous bone invasion.
  - Extensive facial nerve tumors.
  - Cholesterol granuloma (only with preoperative facial and hearing impairment).
- Intradural lesions:
  - Large clival and petroclival lesions lying ventral to the brainstem, that is, petroclival meningiomas.
  - Previously irradiated petroclival meningiomas.
  - Residual or recurrent nonacoustic lesions of the posterior fossa with anterior extension into the prepontine cistern, particularly those with encasement of the vertebrobasilar artery or perforating arteries, or both, that is, huge posterior fossa epidermoids
  - Recurrent acoustic neurinomas with facial nerve paralysis.
- *Transdural lesions* invading the petrous apex as en plaque meningiomas, or primary clival or temporal bone lesions with secondary posterior fossa extension as chordomas, chondrosarcomas, and extensive glomus jugulare tumors.
- Some cases of epidermoids.

Surgical Technique

A wide **C**-shaped postauricular incision is made. The incision starts 3 cm above the auricle, curves posteriorly to approximately 4 to 5 cm posterior to the auricular sulcus, and ends inferiorly at the level of the mastoid tip. The skin and subcutaneous tissues are elevated and the muscoloperiosteal layer is incised in a T-shaped pattern. A small Palva flap based anteriorly is outlined.

The external auditory canal is transected and closed as a cul de sac. The anterior skin flap is retracted using skin hooks, whereas the muscoloperiosteal layer is raised and is kept retracted using 1/0 silk sutures.

An extended mastoidectomy is performed, with removal of bone 2 to 3 cm posterior to the sigmoid sinus and over the middle fossa dura. The external auditory canal (posterior and superior walls) is drilled and the facial nerve is skeletonized. The inferior tympanic bone is also drilled.

The labyrinthectomy is performed and the internal auditory canal is identified. Bone superior and inferior to the internal auditory canal is drilled, creating two deep troughs around the canal.

The retrofacial air cells are drilled. The anterior wall of the external auditory canal and the tympanic bone are thinned out. The internal carotid artery is identified in front of the cochlea.

The cochlea is drilled. The internal carotid artery is better identified. All the bone inferior and superior to the internal auditory canal is completely removed.

In case of a modified transcochlear approach, the facial nerve is freed from the third to the fist portion and posteriorly rerouted together with all the contents of the internal auditory canal.

For intradural cases, the dura is next opened and the pathology is dealt with.

The surgical technique has been shown in ▶ Fig. 10.47, ▶ Fig. 10.48, ▶ Fig. 10.49, ▶ Fig. 10.50, ▶ Fig. 10.51, ▶ Fig. 10.52, ▶ Fig. 10.53, ▶ Fig. 10.54, ▶ Fig. 10.55, ▶ Fig. 10.56, ▶ Fig. 10.57, ▶ Fig. 10.58, ▶ Fig. 10.59, ▶ Fig. 10.60, ▶ Fig. 10.61, ▶ Fig. 10.62, ▶ Fig. 10.63, ▶ Fig. 10.64, ▶ Fig. 10.65, ▶ Fig. 10.66, ▶ Fig. 10.67, ▶ Fig. 10.68, ▶ Fig. 10.69, ▶ Fig. 10.70.

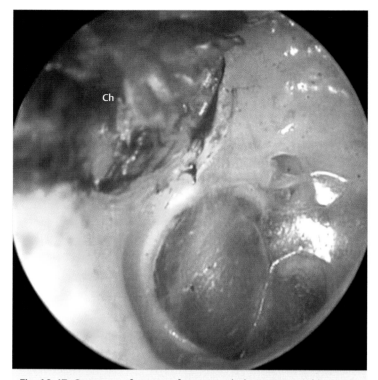

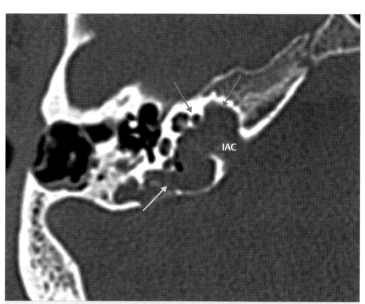

Fig. 10.48 CT scan of the same case, axial view. The cholesteatoma engulfs the labyrinth (*yellow arrow*) and the basal turn of the cochlea (*green arrow*), reaching the petrous apex (*red arrow*) and the internal auditory canal (IAC).

Fig. 10.47 Otoscopy of a case of massive cholesteatoma (Ch) is shown. The patient underwent canal wall down tympanoplasty elsewhere, and the mastoid cavity is filled with debris. No cholesteatoma is seen in the tympanic cavity. Audiometry showed moderate to severe mixed hearing loss. Facial nerve function was normal (grade I House–Brackmann scale), so a transotic approach was performed.

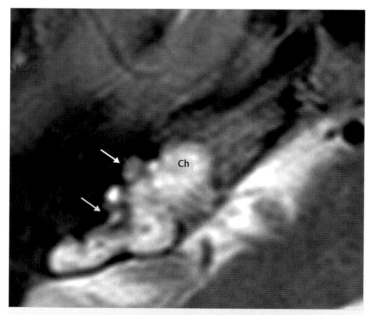

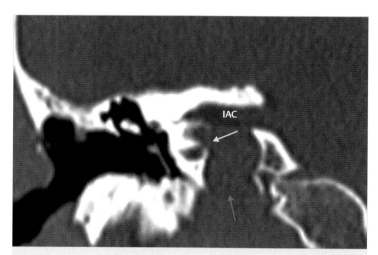

Fig. 10.50 CT scan of the same case, coronal view. The cholesteatoma invades the labyrinth (*yellow arrow*), the jugular bulb (*green arrow*), and the roof of the internal auditory canal (IAC).

Fig. 10.49 MRI (T2W), axial view. The cholesteatoma (Ch) has advanced far medially, eroding the posterior labyrinth to reach the petrous apex. The apical turn of the cochlea (*white arrow*) and the posterior semicircular canal (*yellow arrows*) seem spared.

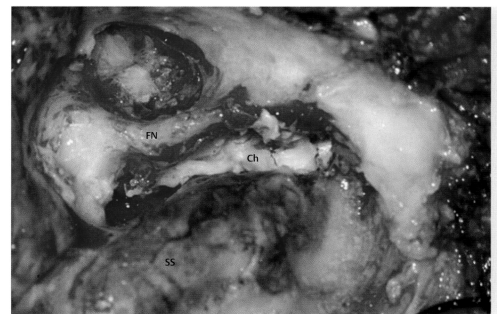

Fig. 10.51 Intraoperative image. Blind sac closure of the external auditory canal, removal of the tympanic membrane and the ossicles, and extended mastoidectomy have been performed. Further removal of the bone exposed huge cholesteatoma located medially to the labyrinth. The sigmoid sinus is exposed to enhance access to the digastric ridge. Ch, cholesteatoma; FN, facial nerve; SS, sigmoid sinus.

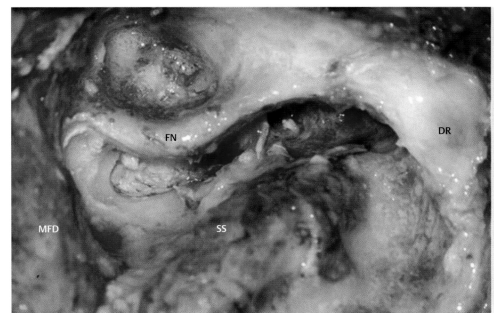

Fig. 10.52 Intraoperative image. The drilling is advanced superiorly by removing lateral and posterior semicircular canals. The cholesteatoma goes medial to the labyrinth toward the internal auditory canal. Facial nerve is well skeletonized. DR, digastric ridge; FN, facial nerve; MFD, middle fossa dura; SS, sigmoid sinus.

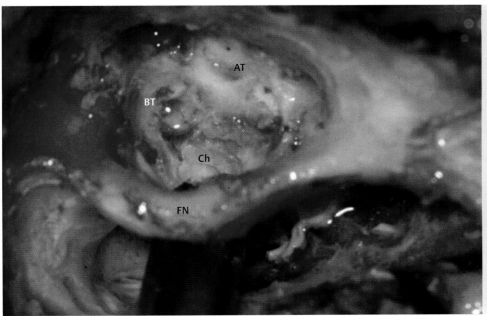

Fig. 10.53 Intraoperative image. The cholesteatoma has been removed from the labyrinth and the subfacial space. The cholesteatoma invading the modiolus is seen. AT, apical turn of cochlea; BT, basal turn of cochlea (upper pole); Ch, cholesteatoma; FN, facial nerve.

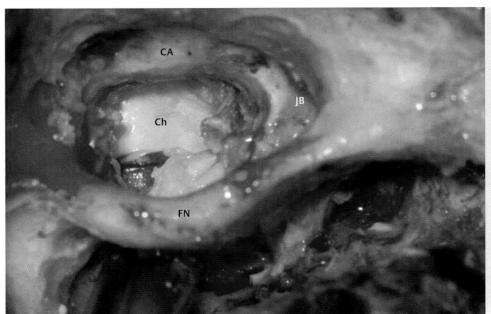

Fig. 10.54 Intraoperative image. Cochlea has been completely removed. Debris of the cholesteatoma filling the petrous apex is partially evacuated. The position of the jugular bulb located comparatively inferiorly permits access to the petrous apex from the area under the facial nerve. CA, internal carotid artery; Ch, cholesteatoma; FN, facial nerve; JB, jugular bulb.

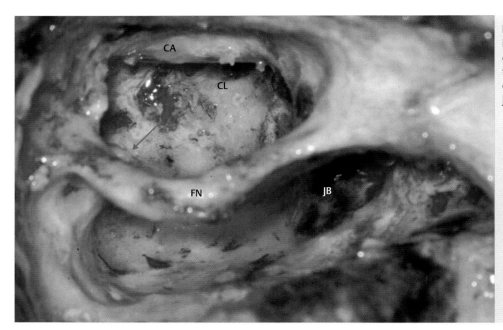

Fig. 10.55 Cleaning of the area anterior to the internal auditory canal (*arrow*) has been accomplished. The clivus is exposed. The cavity is free from the cholesteatoma. CA, internal carotid artery; FN, facial nerve; CL, clivus; JB, jugular bulb.

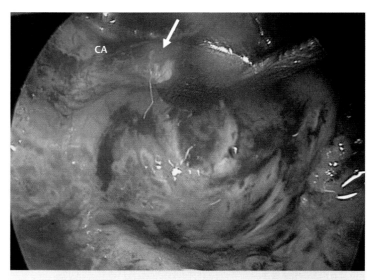

Fig. 10.56 With a 30-degree endoscope, the area under the internal carotid artery (CA) could be explored to check the presence of any residual pathology. In this case, a small piece of skin is detached from the bony wall of the artery.

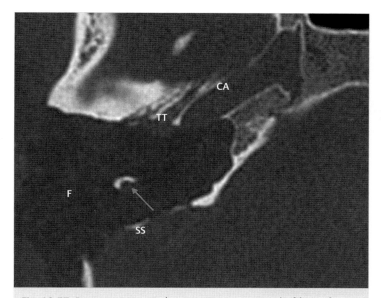

Fig. 10.57 Postoperative CT shows extensive removal of bone from the petrous apex. The mastoid segment of the facial nerve is left in the fallopian canal (*arrow*). The posterior fossa dura is partially exposed, and the carotid artery is uncovered posterolaterally. CA, carotid artery; F, abdominal fat; SS, sigmoid sinus; TT, tensor tympani.

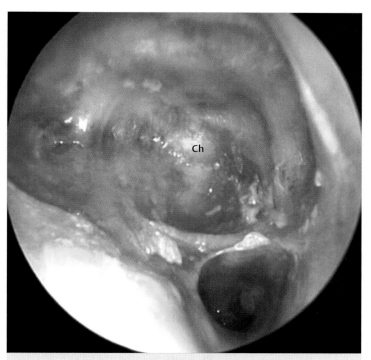

Fig. 10.58 Otoscopy of a case of massive PBC. The patient underwent six tympanoplasties elsewhere. A huge cavity is seen with the presence of a whitish mass strongly suggestive of a recurrent cholesteatoma (Ch). The patient complained of recurrent otorrhea and hearing loss (mixed type). Facial nerve function was normal.

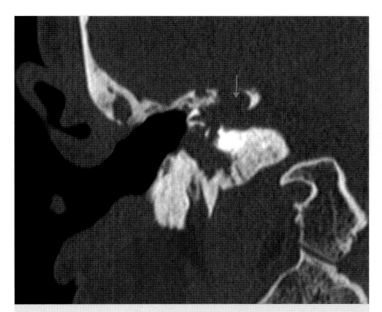

Fig. 10.59 CT scan of the same case, coronal view. Massive PBC with invasion of the labyrinth and the roof of the internal auditory canal (*arrow*).

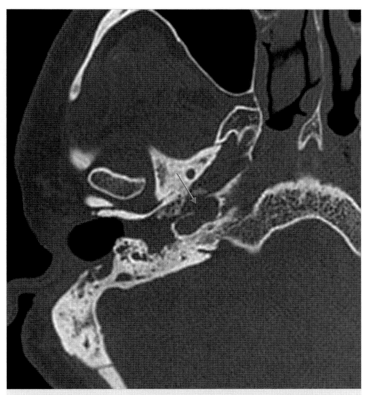

Fig. 10.60 CT scan of the same case, axial view. The cholesteatoma extends anteromedially to the vertical portion of the internal carotid artery. Considering this anterior extension, an infratemporal fossa approach type B was incorporated into the transotic approach for the removal of the disease.

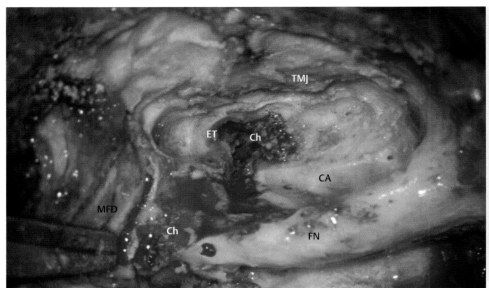

Fig. 10.61 Intraoperative picture. The cholesteatoma has been removed from the tympanic cavity and the mastoid. The labyrinth and the cochlea, involved by the cholesteatoma, have been removed too. The cholesteatoma infiltrates the Eustachian tube and the area anterior to the carotid artery. CA, carotid artery; Ch, cholesteatoma; ET, Eustachian tube; FN, facial nerve; MFD, middle fossa dura; TMJ, temporomandibular joint.

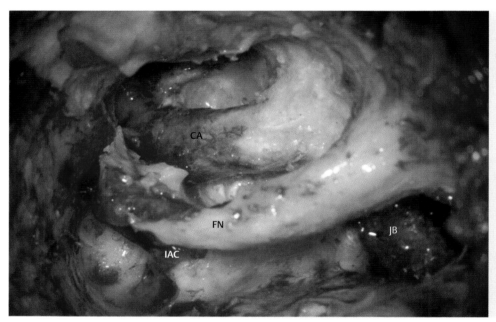

Fig. 10.62 Intraoperative picture. View after complete removal of the cholesteatoma. The carotid artery is under control until its horizontal part (*arrow*). CA, carotid artery; FN, facial nerve; IAC, internal auditory canal; JB, jugular bulb.

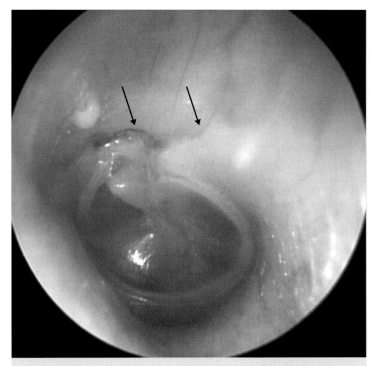

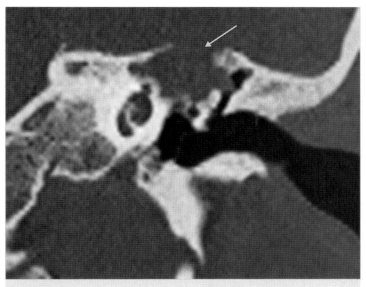

Fig. 10.64 CT scan of the same case, coronal view, shows supra-labyrinthine PBC (*arrow*).

Fig. 10.63 Case of a supralabyrinthine PBC. This 26-year-old female patient was evaluated for left progressive facial palsy for the last 1 year (near total, grade V House–Brackmann scale) and moderate to severe mixed hearing loss. Ten years before, she had head trauma with temporal bone fracture (*arrows*) and temporary left facial nerve palsy. The patient underwent PBC removal through a modified transcochlear approach type A with facial nerve reconstruction.

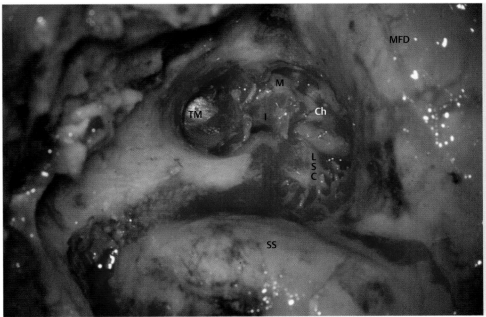

Fig. 10.65 Intraoperative picture. Blind sac closure of the external auditory canal and extended mastoidectomy have been performed. Cholesteatoma is seen in the supralabyrinthine area, infiltrating the middle fossa dura. Ch, cholesteatoma; I, incus; LSC, lateral semicircular canal; M, malleus; MFD, middle fossa dura; SS, sigmoid sinus; TM, tympanic membrane.

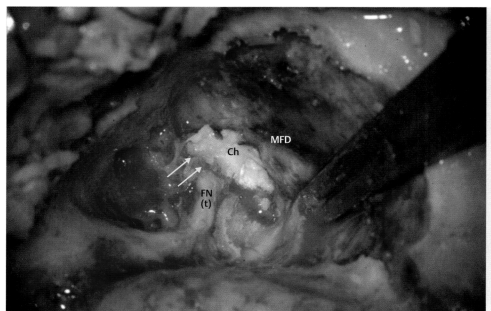

Fig. 10.66 Intraoperative picture. The cholesteatoma involves the supralabyrinthine area toward the internal auditory canal. The second portion of the facial nerve is engulfed by the pathology, leading to interruption of the nerve itself (*arrow*). The labyrinth has been previously drilled. Ch, cholesteatoma; FN (t), tympanic portion of the facial nerve; MFD, middle fossa dura.

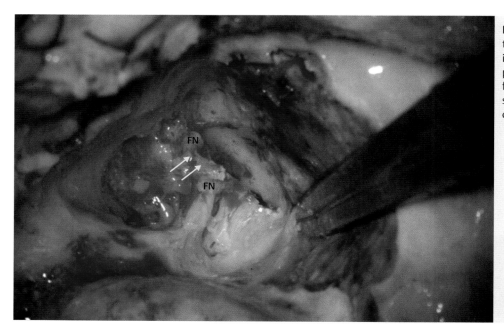

Fig. 10.67 Intraoperative view after removal of the cholesteatoma. The facial nerve (FN) is interrupted on its second portion (*arrow*). The proximal stump of the facial nerve is replaced by fibrous tissue, so a healthy portion of the nerve should be found for the anastomosis with the distal stump.

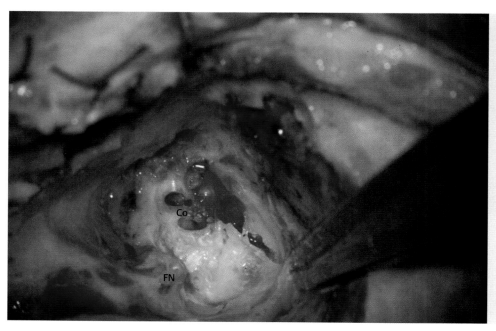

Fig. 10.68 Intraoperative picture. The third and second healthy portions of the facial nerve (FN) are detached from the fallopian canal and rerouted posteriorly. The cochlea (Co) is drilled to reach the fundus of the internal auditory canal and the first portion of the facial nerve.

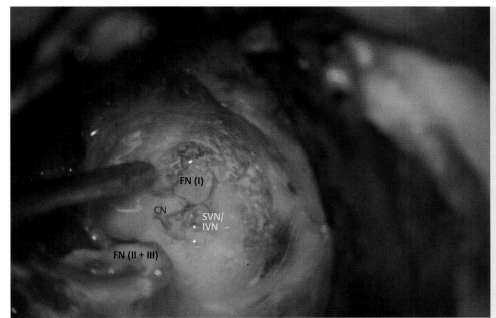

Fig. 10.69 Intraoperative picture after removal of the cochlea and opening of the internal auditory canal. From this view, the first portion of the facial nerve (FN I) is just superior to the cochlear nerve (CN) and anterior to the vestibular nerves (SVN/IVN). The facial nerve, in its second and third portion (FN II + III), has been posteriorly rerouted.

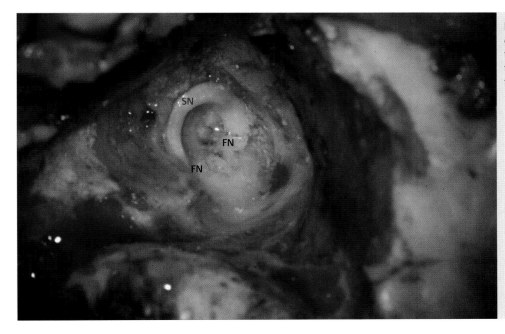

Fig. 10.70 Intraoperative picture. A sural nerve graft (SN) is used to restore continuity of the facial nerve. The two ends are fixed with temporalis fascia and fibrin glue. The cavity is further obliterated with abdominal fat.

10.1.2 Problems in Surgery

Hearing preservation. Hearing preservation would be important in exceptional cases, that is, bilateral PBCs or in a PBC of the only hearing ear. However, in the era of BAHA, Cochlear Implants. and Vibrant Soundbridge, even these cases can be treated successfully with hearing rehabilitation. If the cochlea is not destroyed beyond what is essential for the clearance of the disease, a cochlear implant should be used in ears with an accessible cochlear lumen even after labyrinthectomy. Another option is a BAHA if bone conduction is preserved in the ipsilateral ear.

Facial nerve. Facial nerve lesions may vary from simple erosion of the fallopian canal to total interruption of the nerve with fibrous tissue interposition. Management depends on three principal factors: preoperative status, degree of facial nerve involvement, and the extent of the lesion. In cases where the preoperative facial nerve function is good, a surgeon can be optimistic about a favorable facial nerve outcome depending on the extension of the pathology.

- *Decompression*: If there is a compression of the nerve with preserved anatomical integrity, then decompression of the nerve should be performed.
- *Rerouting*: When the lesion is present medial to the facial nerve and complete control over the lesion is hampered due to the position of the nerve, then rerouting of the facial nerve is undertaken, which could be partial or complete.
- *End-to-end anastomosis*: If there is a discontinuity of the nerve or a fibrous tissue interposition, the affected segment should be excised and a tension-free end-to-end anastomosis should be performed.
- *Nerve grafting*: Whenever the nerve segment lost is long and a tension-free end-to-end anastomosis is not possible, continuity of the nerve can be restored using a nerve graft. We prefer a sural nerve for grafting purposes.

- *Facial-hypoglossal or facial-trigeminal (masseteric nerve) anastomosis*: In patients with long duration of facial palsy (> 12 months).

Internal carotid artery. The PBC may involve the internal carotid artery in the vertical and/or the horizontal parts. In this situation, a complete control over the artery is important prior to attempting its removal. A modified transcochlear approach type A/transotic approach is used for involvement of the vessel in the vertical part, whereas an infratemporal fossa type B/modified transcochlear approach type B is used for involvement of vertical and horizontal parts. In case of a lesion extending into the petrous apex, clivus, sphenoid sinus, and the rhinopharynx, it is important to perform a complete control of the internal carotid artery to mobilize the artery if necessary. PBC are less aggressive in terms of arterial involvement and are easier to dissect as compared with other tumors (i.e., tympanojugular paragangliomas). The internal carotid artery has a thick adventitia which resents the dissection of the matrix but it requires extreme caution and surgical skill to clear it.

Sigmoid sinus and jugular bulb. Dealing with the jugular bulb in cases where it is involved is a well-thought-out strategy. Preoperative imaging must be carefully analyzed for two aspects: the relationship of the lesion with the jugular bulb and the patency of the contralateral venous drainage system by MR venography. In the presence of a hypoplasia of the contralateral venous system, sacrifice of the bulb means occlusion of the main venous drainage of the brain, with the consequent risk of benign intracranial hypertension or venous infarction of the temporal lobe. In such cases, damage to the jugular bulb or the sigmoid sinus must be avoided at all cost. The involvement of the sigmoid sinus and the jugular bulb presents a problem in matrix removal due to the thin wall and the fragility of these structures. In such cases, it is important to control the internal jugular vein in the neck prior to the dissection of the matrix. The ligation of the internal jugular vein in the neck and the sigmoid sinus packing (extraluminal and intraluminal) enables removal of the lateral wall of the dome of the jugular bulb and the sigmoid sinus to clear the matrix in the rare cases of accidental opening of the bulb. This maneuver also helps in preserving the IX, X, and XI cranial nerves. During this procedure, bleeding from the inferior petrosal sinus is controlled with Surgicel packing. In cases where its involvement is suspected, it is always advisable to ensure preoperatively the patency of the contralateral cerebral vein.

Dura. The matrix is often adherent to the dura of the middle and posterior fossa. Bipolar coagulation of all the suspected portions of the dura mater can be performed to destroy all the possible remnants of the matrix. We have been using bipolar coagulation in all cases to devitalize the epithelium, and also other authors who have used the same technique agree with us. Bipolarizing large areas of the dura does not lead to any dural necrosis if carefully performed. Long-term follow-up has shown that this maneuver is safe and adequate for complete control. There is a risk of opening the dura while removing the adherent matrix, causing an intraoperative CSF leak.

CSF leak. CSF leaks resulting from dural tears do not need special repair but can be swiftly managed by inserting free muscle plugs into the subarachnoid space through the defect and cavity obliteration with fat. CSF leak from the internal auditory canal can be treated by adopting a translabyrinthine approach.

Examination of hidden areas. Once the removal of the disease has been achieved, it is useful to carry out an endoscopic examination of the cavity with a 30-degree rigid endoscope to visualize the hidden areas that might not be accessible to the microscope. In some cases, epithelium missed by the conventional technique can be found on endoscopic examination. In our experience, if the approach is correct this technique is rarely required.

Residual lesions or recurrences. After complete eradication of the disease, it is mandatory to obliterate the cavities with autologous abdominal fat. The major disadvantage of cavity obliteration is that the recurrence cannot be directly visualized and detected. Therefore, it is mandatory to follow up these patients radiologically. We perform a high-resolution CT scan and a cerebral MRI (T1 W and T2 W images with fat suppression, diffusion-weighted images, non–echo planar imaging [EPI]) with gadolinium enhancement every year for at least 10 years.

Summary

When a patient presents with hearing loss (sensorineural or mixed) and/or facial nerve paralysis with or without a retrotympanic mass, the probability of a PBC should be considered. In such cases, it is necessary to perform a high-resolution CT scan of the temporal bone. The ideal treatment for PBC is radical surgical removal, although destruction of the labyrinth and rerouting of the facial nerve may be required. The status of the contralateral ear must also be considered. The transotic and modified transcochlear approaches are the most appropriate for the removal of PBC. These approaches offer direct lateral access to the petrous bone and allow the removal of all types of PBC with their possible extension into the clivus, sphenoid sinus, or intradural space. In addition, they have the advantage of minimizing the occurrence of CSF leak and allow control of the different vital structures, including the internal carotid artery. Closure of the external auditory canal as a cul de sac and obliteration of the operative cavity with abdominal fat avoid the risk of infection and the need for frequent toilet of a very deep cavity. The advances in hearing rehabilitation has given further options in cases with preserved cochlea and/or preserved bone conduction. The middle cranial fossa approach can be used in few cases with small supralabyrinthine PBC and noncompromised inner ear function.

Chapter 11

Temporal Bone Paragangliomas

11 Temporal Bone Paragangliomas

Abstract

Paragangliomas are tumors that arise from the paraganglionic system. They originate from the neural crest and are related to the autonomic nervous system. Temporal bone paragangliomas (TBPs) arise either in the adventitia of the jugular bulb or along the course of the Jacobson's or the Arnold's nerve. Otoscopy usually reveals a reddish retrotympanic pulsating mass. A definitive diagnosis is obtained after neuroradiological studies are performed (computed tomography and magnetic resonance imaging scans, digital subtraction angiography). Fisch classification is fundamental in planning the right surgical approach, because it correlates to the grade of involvement of the temporal bone and skull base. *Class A* relates to tumors limited to the middle ear cleft without invasion of the hypotympanum; *Class B* relates to tumors limited to the hypotympanum, mesotympanum, and mastoid without erosion of jugular bulb; *Class C* relates to tumors involving the carotid canal; *Class D* defines only the intracranial tumor extension and should be reported as an addendum to the C stage. The most common presenting symptom of a TBP is hearing loss, with pulsatile tinnitus also affecting the majority of patients. Lower cranial nerve deficits usually develop as a consequence of the progressive invasion of the medial wall of the jugular fossa. In the majority of cases, the treatment is surgical; the type A infratemporal fossa approach is generally used for the removal of class C and D tumors.

Keywords: temporal bone paragangliomas, Fisch classification, infratemporal fossa approach, facial nerve rerouting, pulsatile tinnitus

Paragangliomas are tumors that arise from the paraganglionic system—aggregations of cells found throughout the body associated with vascular and neuronal adventitia. They originate from the neural crest and are related to the autonomic nervous system.

Temporal bone paragangliomas (TBPs) arise either in the adventitia of the jugular bulb or along the course of the Jacobson's nerve (the tympanic branch of the glossopharyngeal nerve) or the Arnold's nerve (the auricular branch of the vagus nerve). The term tympanicum has been applied to those paragangliomas arising on the promontory and remaining confined to the middle ear and mastoid compartments, without erosion of the jugular plate and involvement of the jugular bulb. Jugular paragangliomas have been described as those arising from within the jugular bulb. The exact site of origin is often difficult to determine because paragangliomas can arise from within the canaliculi of the temporal bone, the jugular fossa, and the middle ear cleft, which are in close proximity to each other.

Vagal paragangliomas arise from the nodose ganglion in almost all cases.

Carotid body tumors originate from the carotid body at the carotid bifurcation.

Paragangliomas of the head and neck make up only 3% of all paragangliomas, comprising approximately 0.6% of head and neck tumors and 0.03% of all tumors. The overall incidence of head and neck paraganglioma ranges from 1 in 30,000 to 1 in 100,000, with carotid body tumors making up nearly 60% of head and neck paragangliomas, tympanojugular paragangliomas (TJPs) nearly 40%, and vagal paragangliomas < 5%. The fact that carotid body tumors are far more common than other head and neck paragangliomas is probably due to a higher mass of normal paraganglionic tissue in this area. Carotid body tumors and vagal paragangliomas can be grouped clinically as cervicocarotid tumors.

TJPs constitute the second commonest tumor of the temporal bone and the commonest tumor affecting the jugular fossa. Tympanic paragangliomas are the commonest neoplasm affecting the middle ear. Thus, while rare, these are lesions that are frequently encountered by the skull base and head and neck surgeon.

Paragangliomas can arise both as sporadic and as familial entities, a fact first documented in 1933 by Chase, in a description of bilateral carotid body tumors in sisters. It is now known that 25 to 35% of paragangliomas are associated with recognized genetic defects, most of which are due to hereditary transmission. These defects are usually associated with one of the four familial paraglioma syndromes. This means that approximately 30% of apparently sporadic head and neck paragangliomas are due to one of these defects. Multiple tumors are not uncommon, found in 10 to 20% of sporadic cases and in up to 80% of familial cases.

All subtypes of head and neck paraganglioma show a peak age of presentation in the fourth and fifth decades, with rare incidences of pediatric cases. While the sex ratio is equal for carotid body tumors, females are affected four to six times more than males in TJPs. However, males are more commonly affected in the familial type. All patients with a familial etiology present at a significantly younger age.

Paragangliomas are predominantly benign, slow-growing, highly vascular tumors, but they have a propensity for aggressive local destruction. Due to this clinical behavior, they have the ability to cause significant morbidity, especially when arising in relationship to the skull base with its multitude of associated neurovascular structures.

Because of their generally slow growth and initial absence of symptoms, TJPs are often not detected until they are of significant size. Those arising initially in the tympanic cavity, however, are usually detected at an earlier stage due to the presentation with hearing loss from ossicular chain interference and/or with pulsatile tinnitus. With progression, TJPs most frequently follow a path of least resistance into the middle ear cleft and within the jugular vein. Further spread then occurs through air cell tracts to involve the intrapetrous carotid canal, along the Eustachian tube, into the neck along the carotid sheath, and, in later stages, intracranially. The tumor can also extend along the inferior petrosal sinus. Intracranial spread usually occurs through the medial wall of the jugular foramen. Lower cranial nerve (LCN) involvement occurs later and is usually related to invasion through the medial wall of the jugular bulb. The facial nerve lies in close proximity to the jugular bulb in its vertical segment and is also at risk.

Whether arising in the middle ear or from within the canaliculi or bulb, the most common finding on examination is the presence of a vascular middle ear mass. The classically described blanching of the middle ear component, Brown's sign, is present in 20%. Otoscopy alone is not reliable for assessing extent, most significantly in relation to the degree of hypotympanic extension. Tumors invading the tympanic bone from the jugular fossa can show the classic "rising sun" sign. Paragangliomas can also extend through the tympanic membrane and be confused with an inflammatory polyp, and occasionally otorrhagia can be a significant clinical symptom.

While a paraganglioma is the most common cause of a retrotympanic vascular mass, other pathology must be considered. Obviously, any vascular mass seen on otoscopy, if the margins are not seen in their entirety, involves the jugular bulb until proven otherwise.

A full cranial nerve examination is essential, including upper aerodigestive tract endoscopy and careful palpation of the neck. Silent LCN palsies are present in approximately 10% of patients.

11.1 Clinical Presentation of Tympanic and Tympanomastoid Paragangliomas

Paragangliomas arising in and remaining within the middle ear and mastoid system are termed tympanic and tympanomastoid paragangliomas. In general terms, they are a subtype of TJPs and correspond to the Fisch type A and B classification; they are seen significantly less commonly than are TJPs. These tumors usually present with conductive hearing loss and pulsatile tinnitus at a relatively early stage. They appear to behave in a less aggressive fashion than those arising from the jugular bulb. Interestingly, in our series no tympanic paragangliomas were associated with multiple tumors or with a genetic predisposition.

These tumors are usually otoscopically visible as retrotympanic reddish masses, determination of the degree of extension usually requiring imaging, most importantly to confirm that the jugular plate remains intact. Occasionally, visualization of the retrotympanic mass can be difficult, such as in the presence of tympanosclerosis. Very rarely, presentation is as a polyp occupying the external auditory canal. At presentation, approximately 20% of tympanic paragangliomas have extended to the mastoid air cells. Eustachian tube extension is not uncommon, also occurring in approximately 20% of cases. Ossicular chain involvement is found in around 50%. While rare, direct involvement of the carotid can occur, as can extension downward to invade the jugular bulb.

11.2 Clinical Presentation of Tympanojugular Paragangliomas

TJPs (previously glomus jugulare) are those tumors arising from the paraganglia of the adventitia of the jugular bulb or within the inferior tympanic or mastoid canaliculi. While the term tympanojugular paragangliomas can be used to describe both jugular and tympanic paragangliomas as a single group, those limited to the middle ear and mastoid are usually excluded, as discussed earlier. Treatment outcomes in relation to TJP are highly dependent on the stage of the tumor at diagnosis. A high index of suspicion is required along with the judicious use and review of constantly advancing radiological studies. Accordingly, the goal is to identify these tumors early and, in the age of genetic testing, to selectively use screening to identify presymptomatic lesions.

The most common presenting symptom of a TJP is hearing loss, present in approximately 60 to 80% of cases, with pulsatile tinnitus also affecting the majority of patients. Hearing loss is usually conductive in nature due to a combination of impingement of the ossicles and a middle ear effusion. Therefore, the diagnosis of a paraganglioma should be considered in any patient with pulsatile tinnitus, especially if it is associated with conductive hearing loss. It is important to note that, due to the nonspecific nature of these symptoms, there is an average 2 to 3 years' delay between the onset of symptoms and diagnosis. Sensorineural hearing loss and/or vestibular symptoms depend on the invasion of the inner ear, internal auditory canal, or cerebellopontine angle, while LCN deficits usually develop as a consequence of the progressive invasion of the medial wall of the jugular fossa. Nerve deficits induced by tumor growth generally develop very slowly, allowing progressive compensation, so that the patient is sometimes unaware of the deficit itself. Silent LCN palsies are noted in around 10% of cases. Palsies of the glossopharyngeal and vagus nerves occur in approximately 35 to 40%, those of spinal accessory and hypoglossal nerves occurring in 21 to 30%. The facial nerve is the next most common cranial nerve involved at presentation, with involvement occurring in approximately 10% of TJPs, although it is reported to be as high as 39%. It is important to consider jugular fossa pathology when investigating an isolated, or compound, LCN lesion. Vocal fold paralysis presenting with a change in voice is the most common clinical scenario. Obviously, evidence of a high vagal lesion, such as palatal asymmetry, strongly suggests pathology at the skull base.

11.3 Imaging Characteristics

High-resolution computed tomography (HRCT), with reconstructions in axial and coronal planes, is mandatory in every suspected case of TJP. If jugular foramen involvement is suspected, T1-weighted (T1W), T2-weighted (T2W), and T1 W gadolinium-enhanced sequences with axial, coronal, and sagittal plane reconstruction, along with magnetic resonance angiography (MRA) and magnetic resonance venography (MRV), are the minimum additional imaging studies required. Diagnostic four-vessel angiography is reserved for doubtful cases. The diagnosis of skull base pathology is based on radiological information, not on histopathology from biopsy specimens.

Tympanic paragangliomas appear on CT as small masses located on the surface of the promontory. In class B lesions, the tumor invades the hypotympanum without erosion of the jugular plate. Mastoid opacification is frequently related to fluid accumulation related to Eustachian tube obstruction.

11.3.1 Tympanojugular Paragangliomas

- *CT scan*: On CT, TJPs show characteristic irregular bony erosion (moth-eaten bone). Early changes are represented as an indistinct lateral margin of the jugular fossa, followed by erosion of the caroticojugular crest or jugular spine. The degree of bony involvement is often difficult to assess, however. The most critical initial step is the differentiation between tympanomastoid paragangliomas and small TJPs, with a coronal image being the most helpful. If HRCT confirms that the lesion remains free of the jugular fossa, no further imaging is mandatory; magnetic resonance imaging (MRI) can be very helpful in differentiating tumor from middle ear and mastoid effusions. However, any doubt on any radiological view necessitates further assessment. The degree of bony infiltration can also be difficult to ascertain and it is often underestimated. This is especially the case in poorly pneumatized temporal bones and in the presence of involvement of the petrous apex, clivus, occipital condyle, and hypoglossal canal, because of the bony marrow usually present in these areas.

- *MRI*: MRI provides exquisite detail relating to the soft-tissue relationships in the deep neck spaces as well as intracranially. Around 60 to 75% of cases have intracranial extension at presentation, with the rate of intradural involvement being approximately 30%. Several sequences can be employed to delineate both the tumor and arterial anatomy and venous drainage. Low to intermediate T1 W signal and relatively high T2 W signal are typical for paragangliomas. Small tumors enhance homogeneously, but areas of necrosis and hemorrhage are present with increasing size. A classic "salt and pepper" pattern in lesions larger than 2 cm (in any dimension) is often seen, especially in T2 W images. This is due to areas of brightening on T2-weighting due to areas of slow flow within the tumor, and the presence of large intratumoral vasculature appearing as flow voids. Axial and coronal images are commonly used to evaluate the lesion, but sagittal images allow appreciation of tumor extension as a whole. Dural invasion is not always easy to detect because often the dura is infiltrated and pushed medially; in other instances, there is a true invasion of the posterior fossa. MRI affords information regarding invasion into the marrow spaces of the base of skull with effacement of the normal fatty signal. While each department often uses a different combination of sequences, no longer are only T1 W, T2 W, and contrast studies used. Dual T2 fast spin echo sequences, noncontrast and contrast time-of-flight sequences, and contrast-enhanced MRA and MRV (often with 3D reconstruction) provide further information. Despite these advances, detection of lesions less than 10 mm in size is difficult, except for those arising in the tympanic cavity.
- *Angiography*: Angiography plays a critical role in the management of TJPs, but is rarely necessary for diagnosis. Paragangliomas display a characteristic intense tumor blush and rapid venous diffusion. This allows differentiation in cases where CT and MRI remain equivocal. Just as importantly, it allows detailed analysis of tumor vascular supply and embolization if operative management is planned, as well as assessment of internal carotid artery (ICA) involvement, contralateral cerebral blood flow, and venous drainage.

11.4 Classification: The Modified Fisch Classification System for TJP

Two classification systems are in common use for TJP, that of Fisch and that of Glasscock–Jackson. In terms of describing the involvement of the ICA, the most critical aspect in planning the surgical approach, we recommend use of the Fisch system. There is also a close correlation between Fisch class C and the likelihood of intracranial extension. We have made minor modifications to the Fisch classification to allow precise surgical planning. For this reason, as well as for consistency in reporting, we recommend that the modified Fisch system be used, as outlined in the following.

- *Class A*: tumors limited to the middle ear cleft without invasion of the hypotympanum:
  - A1: tumor completely visible on otoscopic examination (▶ Fig. 11.1).
  - A2: tumor margins not seen on otoscopy (▶ Fig. 11.2).
- *Class B*: limited to the hypotympanum, mesotympanum, and mastoid without erosion of jugular bulb:
  - B1: tumors confined to the middle ear cleft with extension to the hypotympanum (▶ Fig. 11.3).
  - B2: tumors involving the middle ear cleft with extension to the hypotympanum and the mastoid (▶ Fig. 11.4).
  - B3: tumors confined to the tympanomastoid compartment with erosion of the carotid canal (▶ Fig. 11.5).
- *Class C*: TJP subclassification by degree of carotid canal erosion:
  - C1: tumors destroying the jugular foramen and bulb with limited involvement of the vertical portion of the carotid canal (▶ Fig. 11.6).
  - C2: Tumors invading the vertical portion of the carotid canal (▶ Fig. 11.7).
  - C3: Tumors invading the horizontal portion of the carotid canal (▶ Fig. 11.8).
  - C4: Tumors reaching the anterior foramen lacerum (▶ Fig. 11.9)
- *Class D*: defines only the intracranial tumor extension and should be reported as an addendum to the C stage. De, extradural; Di, intradural.
  - De1: tumors with up to 2 cm dural displacement.
  - De2: tumors with more than 2 cm dural displacement.
  - Di1: tumors with up to 2 cm intradural extension.
  - Di2: tumors with more than 2 cm intradural extension.
  - Di3: tumors with inoperable intracranial intradural extension.
- *Class V*: subclassification by degree of the vertebral artery involvement:
  - Ve: tumors engulfing the extradural vertebral artery (▶ Fig. 11.10).
  - Vi: tumors involving the intradural vertebral artery.

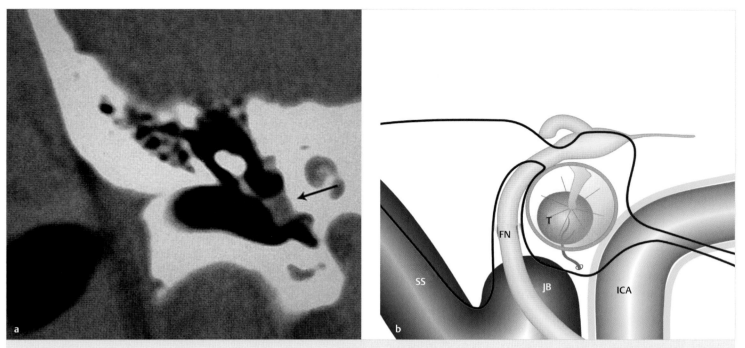

Fig. 11.1 Class A1. Small tumor is clearly seen on the promontory (*arrow*). Tumor margins do not involve the annulus. (a) CT. (b) Schematic illustration. FN, facial nerve; ICA, internal carotid artery; JB, jugular bulb; SS, sigmoid sinus; T, tumor.

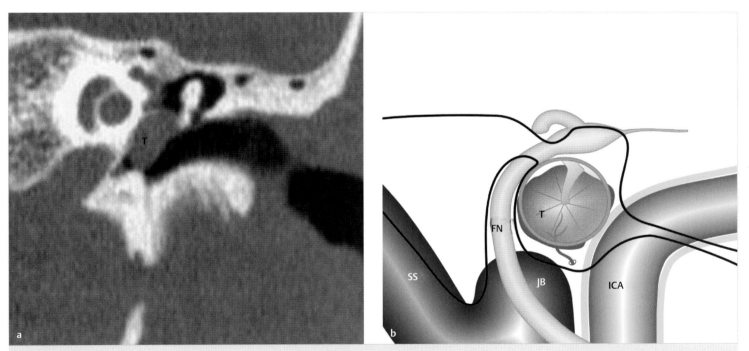

Fig. 11.2 Class A2. Tumor margins (T) are not seen on otoscopy. (a) CT. (b) Schematic illustration. FN, facial nerve; ICA, internal carotid artery; JB, jugular bulb; SS, sigmoid sinus; T, tumor.

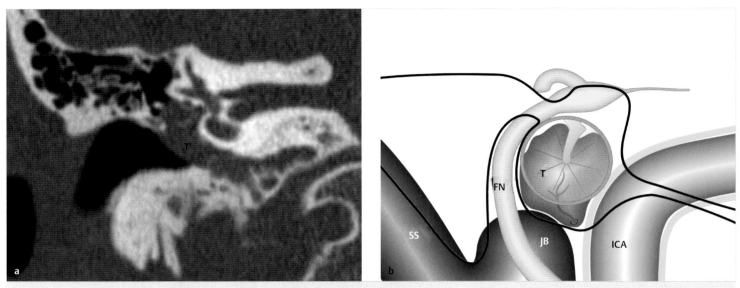

Fig. 11.3 Class B1. Tumor (T) is limited to the middle ear cleft with extension to the hypotympanum but without erosion of the jugular bulb. **(a)** CT. **(b)** Schematic illustration. FN, facial nerve; ICA, internal carotid artery; JB, jugular bulb; SS, sigmoid sinus; T, tumor.

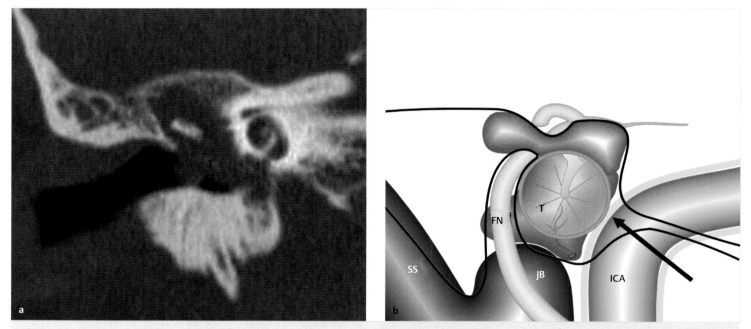

Fig. 11.4 Class B2. Tumor (T) is occupying entire middle ear with extension to the hypotympanum and mastoid. Bony erosion of the promontory, fallopian canal, and ossicles can be noted. Arrow: no erosion of the carotid canal. **(a)** CT. **(b)** Schematic illustration. FN, facial nerve; ICA, internal carotid artery; JB, jugular bulb; SS, sigmoid sinus; T, tumor.

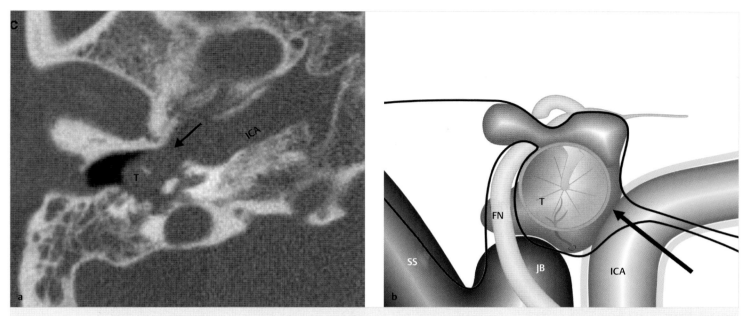

Fig. 11.5 Class B3. Erosion of the carotid canal (*arrow*) can be seen on this slice. (a) CT. (b) Schematic illustration. FN, facial nerve; ICA, internal carotid artery; JB, jugular bulb; SS, sigmoid sinus; T, tumor.

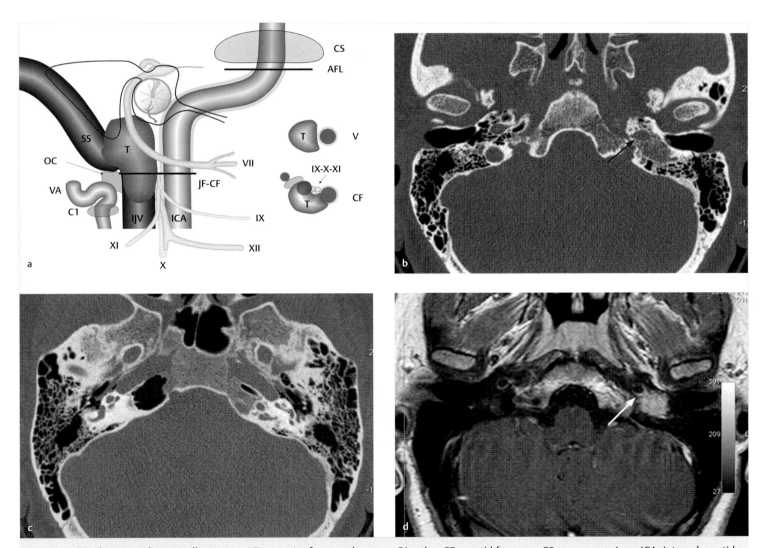

Fig. 11.6 (a) Class C1. Schematic illustration. AFL, anterior foramen lacerum; C1, atlas; CF, carotid foramen; CS, cavernous sinus; ICA, internal carotid artery; IJV, internal jugular vein; JF-CF, jugular foramen–carotid foramen; OC, occipital condyle; SS, sigmoid sinus; T, tumor; V, vertical portion of the internal carotid artery; VA, vertebral artery; VII, facial nerve; IX, glossopharyngeal nerve; X, vagus nerve; XI, spinal accessory nerve; XII, hypoglossal nerve. (b) Class C1 (CT). Note that tumor involvement can be seen in the jugular fossa, and erosion of the carotid foramen of the ICA (*arrow*). (c) Class C1 (CT). The horizontal portion of the carotid canal is not involved. (d) Class C1 (MRI). Tumor extending to but not eroding vertical portion of the carotid canal (*arrow*).

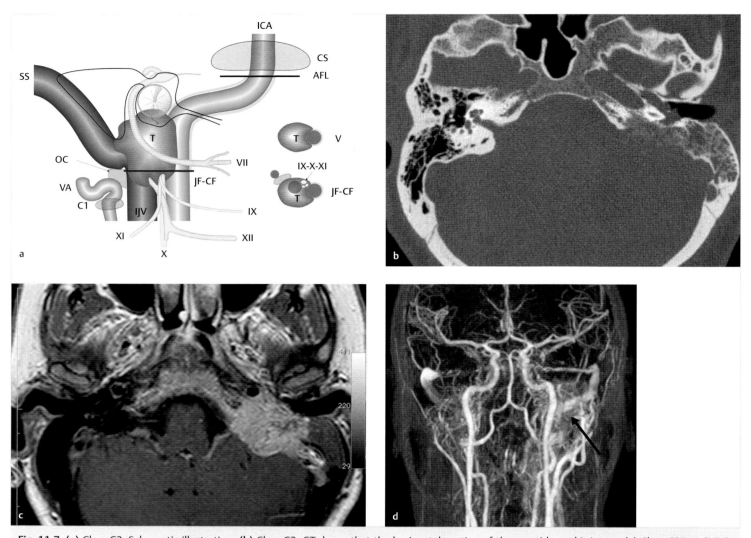

Fig. 11.7 **(a)** Class C2. Schematic illustration. **(b)** Class C2. CT shows that the horizontal portion of the carotid canal is intact. **(c)** Class C2De1 (MRI). Tumor is engulfing the vertical portion of the carotid canal. **(d)** Class C2 (magnetic resonance angiography). Hypervascular area (*arrow*) can be seen lateral to the vertical portion of the carotid artery.

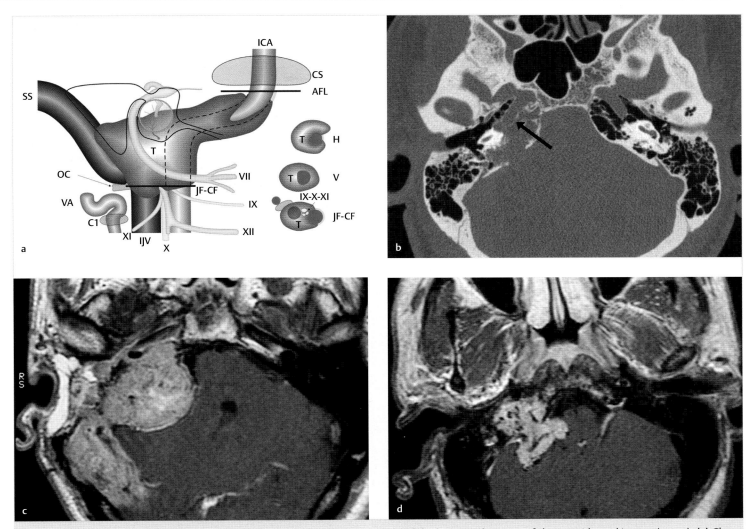

Fig. 11.8 **(a)** Class C3. Schematic illustration. **(b)** Class C3De1 (CT). The erosion of the horizontal portion of the carotid canal is seen (*arrow*). **(c)** Class C3De2 (MRI). MRI shows clearly the involvement of the horizontal portion of the carotid canal and the sigmoid sinus. **(d)** Class C3Di2 (MRI). Large paraganglioma with intradural extension.

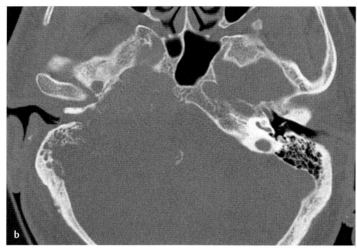

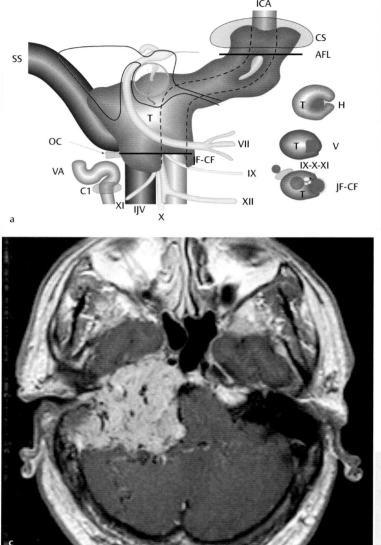

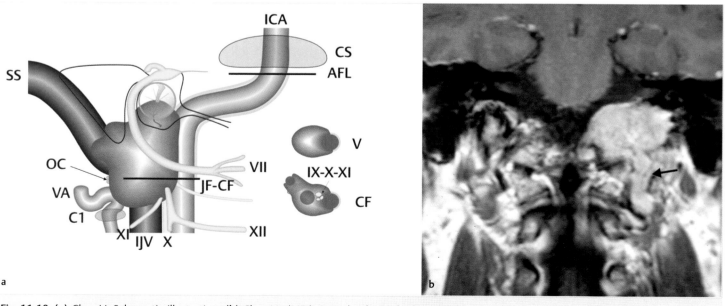

Fig. 11.9 **(a)** Class C4. Schematic illustration. **(b)** Class C4 (CT). The tumor erodes all the temporal bone up to the petrous apex and the clivus, with total engulfment of the carotid artery and the cavernous sinus. **(c)** Class C4Di2 (MRI). MRI of the same case with clear involvement of all the horizontal portion of the carotid artery with extension to the cavernous sinus.

Fig. 11.10 **(a)** Class V. Schematic illustration. **(b)** Class Ve (MRI). Extradural vertebral artery (*black arrow*) involved with the tumor.

11.5 Class A: Tympanic Paragangliomas

Class A type tumors have been shown in ▶ Fig. 11.11, ▶ Fig. 11.12, ▶ Fig. 11.13, ▶ Fig. 11.14, ▶ Fig. 11.15, ▶ Fig. 11.16, ▶ Fig. 11.17, ▶ Fig. 11.18, ▶ Fig. 11.19, ▶ Fig. 11.20, ▶ Fig. 11.21, ▶ Fig. 11.22.

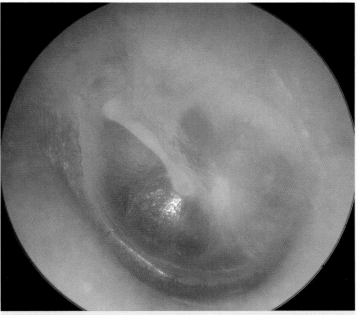

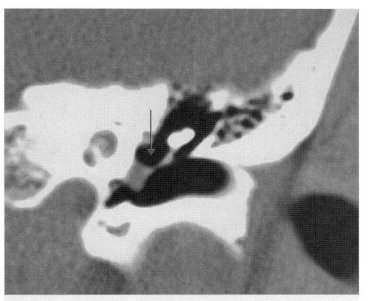

Fig. 11.11 Left ear. Glomus tympanicum or class A tumor. The small red mass behind the anteroinferior quadrant is localized on the promontory and does not extend toward the hypotympanum (see ▶ Fig. 11.12).

Fig. 11.12 CT scan of the case presented in ▶ Fig. 11.7. The lesion is limited to the region of the promontory. There are no visible signs of bone erosion.

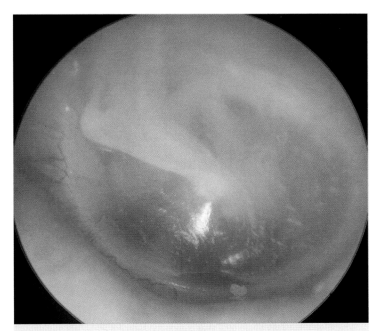

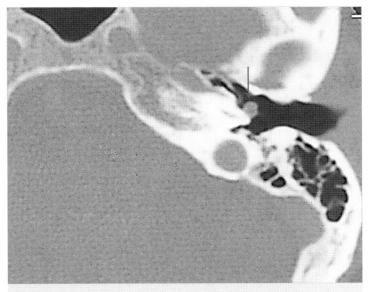

Fig. 11.13 Left ear. Another example of a small class A glomus tumor.

Fig. 11.14 CT scan of the case described in ▶ Fig. 11.13. The tumor is again limited to the promontory.

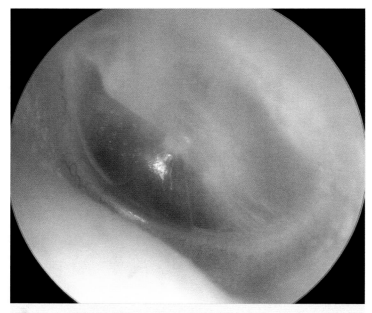

Fig. 11.15 Left ear. This small tympanic paraganglioma is situated in the anteroinferior quadrant of the middle ear near the tubal orifice. Further growth of the tumor can block the tubal orifice, leading to middle ear effusion.

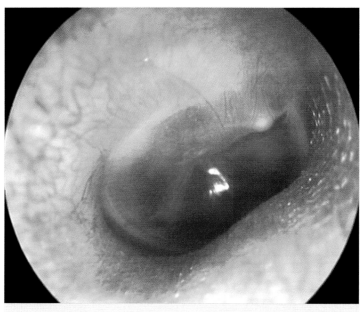

Fig. 11.16 Right ear. Class A1 tumor. The patient complains only on pulsatile tinnitus.

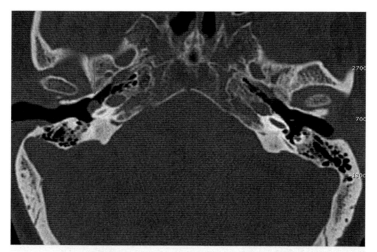

Fig. 11.17 CT scan, axial view, shows the tumor on the promontory.

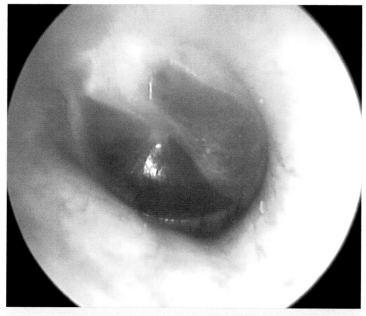

Fig. 11.18 Left ear. The tumor, located on the promontory, slightly extends to the hypotympanic area (see ▶ Fig. 11.18, ▶ Fig. 11.19).

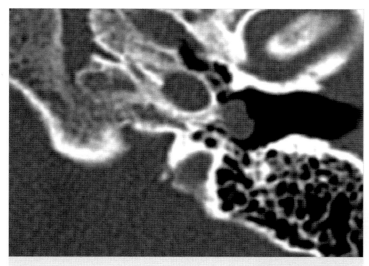

Fig. 11.19 CT scan of the same patient, axial view. The tumor, located on the promontory, is wider than the previous cases.

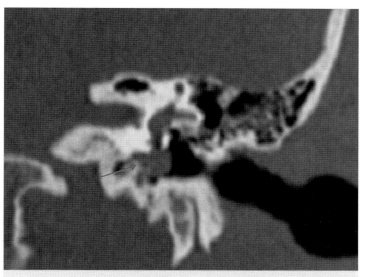

Fig. 11.20 CT scan of the same case, coronal view. Extension of the tumor toward the round window and the hypotympanum is clearly seen (*arrow*).

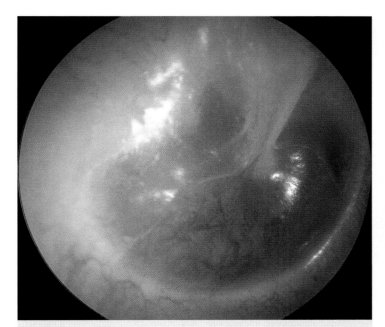

Fig. 11.21 Right ear. Class A2 tympanic paraganglioma. On otoscopy, the tumor margins seem not completely under control.

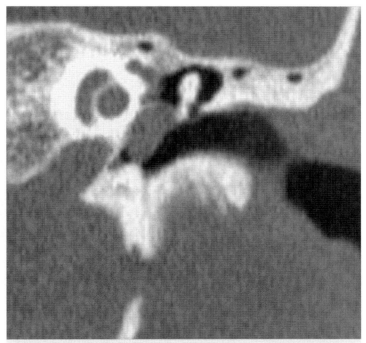

Fig. 11.22 CT scan of the same case.

11.5.1 Surgical Management

- For class A1 tumors, a transcanal approach can be performed safely, as it gives good access to the entire tympanic membrane. When there is limited access due to anatomical variation, these cases are to be treated as class A2.
- For class A2 tumors, a retroauricular transcanal approach is indicated. A modification of the traditional approach is used, removing the entire tympanomeatal flap. After removal of the tumor, myringoplasty is completed with fascia with replace-

ment of the tympanomeatal flap (glove finger flap technique). This technique allows wider access to the tumor by drilling of the bony meatus.

The surgical management of Class A type tumors has been shown in ▶ Fig. 11.23, ▶ Fig. 11.24, ▶ Fig. 11.25, ▶ Fig. 11.26, ▶ Fig. 11.27, ▶ Fig. 11.28, ▶ Fig. 11.29, ▶ Fig. 11.30, ▶ Fig. 11.31, ▶ Fig. 11.32, ▶ Fig. 11.33, ▶ Fig. 11.34, ▶ Fig. 11.35.

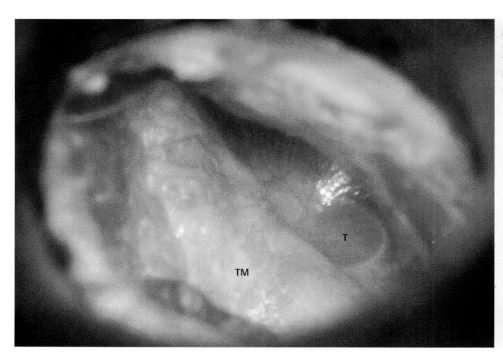

Fig. 11.23 The tympanic membrane is visualized under the largest possible ear speculum. The tumor is touching the tympanic membrane inferior to the umbo. T, tumor; TM, tympanic membrane.

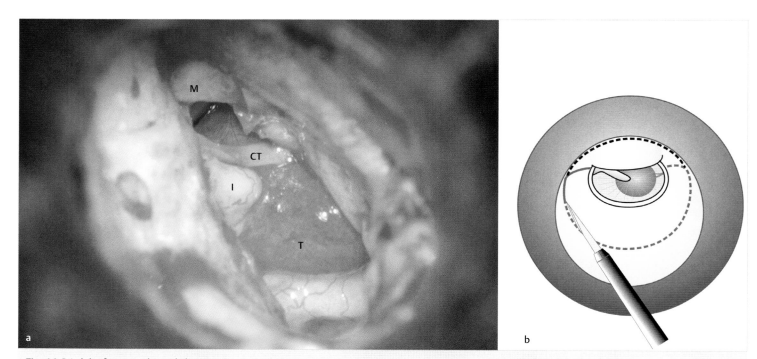

Fig. 11.24 **(a)** After a U-shaped skin incision is made in the posterior meatal skin, the tympanomeatal flap is elevated to expose the tympanic cavity. The tumor seems to originate from the promontory, and extends posterosuperiorly to reach the level of the oval window, anteriorly passing under the handle of the malleus. To visualize the upper pole of the tumor fully, the chorda tympani has been divided and a small atticotomy has been performed with a curette. CT, chorda tympani; I, incus; M, malleus; T, tumor. **(b)** Schematic illustration of the surgical approach.

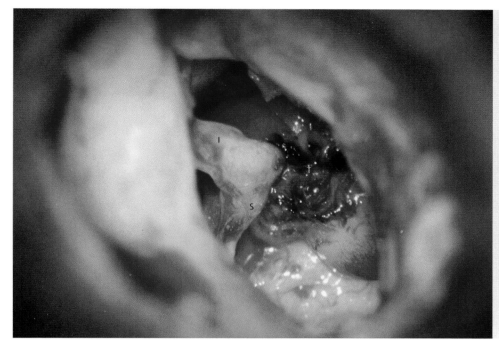

Fig. 11.25 Coagulation of the tumor with fine bipolar forceps should be started from the area away from the important structures to reduce the risk of mechanical and thermal injury. This procedure shrinks the tumor. Piecemeal removal of the tumor facilitates visualization of the tumor. I, incus; S, stapes; T, tumor.

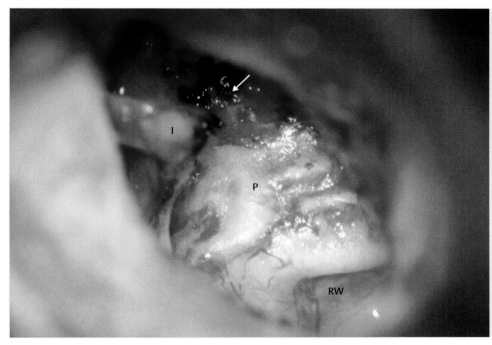

Fig. 11.26 The tumor has been completely removed. The origin of the tumor is located in the area just anteroinferior to the oval window (*arrow*). I, incus; P, promontory; RW, round window niche.

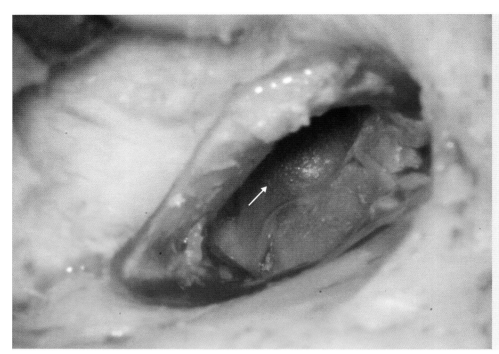

Fig. 11.27 A reddish mass is visible in the anterosuperior quadrant of the tympanic membrane (arrow). Since the anterior margin of the tumor is not visible on otoscopic examination, a retroauricular–transcanal approach is indicated. A lateral incision is visible on the anterior meatal skin for canalplasty.

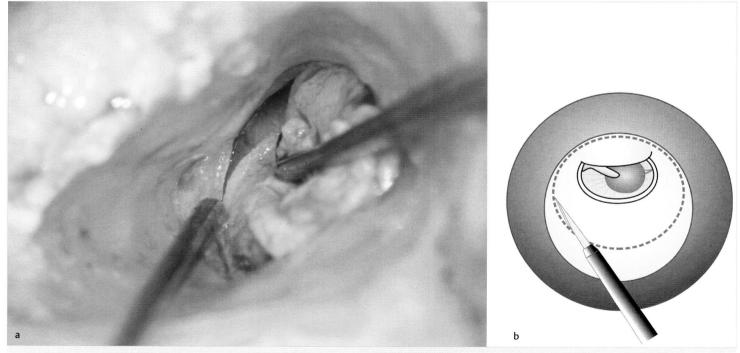

Fig. 11.28 **(a)** After having completed the canalplasty, the tympanomeatal flap is removed carefully. The anterior tympanic annulus, detached from the bony sulcus, can be seen clearly. **(b)** Schematic illustration of the incision line.

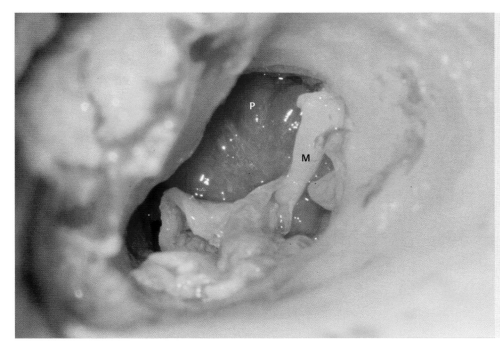

Fig. 11.29 The skin of the external auditory canal with the tympanic membrane is about to be detached from the manubrium. The paraganglioma occupies anterosuperior part of the tympanic cavity, and extends anteriorly toward the Eustachian tube. M, malleus.

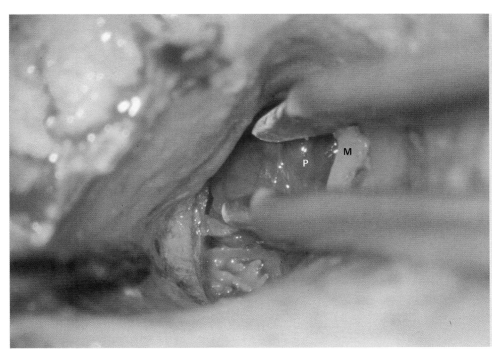

Fig. 11.30 The tumor is coagulated gradually with a bipolar coagulator. The tumor should be managed gently at this point so as not to damage feeding vessels located in the inaccessible portion. M, malleus.

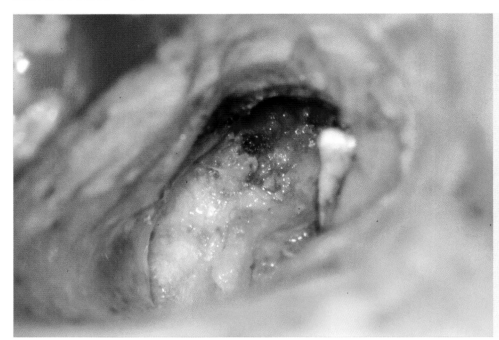

Fig. 11.31 The anteromedial part of the tumor infiltrates the cells in the medial wall of the protympanum.

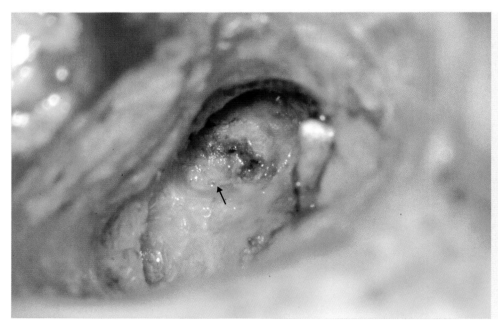

Fig. 11.32 The cells covering the carotid artery (*arrow*) are drilled carefully with a diamond burr, and eradication of the tumor is accomplished.

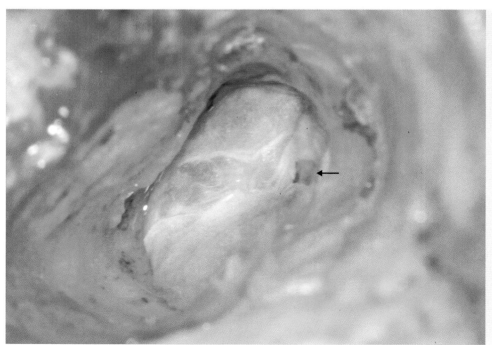

Fig. 11.33 The temporalis fascia is grafted underlay. The handle of the malleus exteriorized in the center of the fascia to avoid lateralization is seen (*arrow*).

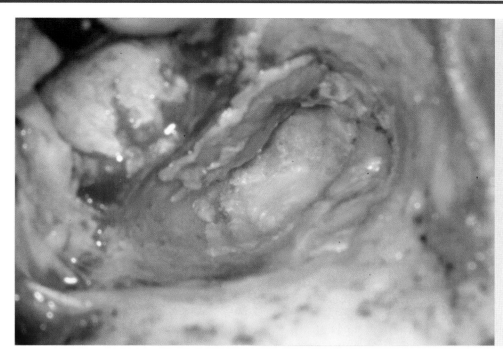

Fig. 11.34 The tympanomeatal flap is replaced in the canal, over the fascia.

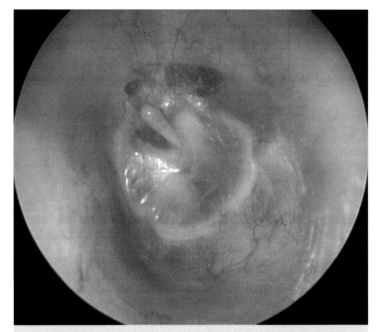

Fig. 11.35 Otoscopy of the same patients 3 months after surgery. The middle ear is free from the disease and the tympanic membrane is not lateralized.

11.6 Class B: Tympanomastoid Paragangliomas

Class B type tumors have been shown in ▶ Fig. 11.36, ▶ Fig. 11.37, ▶ Fig. 11.38, ▶ Fig. 11.39, ▶ Fig. 11.40, ▶ Fig. 11.41, ▶ Fig. 11.42, ▶ Fig. 11.43, ▶ Fig. 11.44, ▶ Fig. 11.45, ▶ Fig. 11.46, ▶ Fig. 11.47, ▶ Fig. 11.48, ▶ Fig. 11.49, ▶ Fig. 11.50, ▶ Fig. 11.51, ▶ Fig. 11.52.

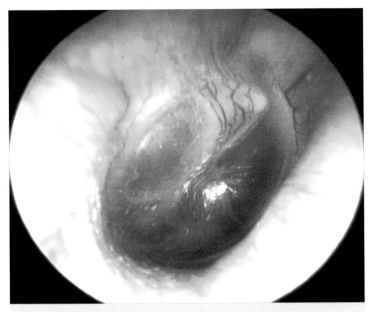

Fig. 11.36 Tympanomastoid (class B paraganglioma). The tumor is confined in the middle ear cleft with extension to the hypotympanum (see ▶ Fig. 11.37).

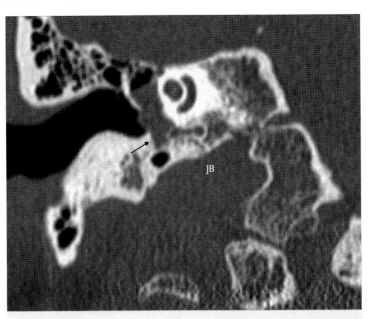

Fig. 11.37 The coronal view of the CT scan shows that the tumor infiltrates the hypotympanic cells (*arrow*) without erosion of the jugular bulb (JB).

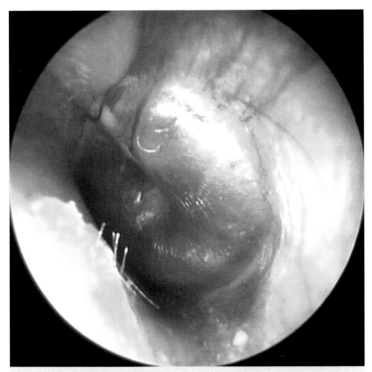

Fig. 11.38 Left ear. Type B2 glomus tumor. The tumor causes bulging of the posterior quadrants of the tympanic membrane.

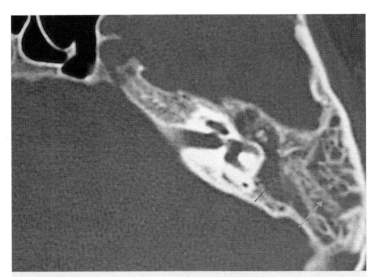

Fig. 11.39 CT scan of the same case, axial view, demonstrates extension of the disease into the mastoid (*red arrow*). Effusion in the mastoid is also present due to retention (*green arrow*).

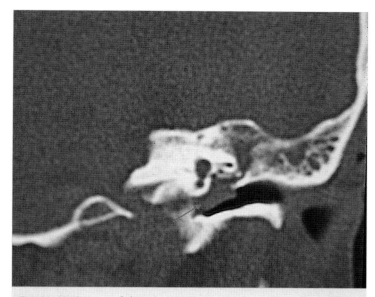

Fig. 11.40 CT scan of the same case, coronal view. The tumor extends to the hypotympanum but does not erode the bone overlying the dome of the jugular bulb (*arrow*).

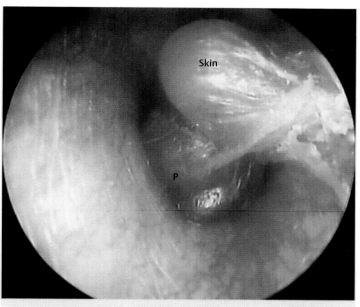

Fig. 11.41 A reddish polypoidal pulsating mass covered with skin, protruding from the tympanic cavity, is visible on otoscopy. P, polyp in the external auditory canal.

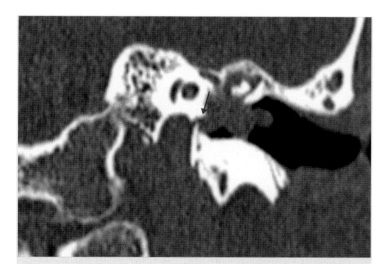

Fig. 11.42 CT scan of the same case demonstrates soft tissue filling the middle ear. No erosion is observed in the jugular bulb. The tumor is classified as class B3 due to a small erosion of the carotid canal indicated by the blue arrow.

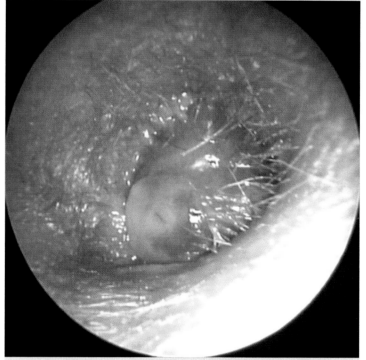

Fig. 11.43 Another case of B3 tumor. The pulsating mass protrudes outside the external auditory canal. Biopsy is absolutely contra-indicated in cases like this.

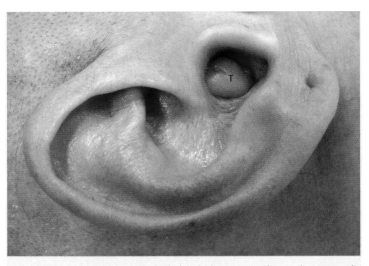

Fig. 11.44 Left ear. B3 tumor (T) that bulges as a polyp in the external auditory canal.

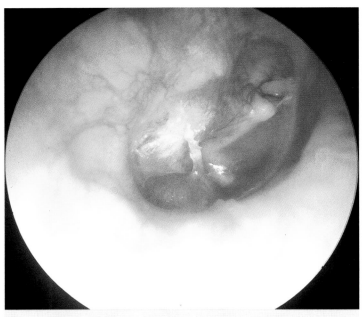

Fig. 11.45 Right ear. Reddish mass protruding from the inferior wall of the external auditory canal.

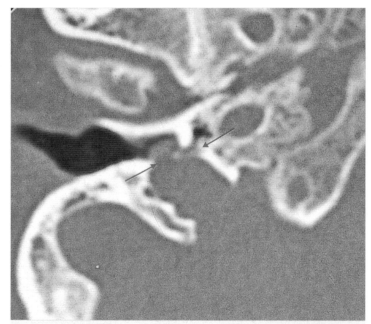

Fig. 11.46 CT scan of the previous case. Axial view demonstrating the erosion caused by the tumor of the bone overlying the jugular bulb. This tumor can be considered an intermediate class between B and C. The tumor is localized in the hypotympanum and extends to the jugular bulb but does not invade it (*arrows*).

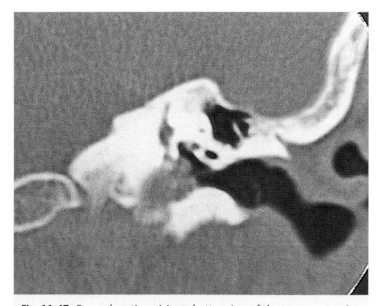

Fig. 11.47 Coronal section giving a better view of the tumor extension toward the jugular bulb. Intraoperatively, no invasion of the bulb was noted and the integrity of the bulb was thus conserved.

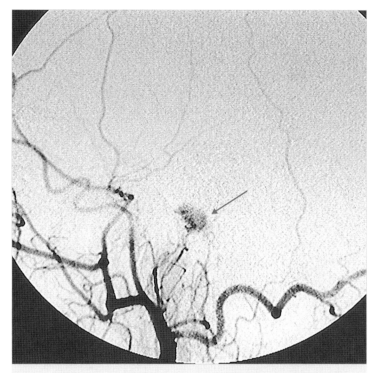

Fig. 11.48 Angiography of the same case. The blood supply of the tumor (*arrow*) is derived from the ascending pharyngeal artery that is a branch of the external carotid artery.

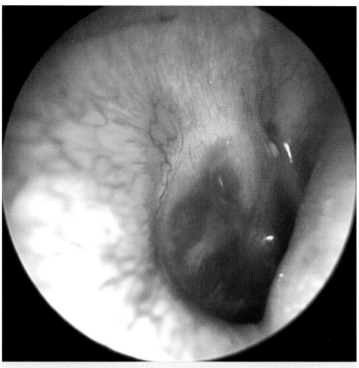

Fig. 11.49 Right ear. The otoscopy shows a reddish pulsating retrotympanic mass suggestive for a paraglioma.

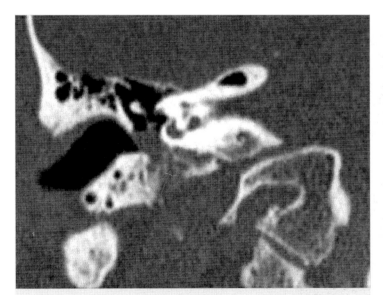

Fig. 11.50 CT scan of the same case, coronal view. The tumor is located in the hypotympanic area and extends to the jugular bulb (*arrow*).

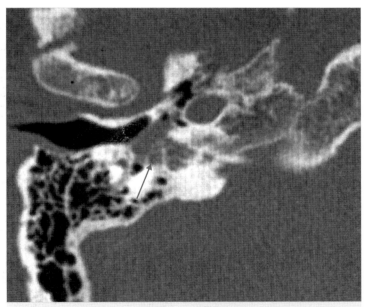

Fig. 11.51 CT scan of the same case, axial view. The tumor slightly infiltrates the mastoid compartment (*arrow*). The vertical portion of the carotid artery is not involved. Even in this case, the tumor can be considered an intermediate class between B and C.

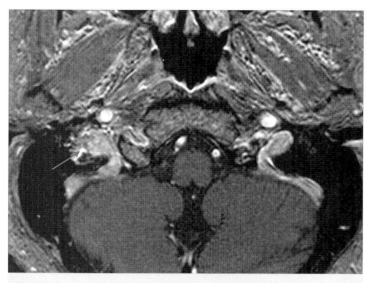

Fig. 11.52 MRI scan (T1W + gadolinium enhancement) of the same case, axial view. There is no clear invasion of the jugular bulb even if the tumor is in close proximity. Considering patient's age (80 years old), we preferred to follow a wait-and-scan protocol with yearly CT and MRI scans. After 2 years of follow-up, the tumor has still not grown.

11.6.1 Surgical Management

- For class B1 tumors, canal wall up mastoidectomy with posterior tympanotomy is performed to access the posterior extension of the tumor in the tympanic sinus and the facial recess. The tympanotomy should be extended inferiorly, with sacrifice of the chorda tympani nerve, to approach the tumor extending to the hypotympanum.
- For class B2 tumors, tympanotomy is extended to access the invasion of the tumor medial to the mastoid segment of the facial nerve.
- For class B3 tumors, a subtotal petrosectomy with drilling of the anterior wall of the external auditory canal and removal of the posterior canal wall is required to access the area around the ICA. In such cases, obliteration of the cavity with abdominal fat and blind sac closure of the external auditory canal is necessary.

The surgical management of Class B type tumors has been shown in ▶ Fig. 11.53, ▶ Fig. 11.54, ▶ Fig. 11.55, ▶ Fig. 11.56, ▶ Fig. 11.57, ▶ Fig. 11.58, ▶ Fig. 11.59, ▶ Fig. 11.60, ▶ Fig. 11.61.

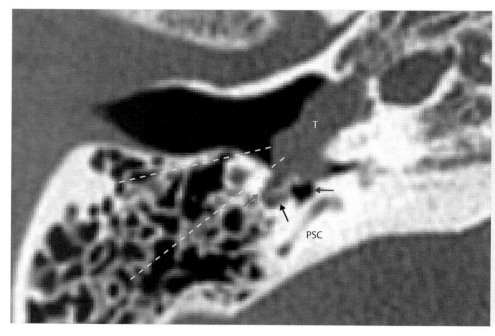

Fig. 11.53 CT scan, axial view, of the case in ▶ Fig. 11.36. Considering the tumor class (B1), a canal wall up tympanoplasty with posterior tympanotomy is planned. The tumor (T) does not reach the mastoid, and the tympanic sinus (*blue arrow*) is free of disease. To expose the hypotympanum, posterior tympanotomy is extended inferiorly, lateral to the facial nerve (*red arrow*) and medial to the tympanic membrane. This is shown as dashed lines. The stapedial muscle (*black arrow*) is located medial to the facial nerve. PSC, posterior semicircular canal.

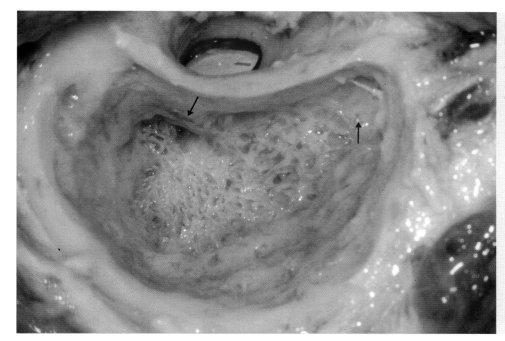

Fig. 11.54 Mastoidectomy is completed. As seen on the preoperative CT scan (▶ Fig. 11.37, ▶ Fig. 11.53), the mastoid is free of disease. The facial nerve runs in the area between the short process of the incus (*black arrow*) and the digastric ridge (*blue arrow*).

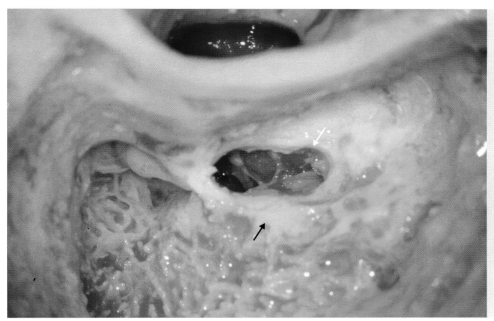

Fig. 11.55 The posterior edge of the tumor is visible through the posterior tympanotomy (*white arrow*). The facial nerve runs in the medial edge of the opening (*black arrow*). A thin bony shell should be maintained so as to avoid any damage.

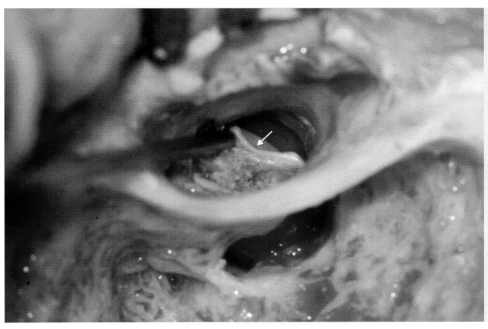

Fig. 11.56 To preserve the tympanic membrane, the fibrous annulus (*arrow*) is carefully detached from the bony annulus; the tympanic cavity is visible. The tumor occupying the tympanic cavity is visible through both the meatus and the posterior hypotympanotomy.

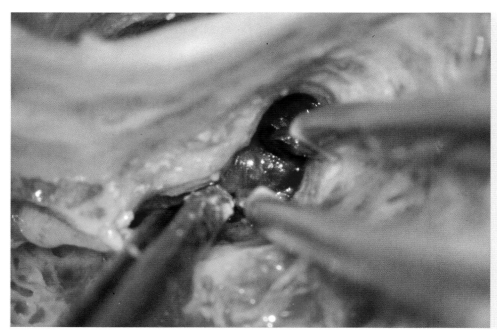

Fig. 11.57 Through the posterior tympanotomy, the tumor is coagulated with a bipolar cautery. Bipolar coagulation is used on the surface of the tumor to avoid bleeding. Never insert the tip of the cautery into the tumor mass. After coagulating the tumor sufficiently, it is removed piecemeal.

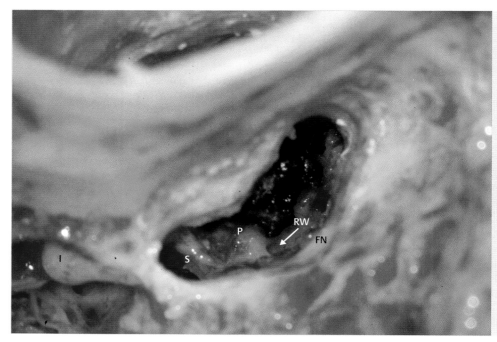

Fig. 11.58 Removal of the tumor from the area inferior to the stapes exposes structures located in the posterior mesotympanum. FN, facial nerve; I, body of incus; P, promontory; RW, round window niche; S, stapes.

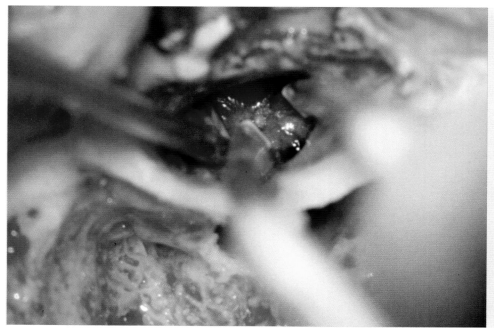

Fig. 11.59 The tumor in the tympanic cavity is coagulated through the meatus with a bipolar cautery. After coagulating the tumor sufficiently, it is removed piecemeal.

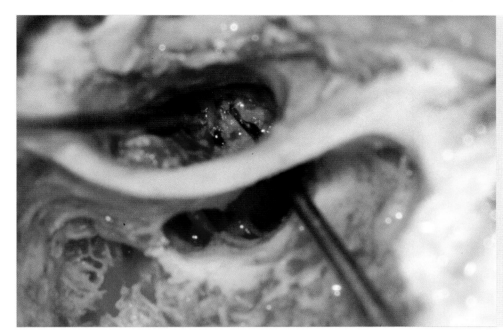

Fig. 11.60 Tumor infiltrating the hypotympanic cells is removed with combined approach, with a dissector inserted through the posterior tympanotomy and a suction tube through the meatus.

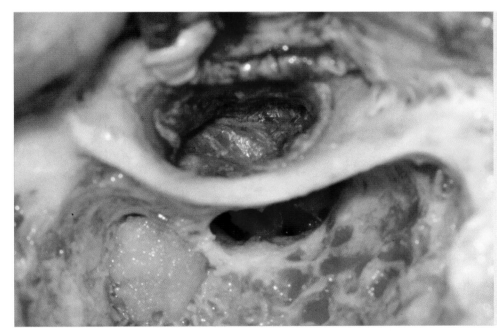

Fig. 11.61 After having removed the whole tumor and packed the middle ear with Gelfoam, the temporalis fascia and the tympanomeatal flap are placed as in ▶ Fig. 11.32, ▶ Fig. 11.33.

11.7 Class C: Tympanojugular Paragangliomas

Class C type tumors have been shown in ▶ Fig. 11.62, ▶ Fig. 11.63, ▶ Fig. 11.64, ▶ Fig. 11.65, ▶ Fig. 11.66, ▶ Fig. 11.67, ▶ Fig. 11.68, ▶ Fig. 11.69, ▶ Fig. 11.70, ▶ Fig. 11.71, ▶ Fig. 11.72, ▶ Fig. 11.73, ▶ Fig. 11.74, ▶ Fig. 11.75, ▶ Fig. 11.76, ▶ Fig. 11.77, ▶ Fig. 11.78, ▶ Fig. 11.79, ▶ Fig. 11.80, ▶ Fig. 11.81, ▶ Fig. 11.82, ▶ Fig. 11.83, ▶ Fig. 11.84, ▶ Fig. 11.85, ▶ Fig. 11.86, ▶ Fig. 11.87, ▶ Fig. 11.88, ▶ Fig. 11.89, ▶ Fig. 11.90, ▶ Fig. 11.91, ▶ Fig. 11.92, ▶ Fig. 11.93, ▶ Fig. 11.94, ▶ Fig. 11.95, ▶ Fig. 11.96, ▶ Fig. 11.97, ▶ Fig. 11.98, ▶ Fig. 11.99, ▶ Fig. 11.100, ▶ Fig. 11.101, ▶ Fig. 11.102, ▶ Fig. 11.103, ▶ Fig. 11.104, ▶ Fig. 11.105, ▶ Fig. 11.106, ▶ Fig. 11.107, ▶ Fig. 11.108, ▶ Fig. 11.109, ▶ Fig. 11.110, ▶ Fig. 11.111, ▶ Fig. 11.112, ▶ Fig. 11.113, ▶ Fig. 11.114, ▶ Fig. 11.115, ▶ Fig. 11.116, ▶ Fig. 11.117, ▶ Fig. 11.118, ▶ Fig. 11.119.

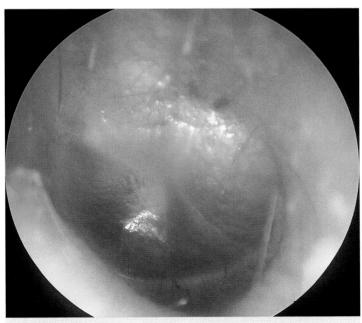

Fig. 11.62 Class C1 glomus tumor. The only complaint of the patient was ipsilateral pulsatile tinnitus of 4 years' duration (see subsequent figures).

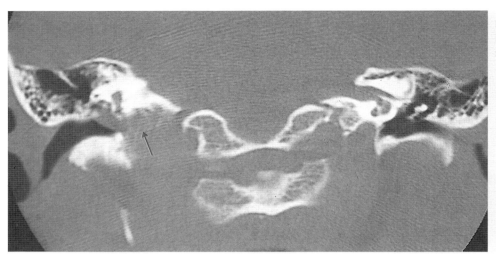

Fig. 11.63 CT scan, coronal view, showing enlargement of the jugular foramen with extension of the tumor into the middle ear (*arrow*).

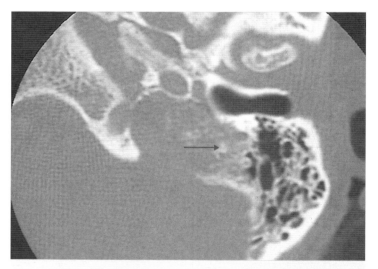

Fig. 11.64 CT scan, axial view. The jugular foramen is enlarged. Irregular erosion of the borders of the jugular foramen can be observed (*arrow*, differential diagnosis with LCNs' schwannoma).

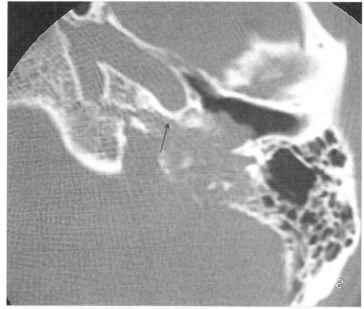

Fig. 11.65 Axial view demonstrates that the horizontal segment of the internal carotid artery is free of tumor (*arrow*).

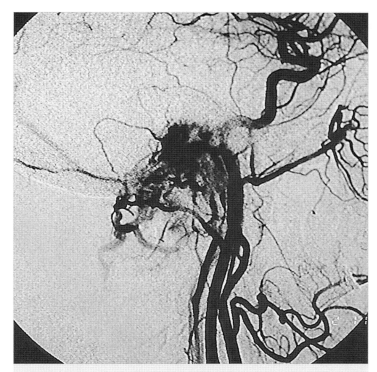

Fig. 11.66 Angiography demonstrating that the blood supply of the tumor comes from the ascending pharyngeal, the occipital, and the posterior auricular arteries.

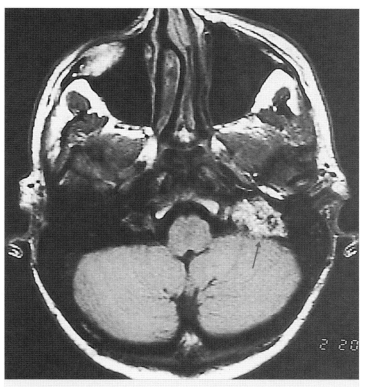

Fig. 11.67 MRI with gadolinium. The tumor is enhancing except for some flow-void zones corresponding to large vascular spaces (*arrow*). This picture is pathognomonic of glomus tumors.

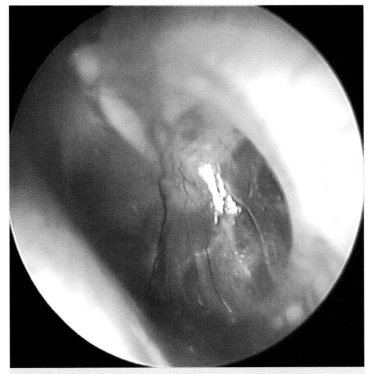

Fig. 11.68 Left ear. Class C1 tumor. A reddish pulsating retrotympanic mass is visible in the inferior quadrants. The patient complained only on pulsatile tinnitus. LCNs' function was normal. Considering patient age (67 years old) and function of LCNs, a "wait-and-scan" protocol was applied.

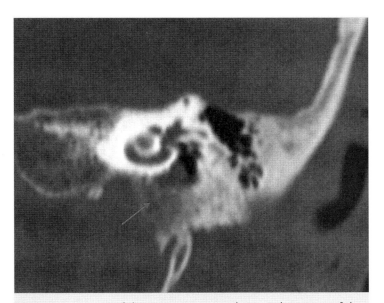

Fig. 11.69 CT scan of the same case, coronal view. Enlargement of the jugular foramen with irregular bone erosion (*arrow*, "moth-eaten" bone).

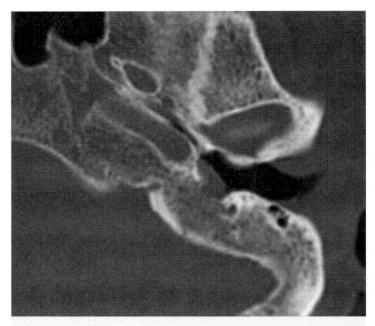

Fig. 11.70 CT scan of the same case, axial view. The horizontal portion of the carotid artery is free from the pathology.

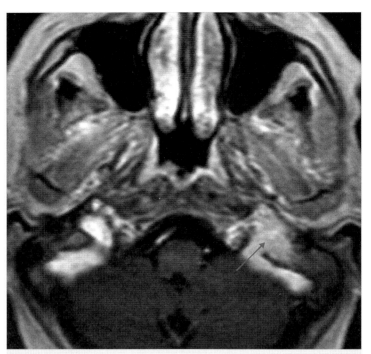

Fig. 11.71 MRI scan (T1W + gadolinium enhancement), axial view. The tumor infiltrates the jugular bulb (*arrow*).

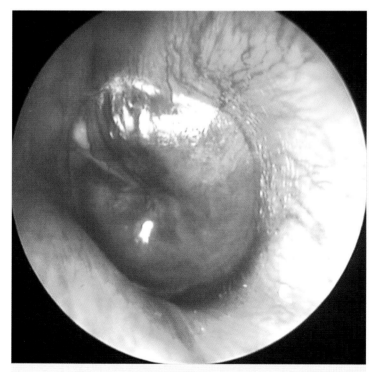

Fig. 11.72 Left ear. Class C1 TJP. This 70-year-old female patient complained only of hearing loss. The CT scan revealed the presence of a tumor extended to the area of the Eustachian tube, resulting in middle ear effusion. Considering the absence of LCNs dysfunction, the patient has been followed up just with yearly CT and MRI scans.

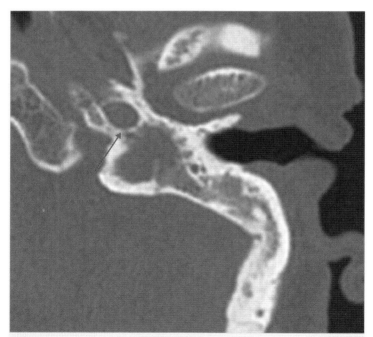

Fig. 11.73 CT scan of the same patient, axial view. The tumor involves the jugular foramen area but does not invade the vertical portion of the carotid artery (*arrow*).

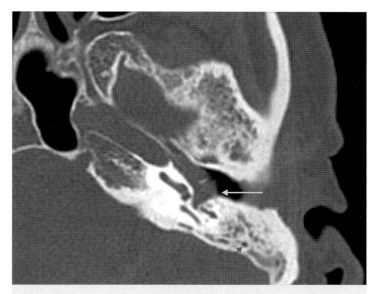

Fig. 11.74 CT scan of the same patient, axial view. The middle ear is filled with the tumor (*yellow arrow*) and the area of the Eustachian tube is blocked, resulting in middle ear effusion (*red arrow*, opacification of mastoid air cells).

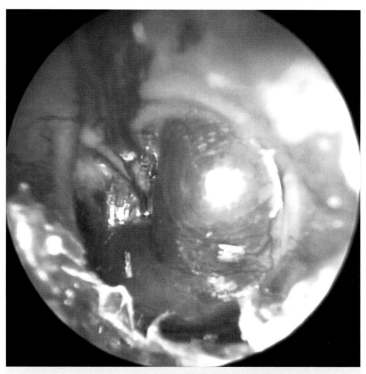

Fig. 11.75 Left ear. Class C1 TJP. This female patient (50 years old) underwent surgical removal of the disease through an infratemporal fossa type A approach. Function of cranial nerves IX and X worsened immediately after surgery. Good contralateral compensation was achieved with swallowing and speech rehabilitation with no need for further pharyngolaryngeal surgery. At the last clinical follow-up, facial nerve function is grade II House–Brackmann scale (mild dysfunction).

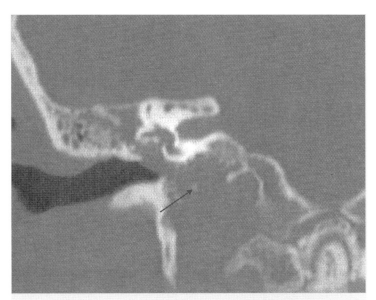

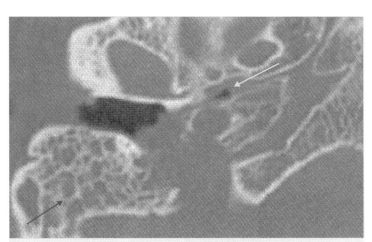

Fig. 11.77 CT scan, axial view, of the same case. Obstruction of the Eustachian tube is present (*yellow arrow*), resulting in middle ear and mastoid effusion (*red arrow*).

Fig. 11.76 CT scan, coronal view, of the same case. The jugular foramen is enlarged by the tumor (*arrow*), which fills the middle ear.

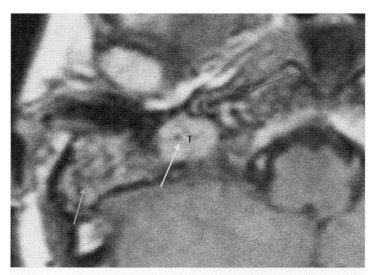

Fig. 11.78 MRI scan (T1W + gadolinium enhancement), axial view, of the same case. The tumor (T) does not involve the horizontal portion of the carotid artery (*red arrow*). Intratumoral flow voids (*yellow arrow*) and mastoid effusion (*green arrow*) are also visible.

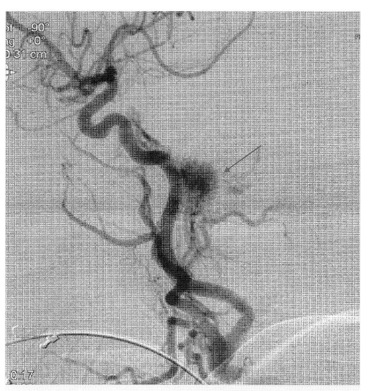

Fig. 11.79 Angiography of the same case. The blood supply of the tumor (*arrow*) is derived from the ascending pharyngeal artery.

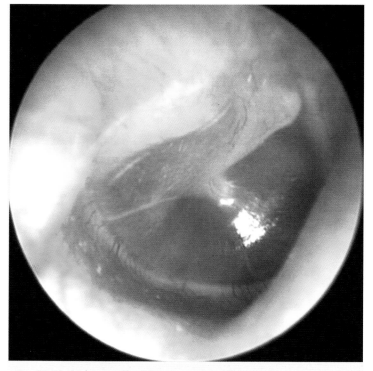

Fig. 11.80 Right ear. Class C1 tumor. A reddish retrotympanic mass is visible in the inferior quadrants

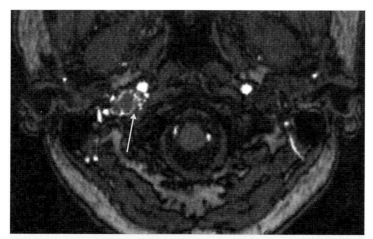

Fig. 11.81 Angio-MRI scan of the same case. The tumor (*yellow arrow*) invades the jugular foramen with slight involvement of the vertical portion of the carotid artery.

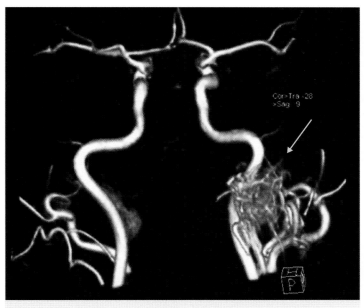

Fig. 11.82 Color 3D angio-MRI showing the tumor (*arrow*).

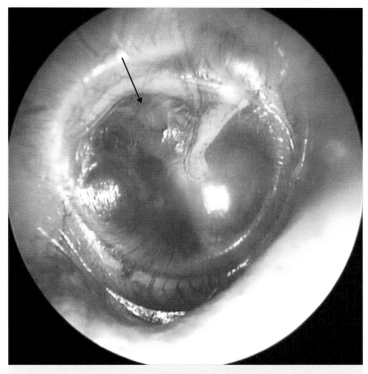

Fig. 11.83 Otoscopy of another case of C1 class tumor. The tympanic membrane is retracted due to poor ventilation of the middle ear, resulting in myringostapediopexy (*arrow*).

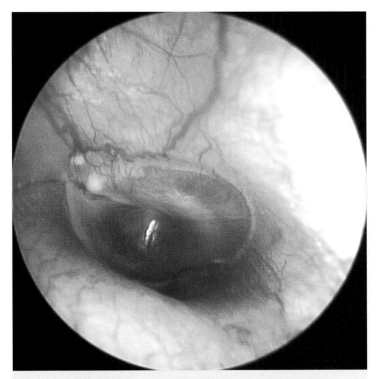

Fig. 11.84 Left ear, class C2 tumor. Note the reddish retrotympanic mass in the posteroinferior portion of the tympanic membrane.

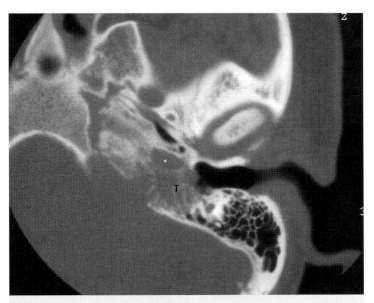

Fig. 11.85 CT, axial view. Infiltration of bone surrounding the ICA (*asterisk*) is seen extending toward the genu. T, tumor.

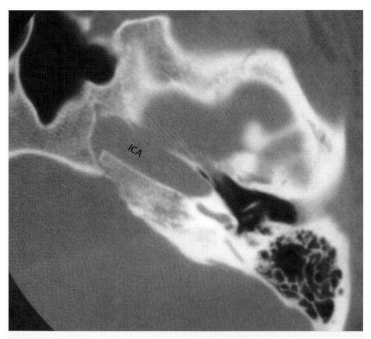

Fig. 11.86 The horizontal segment of the ICA appears free of tumor.

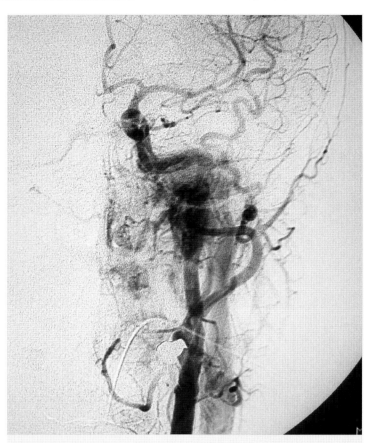

Fig. 11.87 Angiography before tumor embolization, revealing a characteristic tumor blush and rapid venous drainage, with evidence of a patent jugular vein.

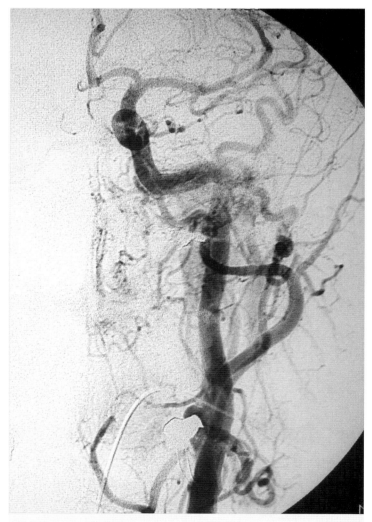

Fig. 11.88 Angiography after tumor embolization. Despite significant reduction in tumor vascularity, tumor blush can still be seen adjacent to the distal vertical carotid. In class C tumors, preoperative embolization is fundamental in reducing intraoperative bleeding. Therefore, it should always been performed before surgical treatment.

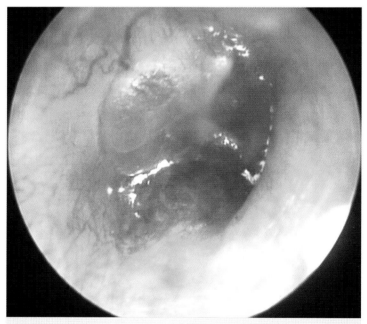

Fig. 11.89 Right ear. Class C2 tumor. The patient (65 years old) has no other symptoms than hearing loss (conductive, moderate) and pulsatile tinnitus. LCNs function is normal. A "wait-and-scan" protocol was adopted. For the last 3 years, the tumor has not shown any growth.

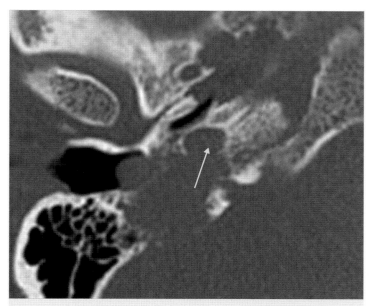

Fig. 11.90 CT scan, axial view. The tumor invades the vertical portion of the carotid canal (*arrow*).

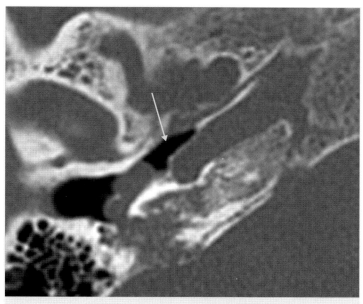

Fig. 11.91 CT scan, axial view. The tumor does not involve the horizontal portion of the internal carotid artery (*arrow*).

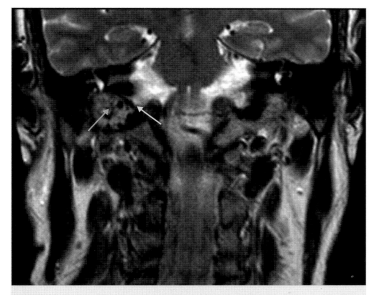

Fig. 11.92 MRI (T2W), coronal view. Flow voids are visible within the tumor (*green arrow*), which is close to the area of the LCNs (*yellow arrow*).

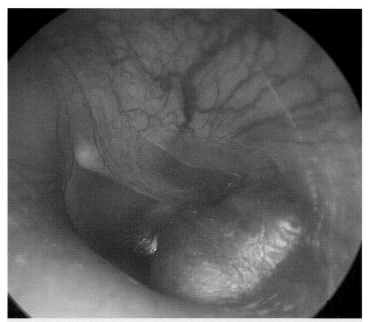

Fig. 11.93 Class C2 De2 TJP of the left ear. The patient complained of pulsatile tinnitus and hearing loss, and 2 months before presentation the patient started to suffer from dysphonia, dysphagia, and hypoglossal paresis due to compression by the slowly growing tumor.

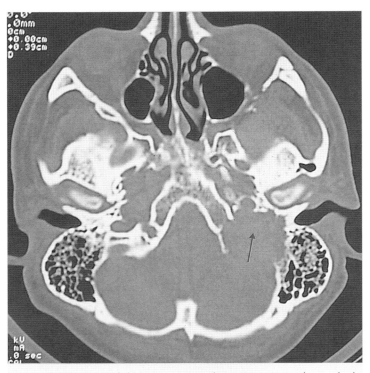

Fig. 11.94 CT scan of the case presented in ▶ Fig. 11.93. The marked erosion of the jugular foramen and the vertical portion of the carotid canal can be appreciated (*arrow*).

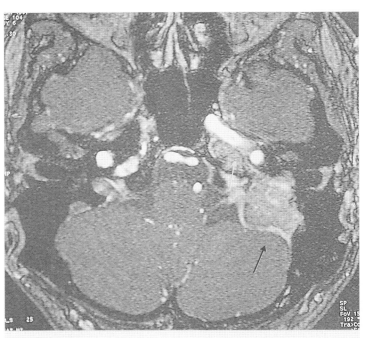

Fig. 11.95 MRI demonstrating tumor in contact with the medial aspect of the horizontal carotid artery (yellow arrow) and the posterior fossa dura (*red arrow*) without infiltrating it.

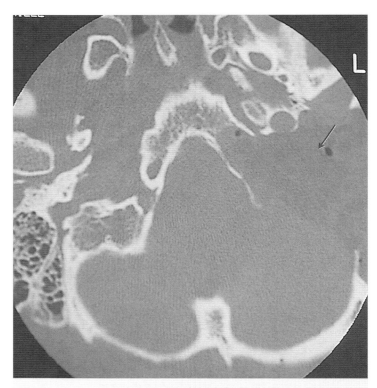

Fig. 11.96 Postoperative CT scan demonstrating tumor removal (arrow) using an infratemporal fossa approach type A.

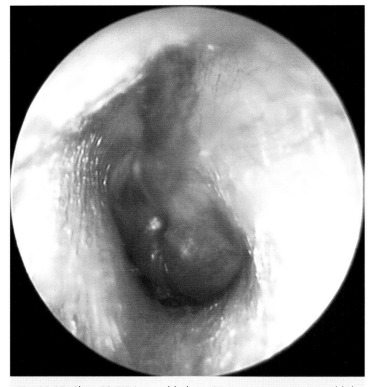

Fig. 11.97 Class C2 TJP in an elderly patient. A retrotympanic reddish mass is visible in the inferior quadrants. Retraction of the anterior quadrants of the tympanic membrane is also present due to middle ear dysventilation. LCNs function was slightly affected (left vocal fold paralysis with good contralateral compensation), so a wait-and-scan protocol was adopted.

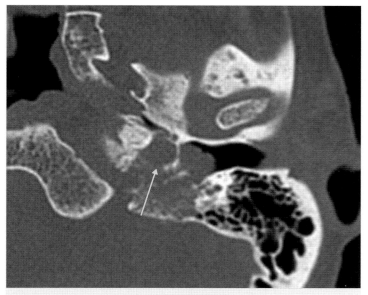

Fig. 11.98 CT scan, axial view, of the same case. The tumor erodes the vertical portion of the carotid canal (arrow).

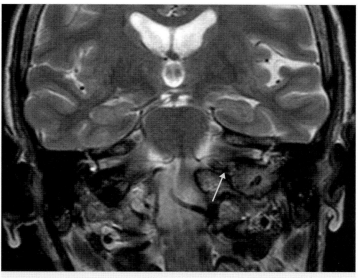

Fig. 11.99 MRI scan (T2W). The tumor is close to the area of the LCNs (*arrow*).

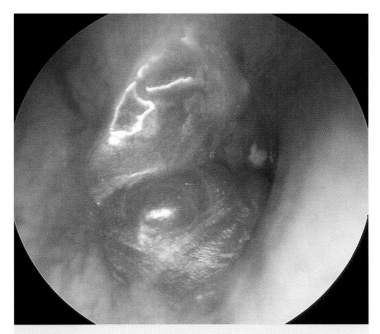

Fig. 11.100 Right ear. Class C3 Di2 tumor. The patient complained of pulsatile tinnitus and mixed hearing loss of 12 months' duration.

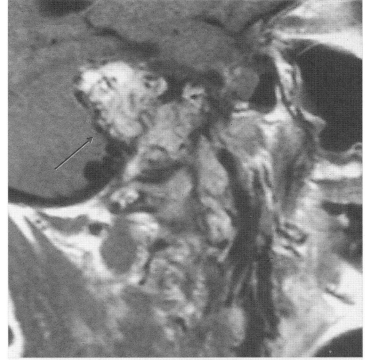

Fig. 11.101 MRI, sagittal view, demonstrating intradural extension of the tumor (*arrow*).

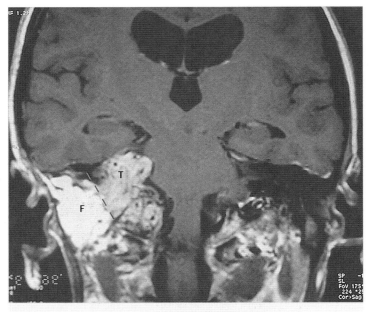

Fig. 11.102 MRI, coronal view, after first-stage removal of the extradural component of the tumor using an infratemporal fossa approach type A. The fat (F) obliterating the operative cavity can be seen. The intradural tumor residue (T) is also observed. Staging is necessary in such cases to avoid communication between the subarachnoid space and the wide open neck spaces.

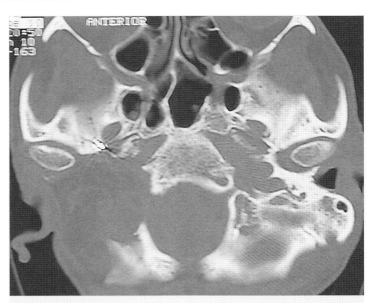

Fig. 11.103 Postoperative CT scan after the second-stage removal of the tumor through a petro-occipital trans-sigmoid approach.

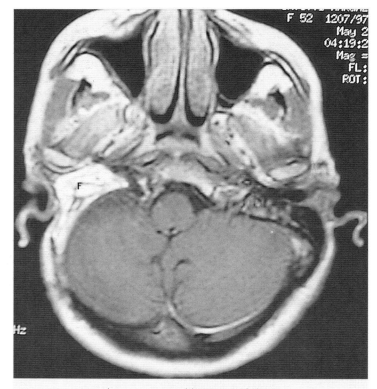

Fig. 11.104 MRI demonstrating obliteration of the operative cavity with abdominal fat (F).

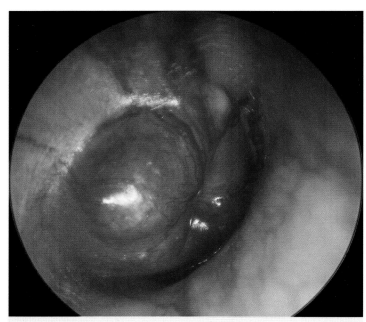

Fig. 11.105 Right ear. Class C3 Di2 tumor. The patient complained of ipsilateral total hearing loss, diplopia, grade IV facial paralysis, and dysphonia (see subsequent figures).

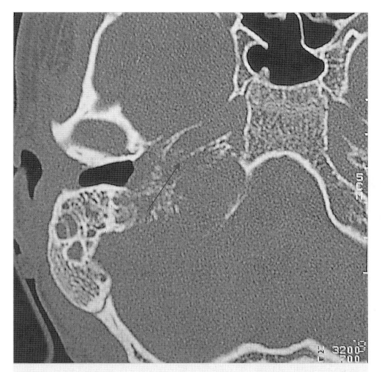

Fig. 11.106 CT scan axial section demonstrating the involvement of the jugular foramen and the horizontal segment of the internal carotid artery (*arrow*). The artery was closed preoperative with a balloon.

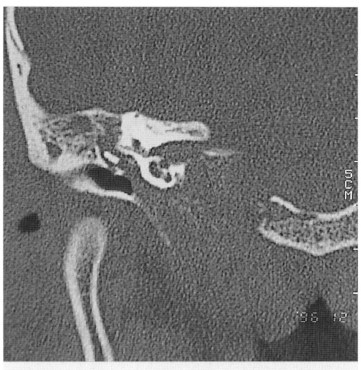

Fig. 11.107 CT scan, coronal section. The tumor involves the internal auditory canal (*arrow*).

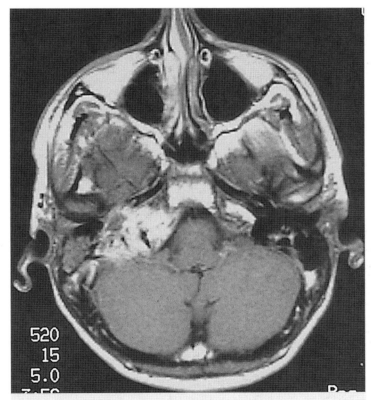

Fig. 11.108 MRI, axial view giving a global idea of the extra- and intradural extension of the tumor.

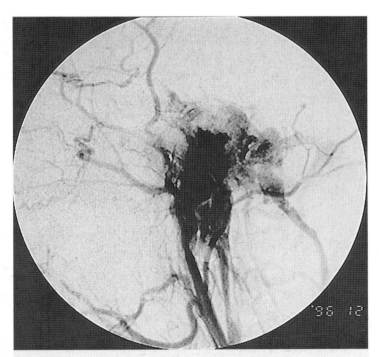

Fig. 11.109 Angiography before embolization.

233

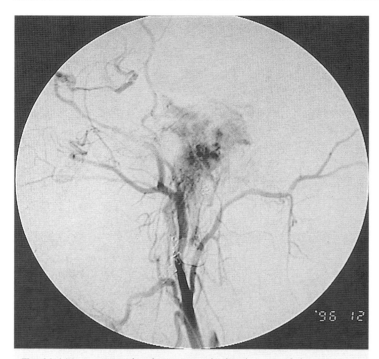

Fig. 11.110 Angiography showing marked reduction of the tumor vascularity following embolization.

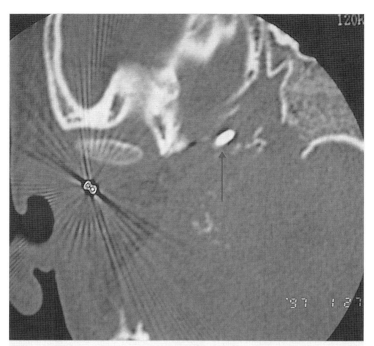

Fig. 11.111 CT scan performed after first-stage removal of the extradural part of the tumor using an infratemporal fossa approach type A. Staging is necessary to avoid communication between the subarachnoid spaces and the neck spaces. The balloon used for the closure of the internal carotid artery can be seen (*arrow*).

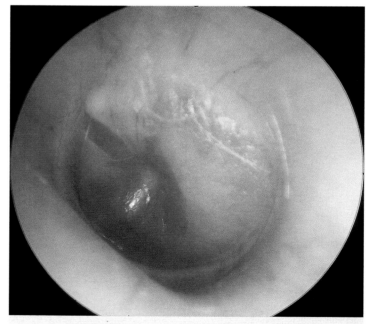

Fig. 11.112 Left ear. Class C2 Di2 glomus jugulare tumor. The patient complained of hearing loss and pulsatile tinnitus of 2 years' duration. He also complained of dysphonia, dysphagia, paralysis of the left half of the tongue, and paresis of the lower face.

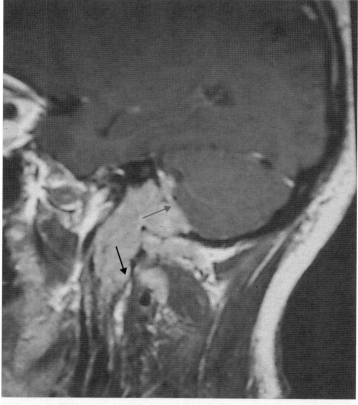

Fig. 11.113 MRI, sagittal view, demonstrating the intradural extension of the tumor (*red arrow*) as well as the inferior extension toward C1 and C2 (*black arrow*).

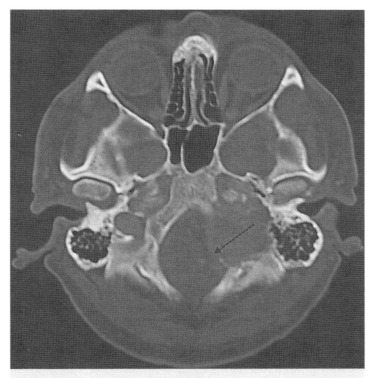

Fig. 11.114 Preoperative CT scan. The jugular foramen is enlarged, with involvement of the foramen magnum (*arrow*).

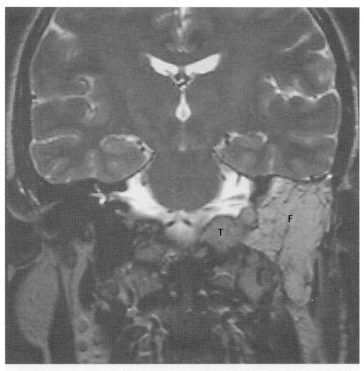

Fig. 11.115 MRI with gadolinium after removal of the extradural part using an infratemporal fossa approach type A. Fat is seen obliterating the operative cavity (F). The intradural tumor residue at the level of the foramen magnum is noted (T).

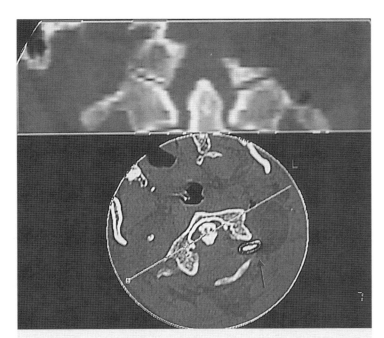

Fig. 11.116 CT scan following the second-stage removal of the intradural portion of the tumor using an extreme lateral approach. The balloon used to close the vertebral artery is visible (*arrow*).

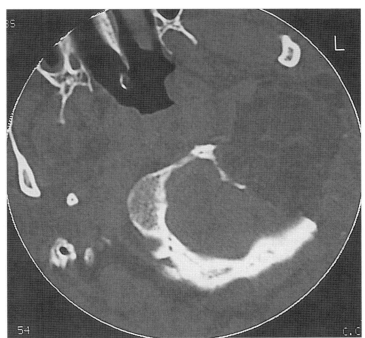

Fig. 11.117 CT scan following the second-stage removal of the intradural portion of the tumor. The removal of a large part of the left occipital condyle is also shown.

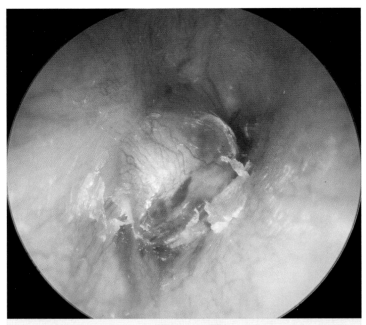

Fig. 11.118 Another example of a large class C3 Di2 glomus tumor.

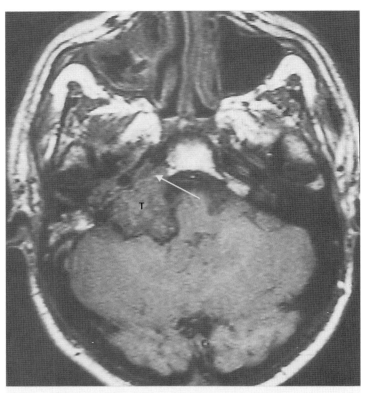

Fig. 11.119 MRI of the case in ▶ Fig. 11.118. T, tumor; *arrow*, horizontal internal carotid artery.

11.7.1 Surgical Management

Because of their unique location, these tumors pose certain problems: (1) the possibility of injury to the LCNs; (2) the fact that the facial nerve is centered on and is closely related to the jugular bulb. These tumors spread to five different "compartments": medially intradural; anteriorly intrapetrous along the ICA; inferiorly extradural to the neck along the LCNs; posteriorly along the sigmoid sinus; posteroinferiorly toward the occipital condyle and the vertebral artery. Young patients with impairment of the vagus nerve should be treated surgically. It must be acknowledged, however, that further LCN injury is likely. Most young patients with intact cranial nerve function should be treated surgically. Radiological assessment revealing patency of the jugulosigmoid system and/or absence of intradural invasion indicates a good prognosis for preservation of LCN function, because both are indicative of absence of infiltration of the medial aspect of the jugular bulb. Assessment of tumor infiltration is not always straightforward, but the presence of intradural tumor essentially means that this barrier has been crossed and sacrifice of the LCNs is necessary if total resection is to be performed.

Another option is to allow the pathology to gradually paralyze the LCNs, especially in cases where the likelihood of neural preservation is low. Compensation tends to occur preoperatively and radical resection can proceed without the concern for neural conservation. However, even in cases of a well-compensated preoperative neural deficit, sacrifice of the nerves produces a further worsening of the situation, probably due to section of residual functioning fibers maintaining a degree of tone. Compensation following acute compound LCN palsies is particularly difficult in elderly patients and normal LCN function should be considered a relative contraindication for surgery in patients older than 60 years. The same is true for patients with coexisting respiratory

problems. Despite our usual approach to achieving surgical cure, in case of advanced age or poor medical status, there is rarely an indication for radical surgical removal. Radiological follow-up often represents the best treatment in these cases. Radiotherapy is reserved for patients whose follow-up documents significant growth. Occasionally resection of the middle ear and mastoid components with a blind sac closure of the external auditory canal provides excellent control in elderly patients with troublesome otorrhagia.

Surgical removal of TJPs implies sacrifice of the jugular bulb. Usually, the venous pathway is already occluded by the tumor and it may be resected without any consequence. However, in particular cases, the bulb is still patent or the compensation has occurred through collaterals, such as the posterior condylar vein, that have to be sacrificed as well; when it happens in the presence of hypoplasia of the contralateral venous system, sacrifice of the bulb means occlusion of the main venous drainage of the brain, with the consequent risk of benign intracranial hypertension or venous infarction of the temporal lobe. In this situation, it is advisable to wait until the occlusion of the bulb by the tumor growth before planning the surgery.

The ICA is involved in the majority of TJPs; this requires angiographic assessment of the degree of involvement, and often consideration of preoperative neuroradiological management of the artery is required to enable safer surgical removal. The risks of preoperative management must be weighed against the risk of intraoperative injury. The patients' age and comorbidities must also be considered. The vertebral artery can also be involved in some complex cases; complete resection requires consideration of the consequences of closure of this artery. The presence of intradural extension is problematic. Single-stage removal creates a high risk of postoperative cerebrospinal fluid (CSF) leakage as a connection is created between the subarachnoid and the neck space during tumor extirpation. We therefore use the following strategy:

- Di1 tumors: only small tumors (< 2 cm) are removed in a single stage. The dura is closed with a muscle plug or abdominal fat.
- Di2 tumors: staged removal is performed. The extradural part is removed first, followed by a second stage after 4 or 6 months for the intradural part.

At our center, we have developed an algorithm for management of TJPs according to the modified Fisch classification:

- C1 tumors: In the case of elderly patients with normal LCNs, a "wait-and-scan" policy is the best option. If elderly patients have paralysis of the LCNs, there are three choices: one is the "wait-and-scan" policy; another is subtotal removal followed by radiotherapy; and the final one is radiotherapy alone. For young patients with normal function of the LCNs, tumor removal via infratemporal fossa approach type A (ITFA) is recommended with preservation of the medial wall of the jugular bulb if it is not infiltrated.
- C2 tumors: In the case of elderly patients, a "wait-and-scan" policy is recommended; but if the tumor grows, subtotal removal or radiotherapy can be considered as treatment options. For young patients, tumor removal via ITFA is preferred with or without preservation of the medial wall of the jugular bulb.
- C3 De1/2 tumors (elderly patients, > 65 years old): First, they are followed up with imaging. If this shows any sign of growth, subtotal removal is recommended, which may be followed by radiotherapy.
- C3 De1/2 tumors (young patients): Surgery such as ITFA should be considered. To remove total tumor, either balloon occlusion of the ICA or stenting of the ICA as preoperative endovascular treatment is usually necessary.
- C3 Di1/2 tumors (young patients): Preoperative endovascular treatment such as either balloon occlusion of the ICA or stenting of the ICA is usually necessary. To prevent postoperative CSF leakage, staged tumor removal is essential. At the first stage, ITFA is performed, and at the second stage intradural removal is completed.
- C4 tumors: To prevent postoperative CSF leakage, staged tumor removal is essential. At the first stage ITFA/B is performed, and at the second stage the removal of intradural lesion is completed except for an unresectable lesion. Radiotherapy is given for the remnant of tumor.
- C4 tumor and ICA involvement: Either balloon occlusion of the ICA or stenting of the ICA is performed. At the first stage, the extradural lesion is resected, and at the second stage the intradural lesion is removed. If the ICA is at risk (making balloon or stenting impossible), subtotal removal is indicated, leaving tumor attached to the ICA, with eventual radiotherapy if clear growth is demonstrated on follow-up.

Surgical management of TJPs will result in maximal conductive hearing loss, as an integral part of the ITFA is a blind sac closure. Most tumors, however, present with a degree of hearing loss, and rehabilitation is efficiently achieved through the use of a BAHA (bone-anchored hearing aid.) The other consequence of an ITFA is mild facial asymmetry (House–Brackmann grade II in the majority of cases), due to the need to mobilize the facial nerve. In particular in patients enrolled in a wait-and-see policy, the

development of a facial weakness may be an indication for partial removal with the aim of decompressing or grafting the facial nerve. ▶ Table 11.1 shows the authors' experience in treating these tumors.

Table 11.1 Gruppo Otologico experience in management of temporal bone paragangliomas (382 cases, 1988–2012, published data)

Temporal bone paragangliomas managed at the Gruppo Otologico	
Class management	No. of patients (%)
A	80
Surgery	80 (100%)
B	65
Surgery	65 (100%)
C, D, and V	237
Surgery	182 (77%)
Wait and scan	46 (19%)
Surgery followed by radiotherapy	7 (3%)
Wait and scan followed by radiotherapy	1 (0.5%)
Radiotherapy	1 (0.5%)

11.8 Type A Infratemporal Fossa Approach

The key point of this approach is the anterior transposition of the facial nerve, which provides optimal control of the infralabyrinthine and jugular foramen regions, as well as the vertical portion of the ICA.

Indications

The main indication for this approach is lesions of the jugular foramen—type C and D tympanojugular paragangliomas. We do not use this approach for neuromas or meningiomas of the jugular foramen, which we manage using the petro-occipital transsigmoid approach, with preservation of the middle ear function and without anterior transposition of the facial nerve.

11.8.1 Surgical Technique

A postauricular skin incision is performed. A small, anteriorly based musculoperiosteal flap is elevated to help in closure afterwards. The skin of the external auditory canal is transected, elevated, and closed using a blind sac.

The facial nerve is identified at its exits from the temporal bone. The main trunk is the perpendicular bisection of a line joining the cartilaginous pointer to the mastoid tip. The main trunk is traced in the parotid until the proximal parts of the temporal and zygomatic branches are identified.

The posterior belly of the digastric muscle and the sternocleidomastoid muscle are divided close to their origin. The internal jugular vein and the external and internal carotid arteries are identified in the neck. The vessels are marked with umbilical tape.

The skin of the external auditory canal, the tympanic membrane, the malleus, and the incus are removed. A canal wall down mastoidectomy is performed, with the removal of the bone anterior and posterior to the sigmoid sinus.

The facial nerve is skeletonized from the stylomastoid foramen to the geniculate ganglion. The last shell of bone is removed using a double-curved raspatory.

The stapes suprastructure is preferably removed after cutting its crura with microscissors. The inferior tympanic bone is widely removed and the mastoid tip is amputated using a rongeur. A new fallopian canal is drilled in the root of the zygoma superior to the Eustachian tube.

Using strong scissors, the facial nerve is freed at the level of the stylomastoid foramen. The soft tissues at this level are separated from the nerve. The mastoid segment is next elevated using a Beaver knife to cut the fibrous attachments between the nerve and the fallopian canal.

The tympanic segment of the nerve is elevated carefully using a curved raspatory, until the level of the geniculate ganglion is reached. A nontoothed forceps is used to hold the soft tissue surrounding the nerve at the stylomastoid foramen and the anterior rerouting is performed. A tunnel is created in the parotid gland to lodge the transposed nerve. The tunnel is closed around the nerve using two sutures. The nerve is fixed to the new bony canal, just above the Eustachian tube, using fibrin glue.

Drilling of the infralabyrinthine cells is completed and the vertical portion of the ICA is identified. The mandibular condyle is separated from the anterior wall of the external auditory canal using a large septal raspatory. To avoid injury to facial nerve, we no longer use the Fisch infratemporal fossa retractor. The anterior wall of the external auditory canal is further drilled, completing the exposure of the vertical portion of the ICA.

The sinus is closed using Surgicel extraluminally and intraluminally. The proximal part of the sigmoid sinus is compressed extraluminally with Surgicel; the sinus is then opened and packed distally and proximally with two large pieces of Surgicel. With this technique, we avoid the use of dural incision, which may lead to a higher risk of CSF leakage postoperatively.

The structures attached to the styloid process are severed. This process is fractured using a rongeur and is then cut with strong scissors. The remaining fibrous tissue surrounding the ICA at its point of entry into the skull base is carefully removed using scissors.

The internal jugular vein in the neck is double-ligated and cut. The vein is elevated superiorly, with care being taken not to injure the related LCNs. If the XI nerve passes laterally, the vein has to be pulled under the nerve carefully to prevent it from being damaged. If necessary (as in the case of TJPs), the lateral wall of the sigmoid sinus can be removed. Removal continues down to the level of the jugular bulb. The lateral wall of the jugular bulb is opened. Bleeding usually occurs from the apertures of the inferior petrosal sinus and the condylar emissary vein. This is controlled by Surgicel packing. If there is limited intradural extension, the dura is opened without injury to the endolymphatic sac.

At the end of the procedure, the Eustachian tube is closed with a piece of muscle. The dural opening is closed with a muscle plug. A transfixing suture is passed into one dural edge, through the muscle plug, and out from the other dural edge, and then tied. The cavity is obliterated using abdominal fat without rotating the temporalis muscle, which is to be sutured over the fat.

Rarely, there may be marked stenosis in the artery, or its wall may be too fragile due to previous radiotherapy or surgery. A balloon occlusion test is mandatory before removal of the carotid is attempted. Recent introduction of preoperative stenting of the carotid artery offers a new option for treating those patients who are likely to need intraoperative management of the ICA. The rationale for stenting of the ICA is to allow easier mobilization of the artery and of the pericarotid portion of the tumor without the risk of uncontrollable hemorrhage from laceration of the arterial wall. At the beginning of our experience, carotid resection was performed more frequently. We have now adopted a less aggressive attitude nowadays, for fear of long-term consequences such as strokes, hemiplegia, and aneurysm of the contralateral ICA.

With large TJPs (C3 involving the horizontal ICA or C4 reaching the anterior foramen lacerum and extending to the cavernous sinus), the approach is combined with a type B or C infratemporal fossa approach for removal of the tumor.

The Type A infratemporal fossa approach is illustrated in ► Fig. 11.120.

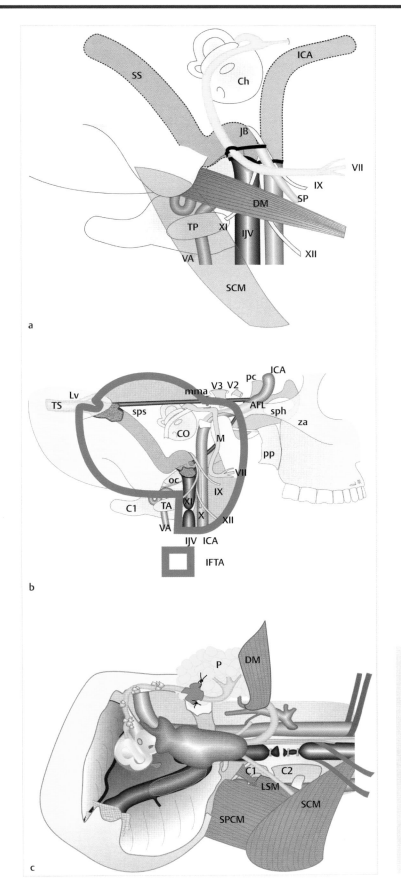

Fig. 11.120 Illustrations for infratemporal fossa approach type A (ITFA). (a) An illustration of obstacles to approaching the jugular bulb. (b) An illustration of the surgical limit in ITFA. (c) An illustration of the surgical view in ITFA. AFL, anterior foramen lacerum; C1, atlas; C2, axis; Ch, cochlea; DM, posterior belly of the digastric muscle; ICA, internal carotid artery; IJV, internal jugular vein; JB, jugular bulb; LSM, levator scapulae muscle; Lv, vein of Labbé; M, mandible; MMA, middle meningeal artery; OC, occipital condyle; P, parotid gland; pc, clinoid process; pp, pterygoid plate; SCM, sternocleidomastoid muscle; SP, styloid process; SPCM, splenius capitis muscle; sph, sphenoid sinus; sps, superior petrosal sinus; TP, transverse process of the atlas; TS, transverse sinus; V2, maxillary branch of the trigeminal nerve; V3, mandibular branch of the trigeminal nerve; za, zygomatic arch; VA, vertebral artery; VII, facial nerve; IX, glossopharyngeal nerve; XI, spinal accessory nerve; XII, hypoglossal nerve.

Summary

Because of the complex anatomy of the temporal bone and the structures at the base of the skull, as well as the invasiveness, rich vascularity, and aggressive behavior of TJPs, surgery for these difficult lesions is problematic. These tumors generally present with hearing loss and pulsatile tinnitus. When the LCNs are invaded, a jugular foramen syndrome becomes manifest.

Otoscopy usually reveals a reddish retrotympanic mass. A definitive diagnosis is obtained after neuroradiological studies are performed. These include an HRCT scan with bony window, MRI with and without gadolinium, and digital subtraction angiography. Radiological studies are essential not only to confirm the diagnosis and define the exact tumor class, but also to properly evaluate these tumors. The neuroradiologist should be able to inform the surgeon about the following:

- Details of the osseous lesion.
- Involvement of the jugular bulb and foramen.
- Exact involvement of the temporal bone.
- The presence of inner ear invasion.
- The relationship between the fallopian canal and the tumor.
- Carotid canal erosion and exact involvement of the ICA.
- Invasion of the petrous apex and clivus.
- Details regarding the relationship between the tumor and surrounding soft tissues, for example:
  - Degree of neck extension.
  - Infratemporal fossa involvement.
  - Intracranial and intradural extension.

Radiology also helps to determine the superior and inferior extension of the tumor, the possibility of other associated lesions (e.g., contralateral glomus or carotid body tumor), and the patency of the contralateral sigmoid sinus and internal jugular vein. In class C and D tumors, selective digital subtraction angiography is essential. Arteriography is performed for both ipsilateral and contralateral internal and external carotids and for the vertebrobasilar system.

A study of the venous phase is also of great importance. Arteriography of the external carotid artery defines the exact feeding vessels for further embolization. In all tumors of class C and D, embolization is fundamental.

Arteriography of the ICA shows vascularization from the caroticotympanic artery and from the cavernous branches of the artery as well as the exact status of arterial invasion by the tumor. Study of the vertebrobasilar system demonstrates the vascularization of intracranial extension of the tumor from muscular, meningeal, and parenchymal (PICA, AICA) branches. Arterial supply from these latter branches indicates a definite intradural extension of the tumor. This study also provides indications for the possibility of embolizing muscular or meningeal branches. When arteriography shows clear involvement of the ICA in its horizontal segment (C3 and C4 tumors), a balloon occlusion test to evaluate the collateral circulation and the possibility of sacrificing the artery is necessary. In some selected cases, when the temporary balloon occlusion test is negative, it might be necessary to perform a permanent closure of the artery 30 to 40 days before operation. Recent introduction of preoperative stenting of the carotid artery offers a new option for treating those patients who are likely to need intraoperative management of the ICA.

In 1978, Fisch classified these lesions into four types: A, B, C, and D. He introduced the type A infratemporal fossa approach for the management of tumors localized in the jugular foramen that were considered inoperable at that time due to the presence of the facial nerve in the middle of the operative field and the inaccessibility of the ICA and petrous apex. To overcome these obstacles, Fisch proposed anterior rerouting of the facial nerve, giving direct access to the whole intratemporal course of the ICA as well as an excellent control of the large venous sinuses. Hearing loss is the only permanent postoperative deficit in this approach and is the result of obliteration of the middle ear.

The type A infratemporal fossa approach is generally used for the removal of class C and D tumors.

In cases with intradural extension, exceeding 2 cm in diameter, staging is indicated where the intradural part is removed in a second stage 6 to 8 months after the first operation. This surgical strategy avoids the high risk of having postoperative CSF leak should a single-stage removal be attempted. The reason for such a risk is the need to resect a wide area of the dura infiltrated by the tumor, and hence the subarachnoid space becomes widely connected to the open neck spaces. Using the staging strategy, we never experienced any CSF leak in our cases.

To sum up, the infratemporal fossa approach offers a wide access to the lateral skull base. The adequate exposure and systematic management of the important arteries and venous sinuses greatly reduces the intraoperative hemorrhage. An accurate preoperative study of the tumor extension, the preoperative tumor embolization, and the eventual closure of an invaded ICA (when feasible) by the neuroradiologist are prerequisites for successful surgery. Therefore, the collaboration between the neuroradiologist and the skull base surgeon is of paramount importance. Lesions of the skull base are rare and very difficult to treat. Management of such cases should be restricted to specialized centers to avoid any serious problems.

Chapter 12

Rare Retrotympanic Masses

12 Rare Retrotympanic Masses

Abstract

A variety of diseases can present as a mass behind an intact tympanic membrane: tumors and tumor-like conditions (facial nerve tumors, meningiomas of the temporal bone, lower cranial nerve schwannomas, chondrosarcomas of the temporal bone, etc.), anomalous anatomy (high jugular bulb, aberrant carotid artery), etc. Otoscopy plays an important role in detecting these conditions, but radiological investigations (computed tomography and magnetic resonance imaging scans) have to be performed always prior to any surgical procedure (even biopsy) due to their diagnostic role. Management of facial nerve tumors and meningiomas of the temporal bone will be thorough in this chapter.

Keywords: retrotympanic mass, facial nerve tumors, meningioma, chondrosarcoma, lower cranial nerve schwannoma, aberrant carotid, high jugular bulb

12.1 Differential Diagnosis of Retrotympanic Masses

A variety of diseases can present as a mass behind an intact tympanic membrane. A detailed history of the patient, audiological assessment, and proper radiological evaluation are essential to reach a proper diagnosis. ▶ Table 12.1 summarizes the most common conditions causing a retrotympanic mass. For details of each condition, the reader is referred to the relevant chapters.

Table 12.1 Conditions that may present as a retrotympanic mass

Anomalous anatomy
High jugular bulb
Aberrant carotid artery
Tumors and tumor-like condition
Congenital cholesteatoma
Iatrogenic cholesteatoma
Tympanojugular paraganglioma
Facial nerve tumor (neuroma, hemangioma)
Carcinoid tumor
Adenoma, adenocarcinoma
Meningioma (primary or secondary to temporal bone invasion)
Chordoma, chondrosarcoma of the jugular foramen (with temporal bone invasion)
Rhabdomyosarcoma
Miscellaneous
Meningoencephalic herniation

12.2 Meningioma

This condition is depicted in the following figures (▶ Fig. 12.1, ▶ Fig. 12.2, ▶ Fig. 12.3, ▶ Fig. 12.4, ▶ Fig. 12.5, ▶ Fig. 12.6, ▶ Fig. 12.7, ▶ Fig. 12.8, ▶ Fig. 12.9, ▶ Fig. 12.10, ▶ Fig. 12.11, ▶ Fig. 12.12, ▶ Fig. 12.13, ▶ Fig. 12.14, ▶ Fig. 12.15, ▶ Fig. 12.16, ▶ Fig. 12.17, ▶ Fig. 12.18, ▶ Fig. 12.19).

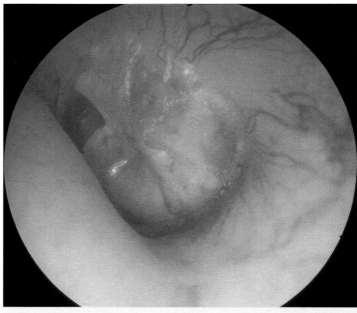

Fig. 12.1 Left ear. This patient presented with dysphagia as her only symptom. A nonpulsating retrotympanic mass was noticed. The mass was whitish rather than the reddish color characteristic of glomus tumor. Computed tomography (CT) scan and magnetic resonance imaging (MRI) demonstrated an en-plaque meningioma invading the posterior surface of the temporal bone.

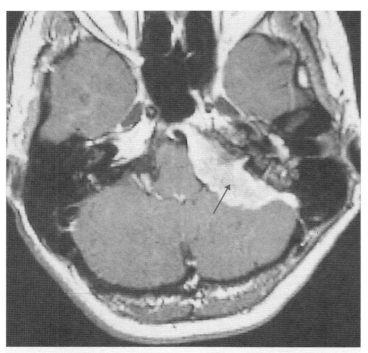

Fig. 12.2 MRI of the case presented in ▶ Fig. 11.2. Large posterior fossa meningioma located along the posterior surface of the petrous bone.

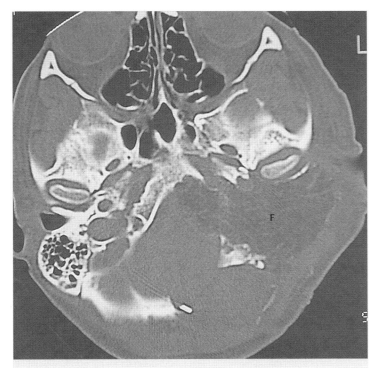

Fig. 12.3 Postoperative CT scan of the case described in ▶ Fig. 12.1. The tumor was removed using a modified transcochlear approach. The surgical cavity was obliterated using abdominal fat (F).

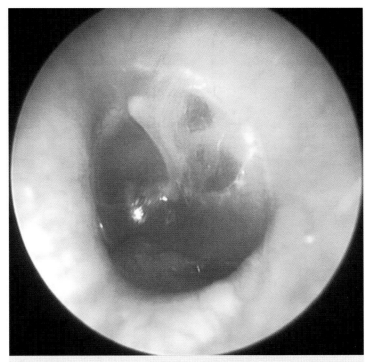

Fig. 12.4 Left ear. Pinkish nonpulsating retrotympanic mass. This 40-year-old patient referred to our clinic for persistent temporal and occipital headache, left hearing loss, and vertigo. Neuroradiological investigations revealed a huge tumor arising from the jugular foramen (see ▶ Fig. 12.5, ▶ Fig. 12.6, ▶ Fig. 12.7), which proved to be a meningioma. The disease was removed through a staged procedure (first stage: removal of the extradural and cervical portion; second stage: removal of the intradural portion).

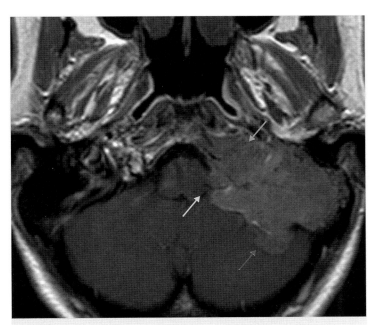

Fig. 12.5 MRI of the same case, axial view (T1W + gadolinium enhancement). The lesion extends to the posterior fossa (cerebellum, *red arrow*; medulla oblongata, *yellow arrow*) and infratemporal fossa (*green arrow*).

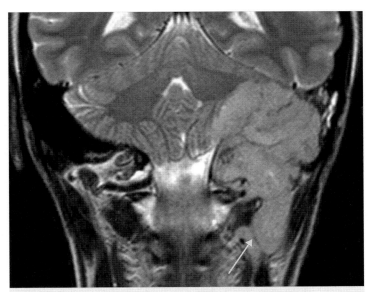

Fig. 12.6 MRI of the same case, coronal view (T2W). Note the cervical extension of the lesion (*arrow*).

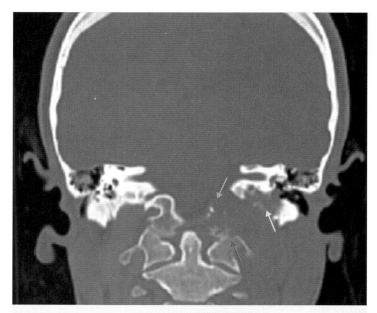

Fig. 12.7 CT scan of the same case, coronal view. Note the massive erosion and involvement of the temporal bone and jugular foramen area (*yellow arrow*). The left jugular tubercle has been completely eroded by the lesion (*green arrow*), which starts to infiltrate even the occipital condyle (*red arrow*). Intratumoral calcifications can be seen.

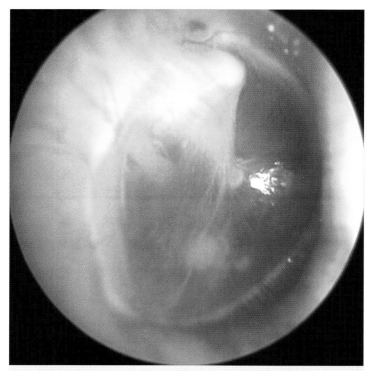

Fig. 12.8 Right ear. Case of an en-plaque meningioma in a 67-year-old patient. The otoscopy shows a reddish nonpulsating retrotympanic mass. Right ear fullness, intermittent pulsatile tinnitus, and dizziness are the only complaints. Considering patient's age, symptoms, the high morbidity related to the surgical treatment, and the slow growing nature of the lesion, a wait-and-scan protocol was adopted. Since 2 years from the diagnosis, the lesion has not yet grown.

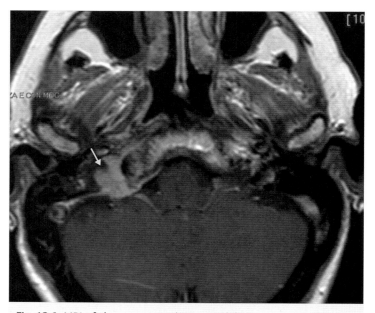

Fig. 12.9 MRI of the same case (T1W + gadolinium enhancement), axial view. The internal carotid artery is enchased by the tumor (*yellow arrow*), which shows broad dural attachment.

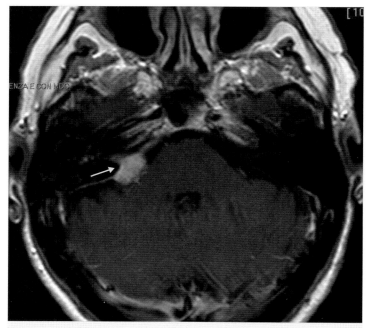

Fig. 12.10 MRI of the same case (T1W + gadolinium enhancement), axial view. The tumor extends in the internal auditory canal and cerebellopontine angle (*yellow arrow*).

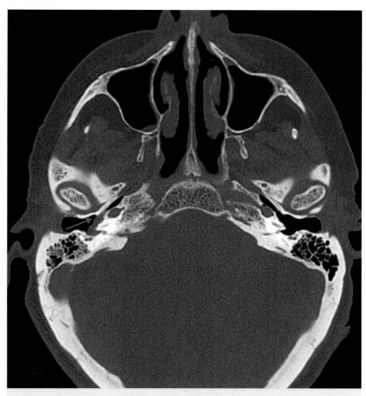

Fig. 12.11 CT scan of the same case, axial view. The tumor extends into the middle ear cleft (*arrow*).

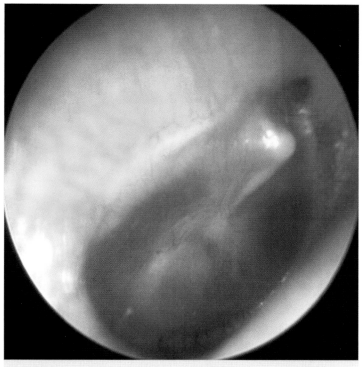

Fig. 12.12 Right ear. Petroclival meningioma. The otoscopy shows a pinkish nonpulsating retrotympanic mass in the anteroinferior quadrants. Eustachian tube is blocked by the tumor, resulting in middle ear effusion (note the opacification of the tympanic membrane).

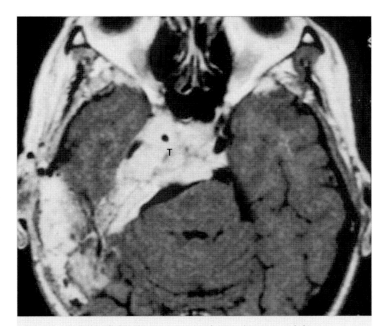

Fig. 12.13 MRI of the same case, axial view (T1W + gadolinium enhancement), shows the extension of the tumor (T).

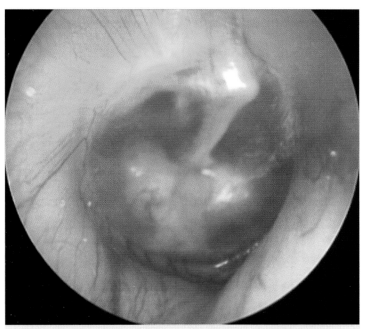

Fig. 12.14 Right huge meningioma extended to the posterior, infratemporal fossae, neck, and contralateral side. This 41-year-old patient refused surgical treatment and died 2 years after radiotherapy.

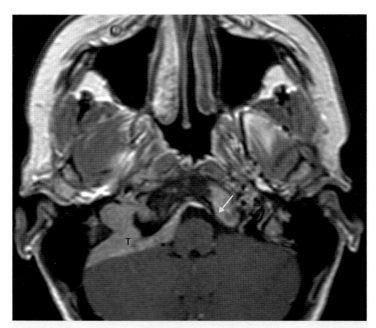

Fig. 12.15 MRI of the same case showing extension of the disease toward the contralateral side (*arrow*). Radical surgical removal of the tumor (T) is impossible due to the involvement of vital structures and the high risk of recurrence.

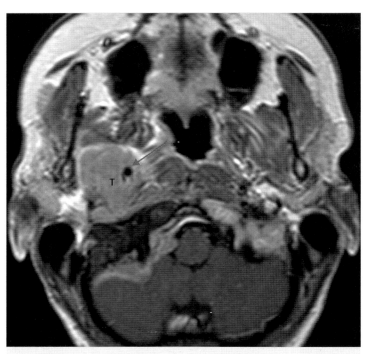

Fig. 12.16 MRI of the same case showing extension of the tumor in the infratemporal fossa. The internal carotid artery is displaced and completely engulfed by the disease (*arrow*).

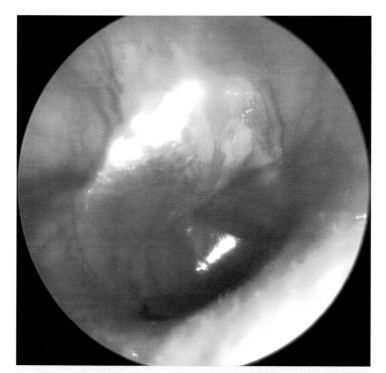

Fig. 12.17 Another case of a skull base meningioma in a 42-year-old female patient presenting with a retrotympanic nonpulsating mass. The tumor, arising from the jugular foramen, was removed through a staged surgery for the presence of wide intradural portion. This avoids the risk of cerebrospinal fluid (CSF) leak in the neck after the first stage (in this case an infratemporal fossa approach type A).

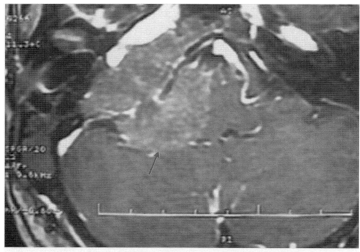

Fig. 12.18 MRI, axial view, of the same case. Note the broad dural attachment of the tumor and its wide intradural portion (*red arrow*).

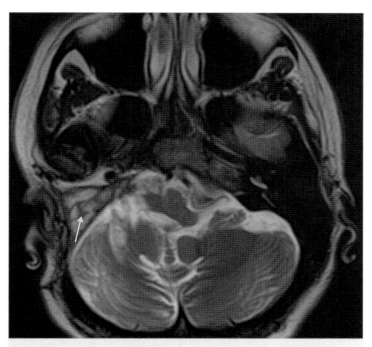

Fig. 12.19 Postoperative MRI (after 2 years from the second stage). The tumor has been completely removed and the cavity is obliterated with abdominal fat (*arrow*).

12.3 Lower Cranial Nerves Neurinoma

This condition is depicted in the following figures (▶ Fig. 12.20, ▶ Fig. 12.21, ▶ Fig. 12.22, ▶ Fig. 12.23, ▶ Fig. 12.24, ▶ Fig. 12.25).

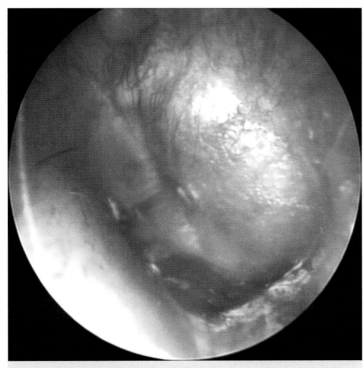

Fig. 12.20 Left ear. Lower cranial nerve neurinoma. Otoscopy shows a retrotympanic bulging. A pinkish mass is visible even in the hypotympanic area. This patient has been managed for 2 years with a wait-and-scan protocol. Due to a tumor growth and the onset of left IX and X cranial nerves palsy, we decided to remove the lesion through a transcochlear-transigmoid approach.

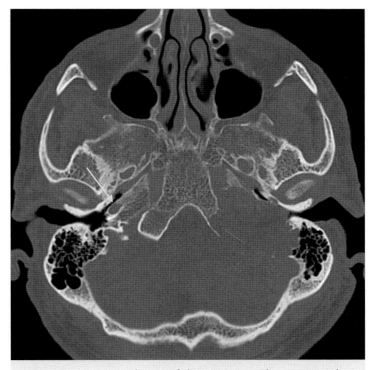

Fig. 12.21 CT scan, axial view, of the same case. The tumor involves the jugular foramen area, engulfing the vertical portion of the internal carotid artery (the yellow arrow shows the level of the free-contralateral artery) and eroding the clivus (*red arrow*).

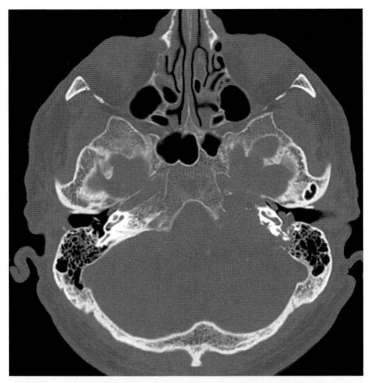

Fig. 12.22 CT scan, axial view, of the same case. Even the medial wall of the horizontal portion of the internal carotid artery is in contact with the tumor (*arrow*).

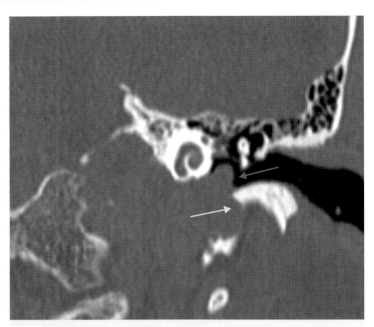

Fig. 12.23 CT scan, coronal view, showing the extension of the tumor in the middle ear cleft (*red arrow*). The tumor spreads from the jugular foramen area eroding the inferior tympanic bone (*yellow arrow*).

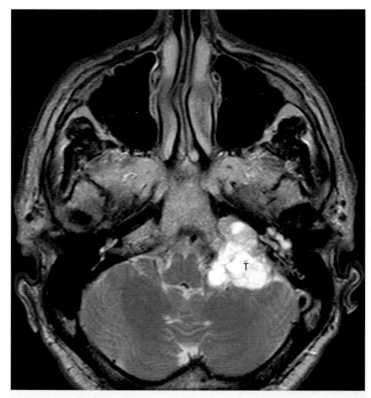

Fig. 12.24 MRI scan of the same case, axial view (T2W). Note the dumbbell-shaped pattern of the tumor (T)

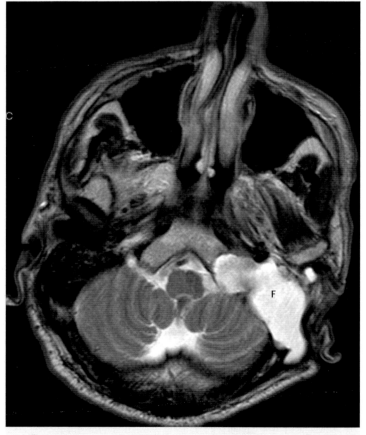

Fig. 12.25 Postoperative MRI of the same case. Total tumor removal has been accomplished. The cavity is obliterated with abdominal fat (F).

12.4 Chondrosarcoma of the Jugular Foramen

This condition is depicted in the following figures (▶ Fig. 12.26, ▶ Fig. 12.27, ▶ Fig. 12.28, ▶ Fig. 12.29, ▶ Fig. 12.30).

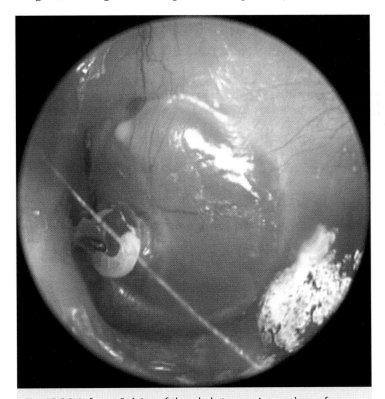

Fig. 12.26 Left ear. Bulging of the whole tympanic membrane for a retrotympanic nonpulsating mass. This 45-year-old female patient underwent transtympanic tube insertion elsewhere for the suspect of a glue ear. One month after tube placement, she developed left IX and X cranial nerves palsy. An MRI showed the presence of a jugular foramen lesion, which proved to be a chondrosarcoma. Chondrosarcomas of the skull are rare slow-growing locally aggressive malignant tumors. These tumors rarely metastasize; therefore, local control represents the goal of therapy. The ideal primary treatment of these tumors is total surgical removal. Radiotherapy may constitute a viable alternative to surgery in selected cases in which there are serious contraindications to surgery as well as in cases with partial excision or with high risk of recurrence. Proton beam radiotherapy, radiosurgery (Gamma knife or Cyber knife), or fractioned radiotherapy is often used as an adjuvant treatment.

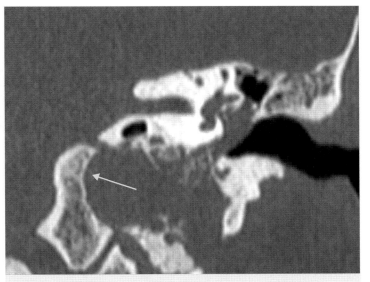

Fig. 12.27 CT scan, coronal view, of the same case. The tumor spreads from the jugular foramen to the middle ear. Irregular bone erosion of the jugular foramen and the occipital condyle (*arrow*) can be observed.

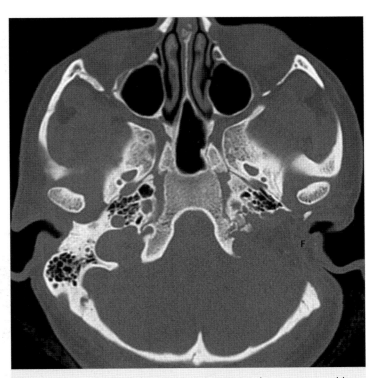

Fig. 12.29 Postoperative CT scan, axial view. Total tumor removal has been accomplished with an infratemporal fossa type A approach. The cavity is obliterated with abdominal fat. The patient underwent adjuvant proton beam radiotherapy.

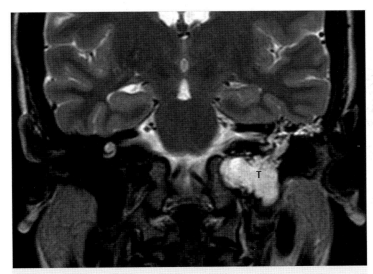

Fig. 12.28 MRI scan, coronal view, of the same case (T2W). The tumor (T) appears as a lobulated ▶ destructive mass.

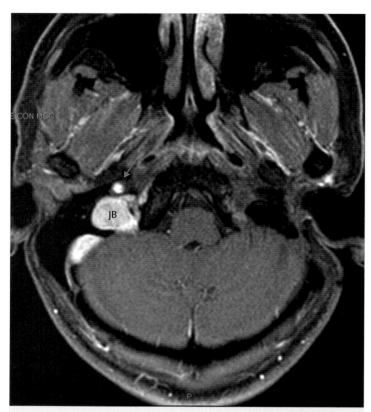

Fig. 12.30 Postoperative MRI scan (3 years after surgery), axial view (T1W + gadolinium enhancement). No recurrence can be observed. The ipsilateral jugular bulb and the vertical portion of the internal carotid artery were closed by the tumor itself preoperatively (JB indicates the bulb on the contralateral side, the arrow indicates the contralateral vertical portion of the internal carotid artery).

12.5 Facial Nerve Tumors

This condition is depicted in the following figures (▶ Fig. 12.31, ▶ Fig. 12.32, ▶ Fig. 12.33, ▶ Fig. 12.34, ▶ Fig. 12.35, ▶ Fig. 12.36, ▶ Fig. 12.37, ▶ Fig. 12.38, ▶ Fig. 12.39, ▶ Fig. 12.40, ▶ Fig. 12.41, ▶ Fig. 12.42, ▶ Fig. 12.43, ▶ Fig. 12.44, ▶ Fig. 12.45, ▶ Fig. 12.46, ▶ Fig. 12.47, ▶ Fig. 12.48, ▶ Fig. 12.49, ▶ Fig. 12.50, ▶ Fig. 12.51, ▶ Fig. 12.52, ▶ Fig. 12.53, ▶ Fig. 12.54, ▶ Fig. 12.55, ▶ Fig. 12.56, ▶ Fig. 12.57, ▶ Fig. 12.58, ▶ Fig. 12.59, ▶ Fig. 12.60, ▶ Fig. 12.61, ▶ Fig. 12.62, ▶ Fig. 12.63).

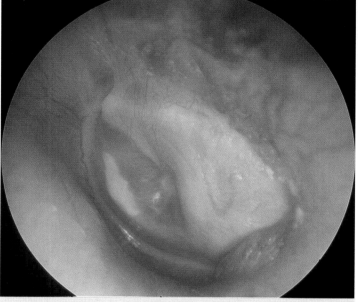

Fig. 12.31 Left ear. A whitish retrotympanic mass is seen causing bulging of the posterior quadrants of the tympanic membrane. A small reddish mass is visible in the posterior inferior regions of the external auditory canal (i.e., lateral to the annulus). The patient complained of left hearing loss and nonpulsating tinnitus of 2 years' duration. In the last 3 months before presentation, left facial nerve paresis started to appear (see subsequent figures).

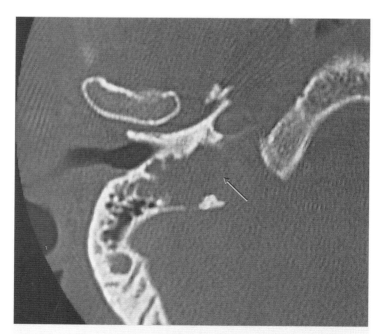

Fig. 12.32 CT scan, axial view, of the case presented in ▶ Fig. 12.31. The tumor is centered on the left jugular foramen (*arrow*).

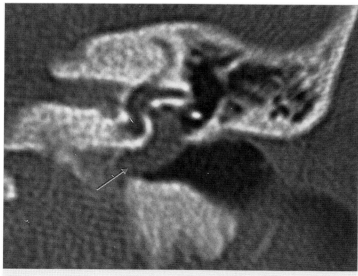

Fig. 12.33 CT scan, coronal view. The mass eroded the bony plate over the jugular bulb extending into the hypotympanum.

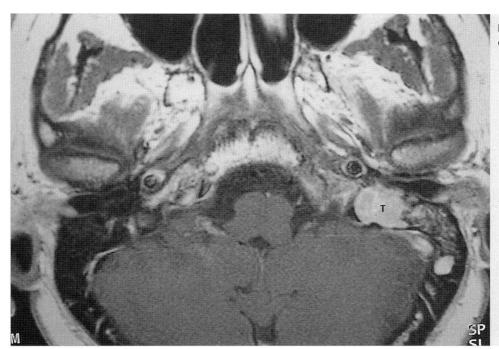

Fig. 12.34 MRI, axial view, shows a mass centered on the jugular foramen (T, tumor).

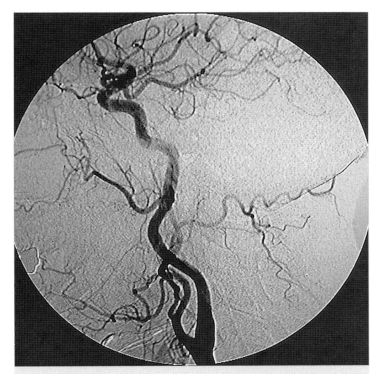

Fig. 12.35 Angiography did not show the characteristic tumor blush of glomus tumors. During surgery, the tumor proved to be a facial nerve neurinoma, as confirmed later by histopathological examination. The tumor was arising from the mastoid segment of the nerve and extended to the jugular bulb.

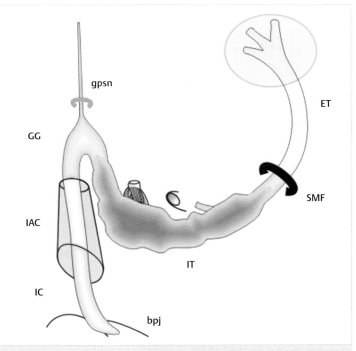

Fig. 12.36 Schematic illustration of the case in ▶ Fig. 12.30. The tumor involves the third (mastoid) portion of the facial nerve. bpj, bulbopontine junction; ET, extratemporal portion of the facial nerve; GG, geniculate ganglion; gpsn, greater superficial petrosal nerve; IAC, internal auditory canal; IC, intracisternal; IT, intratemporal; SMF, stylomastoid foramen.

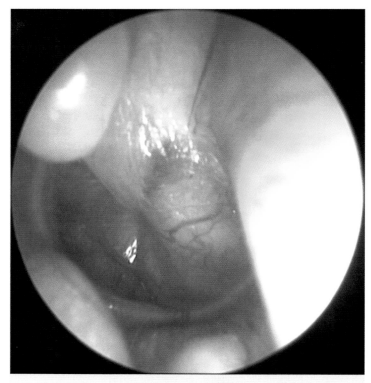

Fig. 12.37 Left ear. Pinkish retrotympanic nonpulsating mass. The patient showed slight worsening of facial nerve function (grade II House–Brackmann scale). Neuroradiological investigations suggested the presence of a facial nerve tumor affecting the mastoid segment. In this case, a wait-and-scan protocol was adopted. Exostoses of the external auditory canal can also be noted.

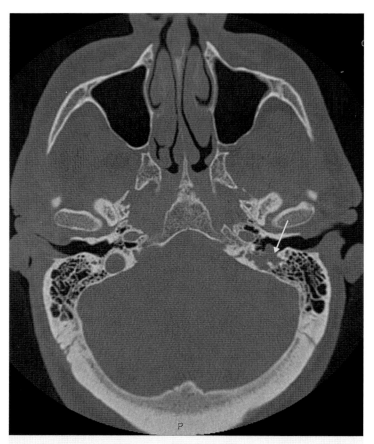

Fig. 12.38 CT scan, axial view, of the same case. A soft-tissue mass corresponding to the area of the third portion of the facial nerve can be noted (*arrow*).

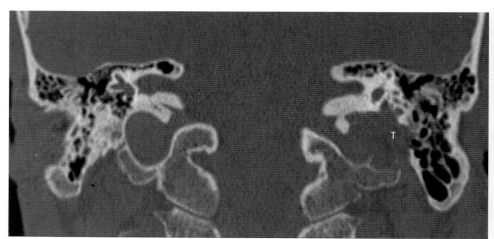

Fig. 12.39 CT scan, coronal view, of the same case. The tumor (T) has caused a marked erosion of the mastoid segment of the fallopian canal.

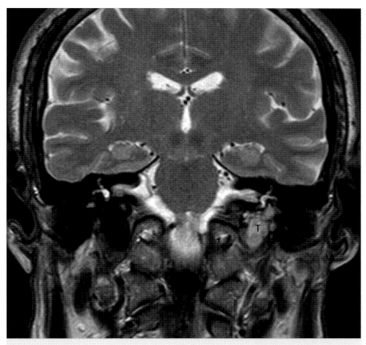

Fig. 12.40 MRI of the same case, coronal view (T2W). The tumor (T) can be noted as a hyperintense mass close to the area of the jugular bulb.

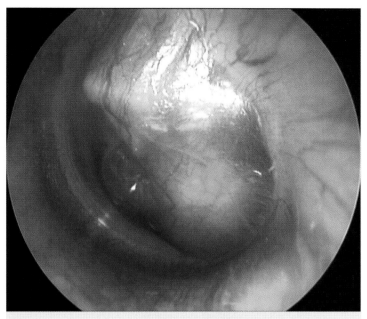

Fig. 12.41 Case similar to that in ▶ Fig. 12.31 and ▶ Fig. 12.37. This child presented with history of facial weakness for the last 18 months.

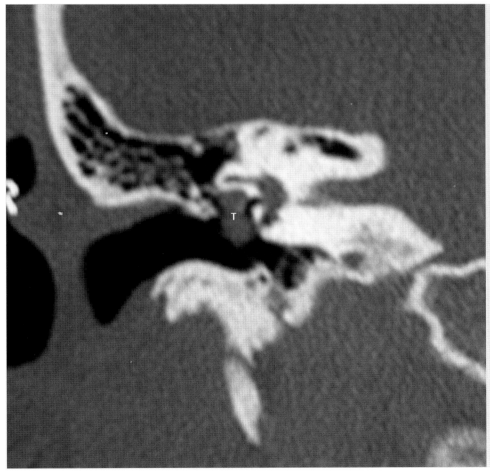

Fig. 12.42 The coronal section CT showed a soft-tissue mass in the location of the tympanic segment of the facial nerve (T).

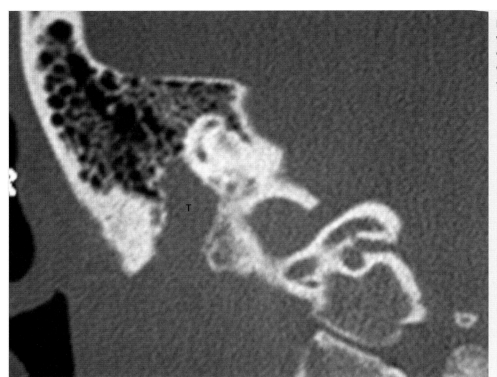

Fig. 12.43 At a more posterior level, the mass was seen to be involving the mastoid segment of the nerve and dilating the canal (T). The operation was planned through a transmastoid approach.

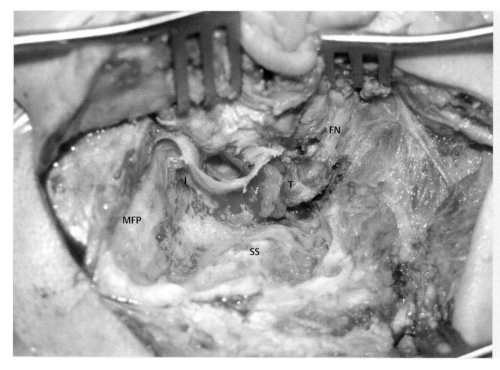

Fig. 12.44 Intraoperative picture. The facial nerve has been decompressed from its tympanic portion to the beginning of the intraparotid portion (FN). The tumor (T) can be seen from the genu medial to the short process of the incus (I) to the beginning of the parotid segment. MFP, middle fossa plate; SS, sigmoid sinus.

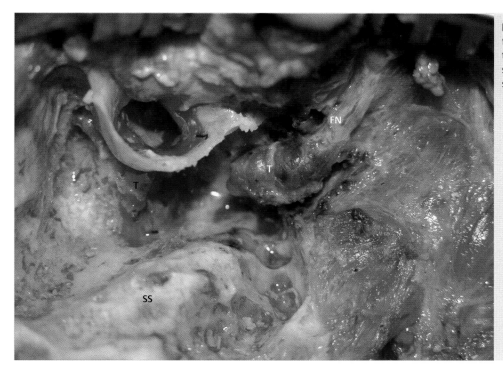

Fig. 12.45 Intraoperative picture. Debulking of the tumor (T) has been started. Notice the tumor remnant at the level of the genu which should also be removed. FN, facial nerve; SS, sigmoid sinus.

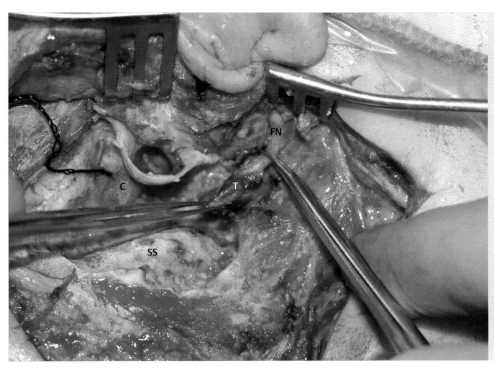

Fig. 12.46 Intraoperative picture. The last piece of the tumor (T) is being cut at an area free of tumor. C, Cottonoid covering the proximal segment of the facial nerve; FN, normal facial nerve tissue; SS, sigmoid sinus.

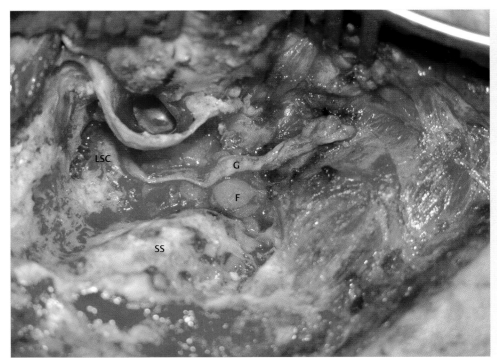

Fig. 12.47 Intraoperative picture. The fat (F) has been used to provide a bed for the graft. An adequate length of greater auricular nerve (G) has been used to bridge the gap between the proximal and distal ends of the facial nerve. Alternatively, a sural nerve graft could be used. The tumor proved to be a facial nerve neurinoma on histopathological examination. LSC, lateral semicircular canal; SS, sigmoid sinus.

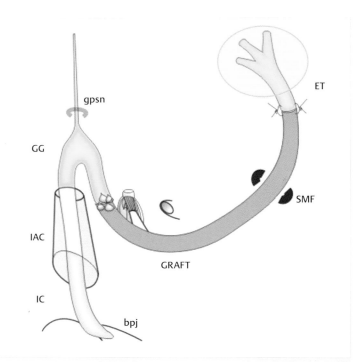

Fig. 12.48 Schematic illustration of repair of an injury involving the mastoid and extracranial segments of the facial nerve as in ▶ Fig. 12.46. For the anastomosis with the extratemporal stump of the facial nerve, fine nylon threads have to be used to suture the nerve ends. For intracranial and intratemporal anastomosis, just fibrin glue and fascia are used. For abbreviations, see ▶ Fig. 12.36.

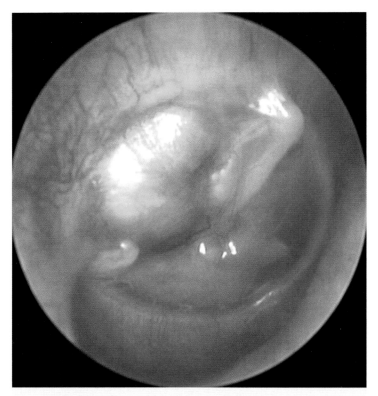

Fig. 12.49 Right ear. Facial nerve tumor involving the geniculate ganglion and the second portion of the facial nerve. This 25-year-old patient showed only conductive hearing loss. So, a wait-and-scan protocol was adopted.

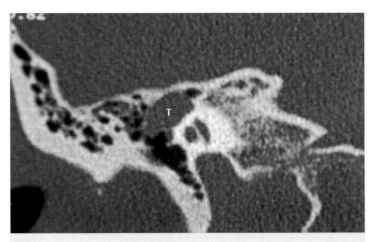

Fig. 12.50 CT scan of the same case, coronal view. The tumor (T) is causing widening of the geniculate ganglion area. The tumor does not erode the cochlea.

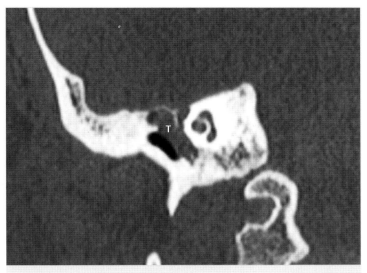

Fig. 12.51 CT scan of the same case, coronal view. The tumor (T) involves even the second portion of the facial nerve. The tumor does not erode the cochlea.

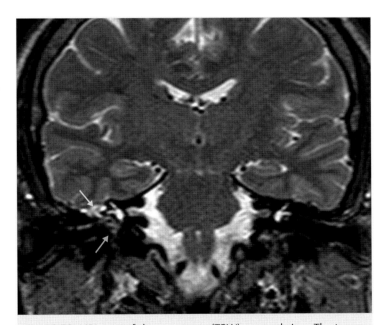

Fig. 12.52 MRI scan of the same case (T2W), coronal view. The tumor is seen in the area of the geniculate ganglion, close to the middle fossa dura plate (*yellow arrow*). Effusion in the middle ear is also evident (*green arrow*).

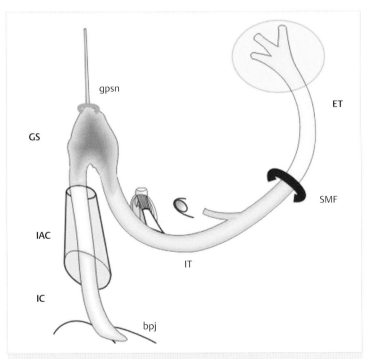

Fig. 12.53 Schematic illustration of the case in ▶ Fig. 12.49. The tumor involves the geniculate ganglion and the tympanic portion of the facial nerve. For abbreviations, see ▶ Fig. 12.36.

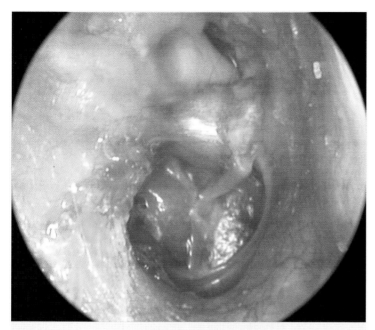

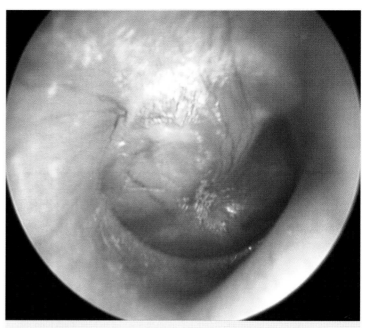

Fig. 12.54 Another case of facial nerve tumor involving the geniculate ganglion area. In this patient, atticotomy has been previously performed elsewhere for the suspect of an epitympanic cholesteatoma. Tympanic membrane atelectasis is also evident. Bone conduction was normal. A combined middle fossa-transmastoid approach was used for tumor removal, considering the onset of facial palsy. After 1 year, the patient showed facial nerve function grade III.

Fig. 12.55 Case similar to that in ▶ Fig. 12.49. This patient had facial nerve palsy (grade IV) and hearing loss due to cochlear involvement.

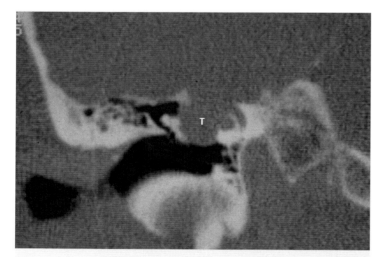

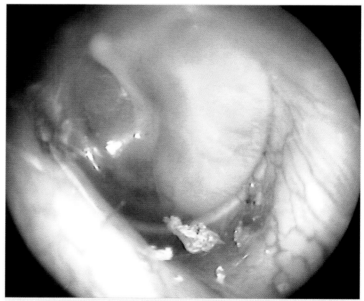

Fig. 12.56 CT of the same patient, coronal view. The tumor (T) erodes the cochlea and the middle fossa dura plate. The patient underwent tumor removal through a transcochlear approach followed by a sural nerve graft anastomosis. After 1 year, the patient achieved a grade III facial nerve function.

Fig. 12.57 Left ear. Another case of facial nerve tumor involving the third portion of the facial nerve. A retrotympanic mass is visible on otoscopy.

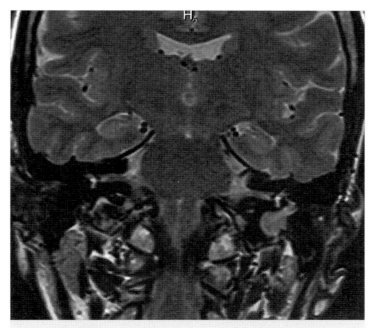

Fig. 12.58 MRI scan, coronal view, of the same case. The tumor (T) is close to the area of the jugular bulb.

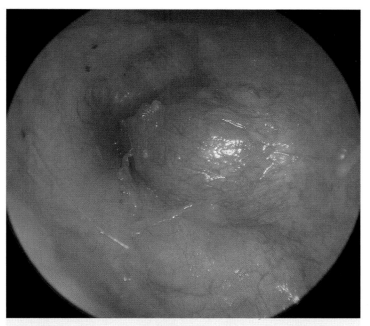

Fig. 12.59 Left ear. Mass protruding into the posterior auditory canal. The patient complained of left mild hearing loss and left facial nerve palsy (grade III) of 6 months' duration.

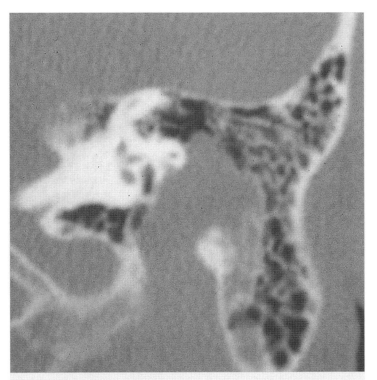

Fig. 12.60 CT scan demonstrated the presence of tumor involving the vertical portion of the facial nerve.

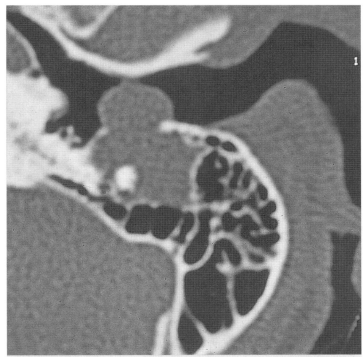

Fig. 12.61 CT scan showed also erosion of the posterior wall of the external canal.

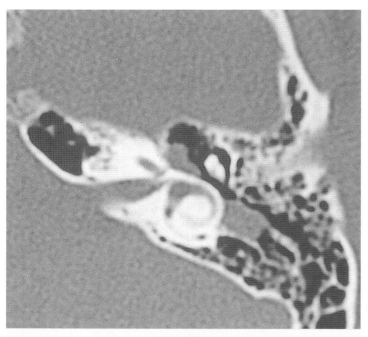

Fig. 12.62 CT scan. The tumor extended to the geniculate ganglion.

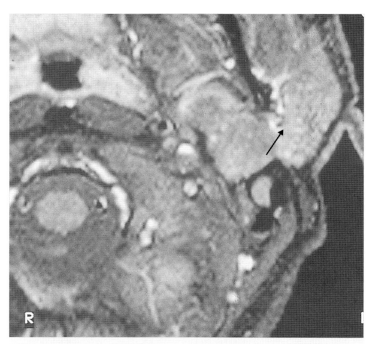

Fig. 12.63 MRI showed a mass extending to the parotid gland area (*arrow*). A combined middle fossa-transmastoid approach with parotid extension was performed. During surgery the tumor proved to be a facial nerve neurinoma extended from the parotid to the intra-labyrinthine segment of the facial nerve. The nerve was reconstructed with sural nerve graft.

12.6 Aberrant Carotid Artery

This condition is presented in ▶ Fig. 12.64 and ▶ Fig. 12.65.

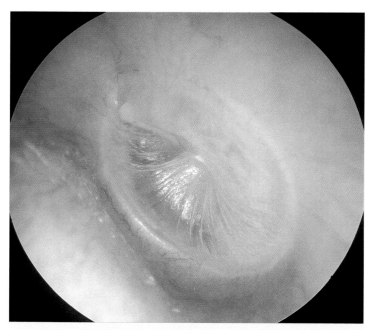

Fig. 12.64 Left ear. A small pulsating reddish area in the anteroinferior quadrant of the tympanic membrane. This picture may be confused with a tympanic paraganglioma.

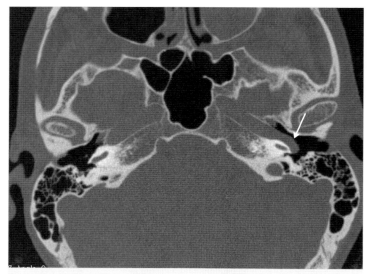

Fig. 12.65 A high-resolution CT scan established the diagnosis of an ectopic internal carotid artery (*arrow*).

12.7 Internal Carotid Artery Aneurysm

This condition is presented in ▶ Fig. 12.66, ▶ Fig. 12.67, ▶ Fig. 12.68, ▶ Fig. 12.69, ▶ Fig. 12.70.

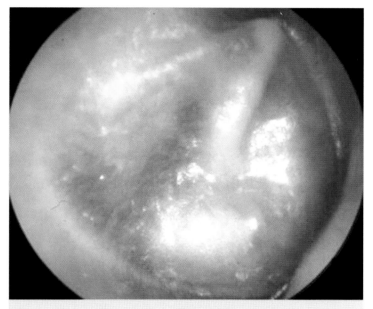

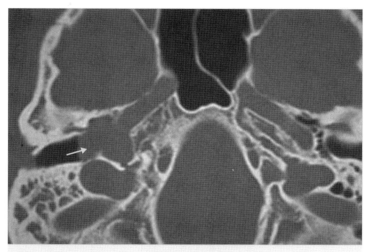

Fig. 12.67 CT scan shows the aneurysm (*arrow*).

Fig. 12.66 Right ear. Retrotympanic pulsating mass in a 45-year-old male patient. The otoscopy was suggestive of tympanojugular paraganglioma. CT and MRI scans showed an aneurysm of the petrosal internal carotid artery. Closure of the artery with coils was further performed. This case emphasize the importance of neuroradiological investigations in case of retrotympanic mass before any surgical treatment.

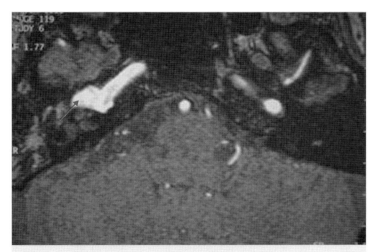

Fig. 12.68 MRI scan shows the aneurysm (*arrow*).

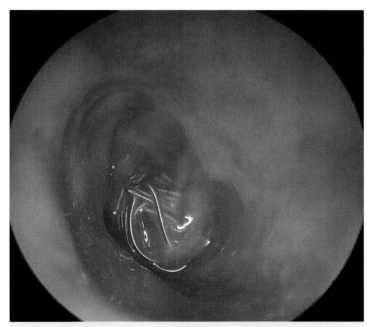

Fig. 12.69 Guglielmi coils used to occlude an intrapetrous internal carotid artery aneurysm.

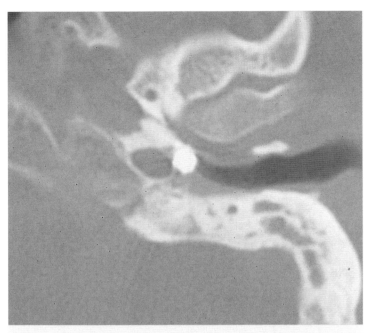

Fig. 12.70 CT scan of the case presented in ▶ Fig. 12.69 demonstrating occlusion of the aneurysm with the coils.

12.8 High Jugular Bulb

This condition is presented in ▶ Fig. 12.71, ▶ Fig. 12.72, ▶ Fig. 12.73, ▶ Fig. 12.74, ▶ Fig. 12.75, ▶ Fig. 12.76, ▶ Fig. 12.77, ▶ Fig. 12.78, ▶ Fig. 12.79, ▶ Fig. 12.80, ▶ Fig. 12.81, ▶ Fig. 12.82.

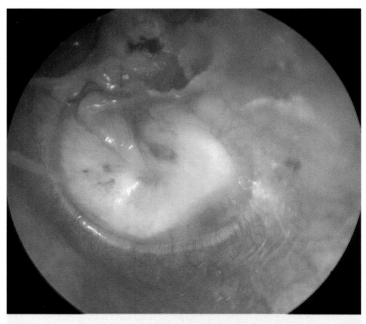

Fig. 12.71 Left ear. Tympanosclerosis involving the whole tympanic membrane. An epitympanic erosion with cholesteatoma is also visible. At the level of the posteroinferior quadrant, a bluish mass is observed. A CT scan (see ▶ Fig. 12.71) proved this mass to be a high jugular bulb.

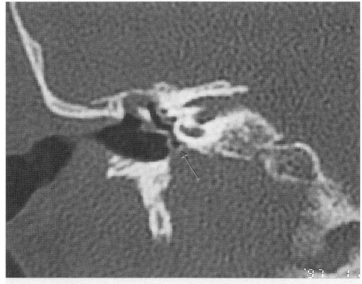

Fig. 12.72 CT scan of the previous case. The uncovered jugular bulb is seen protruding into the middle ear (*arrow*).

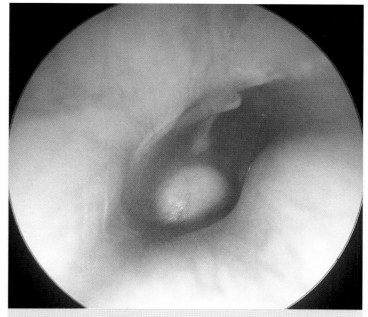

Fig. 12.73 Right ear. Another example of a high jugular bulb covered by a thin bony shell in a young male patient with a skull base malformation (see subsequent figures).

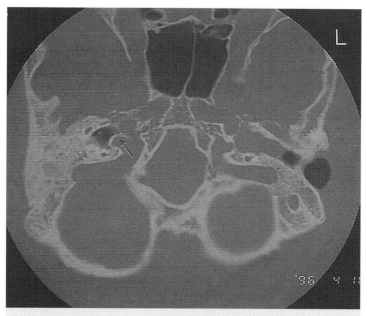

Fig. 12.74 CT scan, axial view. The jugular bulb protrudes into the middle ear (*arrow*).

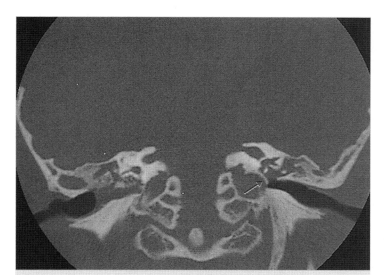

Fig. 12.75 CT scan, coronal view. The high jugular bulb can be observed.

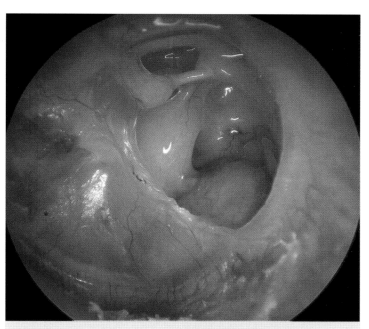

Fig. 12.76 Left ear. A high and uncovered jugular bulb reaching up to the level of the round window is visible through a posterior tympanic membrane perforation.

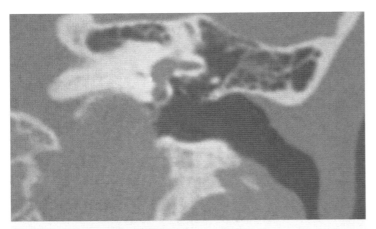

Fig. 12.77 CT scan of the case in ▶ Fig. 12.75.

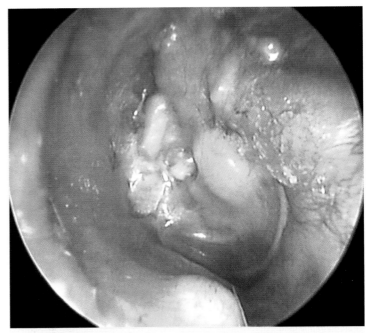

Fig. 12.78 High jugular bulb (*arrow*) in a canal wall down tympanoplasty.

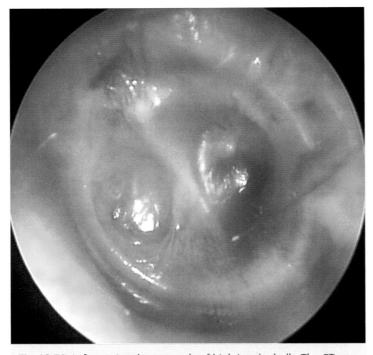

Fig. 12.79 Left ear. Another example of high jugular bulb. The CT scan showed uncovered bulb close to the oval window (see ▶ Fig. 12.80). Middle ear dysventilation with tympanic retraction is also evident.

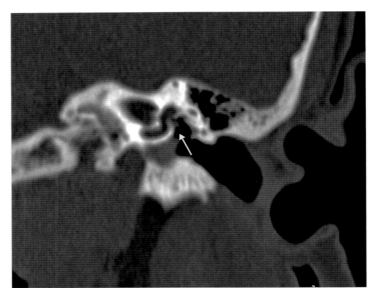

Fig. 12.80 CT scan of the same case, coronal view. Note the proximity of the uncovered bulb to the oval window (*arrow*).

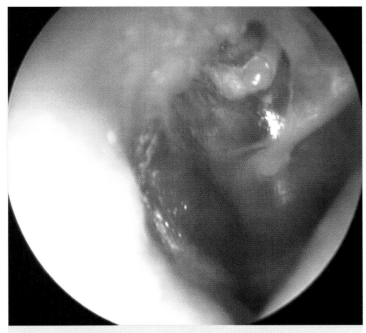

Fig. 12.81 Another case of high jugular bulb. A posterior tympanic retraction pocket with myringoincudopexy is also visible.

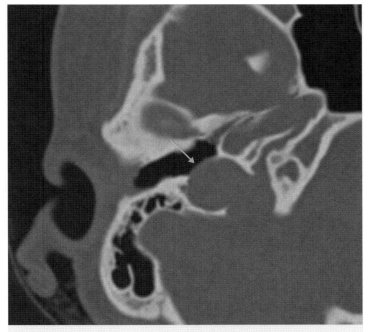

Fig. 12.82 CT scan of the same case, axial view, showing high and uncovered jugular bulb in the middle ear (*arrow*).

Summary: Meningioma

Posterior fossa meningiomas are the second most common tumor of the cerebellopontine angle. These tumors are characterized by a higher morbidity and mortality than acoustic neurinoma.

Surgical removal of these lesions poses many problems because of the deep location, the involvement of vital neurovascular structures, and the large sizes these tumors usually attain before diagnosis. Moreover, they have an aggressive behavior with frequent involvement of the dura and bone. Total removal is fundamental to avoid recurrence and is better achieved in the first operation. Total removal with minimal morbidity can be obtained utilizing an array of approaches that must be adapted to each individual case.

In general, an ideal approach is that which allows total removal with minimal or no brain retraction. The site of the tumor is the most important factor for the choice of the surgical approach. The size of the tumor, the patient's age and general medical condition, and the preoperative status of the cranial nerves are other factors to consider.

Tumors localized posterior to the internal auditory canal in young patients with good preoperative hearing can be removed using a retrosigmoid approach. In the elderly, however, a translabyrinthine approach is preferred to avoid cerebellar retraction. In cases of involvement of the jugular foramen, a POTS approach is adopted.

In small tumors lying anterior to the internal auditory canal, the middle fossa transpetrous approach is utilized. In large petroclival lesions, which pose more difficulties due to their deep location, the intimate relation with the brainstem, and the involvement of vital neurovascular structures, the modified transcochlear approach should be used, irrespective of the preoperative hearing. This approach permits a wide and direct exposure, and a flat angle of vision with no cerebellar or brainstem retraction.

Moreover, it allows the removal of any infiltrated dura or bone.

Though total removal can be obtained in the majority of petroclival meningiomas, it is not always necessary or even safe. Subtotal removal is decided when an arachnoid plane of cleavage between the tumor and the brainstem is absent or when the perforating arteries are at risk of interruption during total tumor removal.

Neuroradiologic evaluation is fundamental to plan surgery. A CT scan with contrast to evaluate the bone, MRI with gadolinium, and in some cases, digital subtraction angiography are of paramount importance in each case.

The neuroradiologist should provide the surgeon with information on the following:
- Anatomical relations of the tumor.
- Tumor consistency.
- Vascularity.
- Peritumoral edema.
- Tumor–brainstem interface.
- Invasion of the dura and bone.
- Relationship between the tumor and the vertebrobasilar and carotid systems.
- Necessity of eventual embolization.

The main blood supply of these tumors comes from large dural arteries. However, significant contributions may also come from pial arteries or from dural branches of the internal carotid and vertebral arteries.

The angiographic data help the neuroradiologist and the skull base surgeon to determine the need for embolization. When indicated, it should be performed a few days before surgery. It not only decreases the intraoperative bleeding, but also produces a certain amount of tumor necrosis, rendering some cases easier to remove.

Close cooperation between the neuroradiologist and the skull base surgeon offers optimal chances for successful management of these challenging tumors.

Summary: Facial Nerve Neurinoma

Tumor involvement of the facial nerve has been estimated to be the cause of facial palsy in 5% of cases. Though uncommon, facial neuromas should be considered in the differential diagnosis of facial nerve dysfunction. Unfortunately, the rarity of facial neuromas and the diversity of their clinical picture, together with the fact that their presentation may mimic other more common pathologies, render the diagnosis of these tumors difficult.

Facial nerve dysfunction is the most common symptom.

It can vary from the classic progressive palsy to sudden or recurrent facial palsy or hemifacial spasm.

In limited cases, the function of the nerve is normal.

Therefore, all patients with progressive facial palsy must be considered to have a tumor until proved otherwise. Moreover, all patients with Bell's palsy persisting for more than 4 weeks and with recurrent facial paralysis should be investigated for the presence of a tumor.

The second most common complaint is hearing loss. Conductive hearing loss is usually associated with tumor involvement of the middle ear with subsequent interference with the ossicular chain.

Sensorineural hearing loss is attributable to inner ear erosion or extension of the tumor into the internal auditory canal.

Most diagnosed tumors are of large size. One reason is that the facial nerve can accommodate tumor expansion to some extent before significant pressure, with subsequent dysfunction, can occur. Another reason is the relatively long duration of symptoms before diagnosis is made. Because of the absence of classic symptomatology in such cases, a higher index of suspicion is needed for early diagnosis. Diagnostic work-up includes audiometric testing, vestibular testing, and auditory brainstem-evoked response. Electrophysiologic testing of facial nerve function in such cases is of little or no benefit. The usefulness of these tests in the diagnosis of facial neuromas has been challenged by other authors (Dort and Fish 1991, Neely and Alford 1974).

Advances in radiologic techniques have aided greatly in the diagnosis of these lesions. The characteristic appearance on CT is that of an enhancing soft-tissue mass, usually in the perigeniculate region, with sharp bony erosion and enlargement of the fallopian canal. High-resolution CT scan is the best method to assess middle and inner ear involvement by tumor.

However, MRI with gadolinium is the best available method for the preoperative assessment of tumor extension, especially of those involving the internal auditory canal, cerebellopontine angle, and/or the parotid region. Both methods are believed to be complementary for the preoperative assessment and the choice of the most suitable surgical approach for removal of these tumors. However, because these tumors show intraneural spread, it is still doubtful whether MRI with gadolinium can show the full extent of the lesion. Therefore, the surgeon should be prepared to expose the whole length of the facial nerve.

Differential diagnosis of these lesions includes acoustic neuroma, congenital cholesteatoma, tympanojugular paraganglioma, facial nerve hemangioma, and parotid tumors. Intradural facial nerve neuromas pose a major diagnostic difficulty, usually being mistaken for acoustic neuromas. Apart from the few cases in which tumor extension to the geniculate ganglion could establish the diagnosis, most of these cases were actually diagnosed intraoperatively.

Congenital cholesteatomas of the petrous bone are uncommon lesions that usually present with hearing loss and facial weakness or paralysis and, therefore, can be mistaken for facial neuromas. Moreover, these lesions appear on CT as smoothly marginated expansile lesions, and on MRI as hypo/isointense on TI and hyperintense on T2 images. Unlike facial neuromas, however, cholesteatomas do not show enhancement following contrast administration, a fact that helps to differentiate between the two lesions.

Treatment generally aims at total removal of the tumor, restoration or preservation of facial nerve function, and conservation of hearing. The surgical approach depends on the extent of the lesion and the preoperative hearing level. There is general agreement that surgical removal is the treatment of choice. There is some controversy, however, regarding facial neuromas and absence of or mild preoperative facial nerve paresis. Some surgeons prefer to delay surgery because the patient is faced with the inevitable postoperative paralysis followed by some degree of recovery that will never be better than grade III House–Brackmann. Patient counseling is important in these cases.

The age at presentation is another factor to be considered. If the patient is young, early surgical resection should be done because these tumors grow inexorably with subsequent intracranial or extratemporal extension, making the approach more difficult and postoperative complications more likely. Moreover, tumor growth causes progressive degeneration and regeneration of facial nerve fibers, leading to collagenization of the distal part of the nerve with consequent poor recovery of facial function following reconstruction. Another reason is that these tumors are potentially invasive: otic capsule erosion may be present in approximately 20% of the cases. On the other hand, in an elderly patient with an absence of or mild facial nerve paresis, facial nerve decompression may suffice if surgery is to be performed.

When total tumor removal involves resection of a long segment of the nerve, a cable graft is usually needed for reconstruction of the facial nerve. The length of the graft and whether it is from the sural or great auricular nerve has no effect on the eventual recovery of facial function.

In summary, facial nerve neuromas are uncommon tumors requiring a high degree of suspicion for their diagnosis. Recent advances in radiological techniques are the cornerstone for the diagnosis and preoperative assessment of these cases, and early surgical resection gives the best prognosis.

Chapter 13

Meningoencephalic Herniation

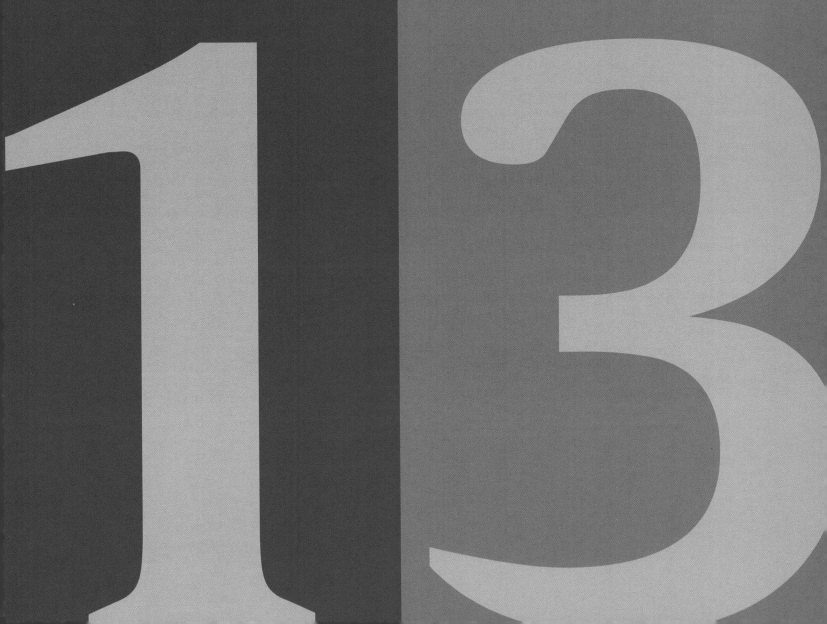

13 Meningoencephalic Herniation

Abstract

Meningoencephalic herniation is the herniation of meningeal and/or encephalic tissue in the middle ear or mastoid. It occurs in connection with infection, previous surgery, head trauma, or congenital tegmental defects. A patient with meningoencephalic herniation has a high risk of developing meningitis and epilepsy due to epileptogenic focus in the herniating tissues.

The patient may present with a pulsatile retrotympanic mass, cerebrospinal fluid leakage, and aphasia. However, the most common manifestation is that of a conductive or mixed hearing loss with a draining ear or serous otitis media. Neuroradiological assessment procedures (computed tomography and magnetic resonance imaging scans) have to be carried out in order to establish a correct preoperative diagnosis. The treatment is surgical and depends on the size of the herniation.

Keywords: meningoencephalic herniation, CSF leak, retrotympanic mass, transmastoid approach, middle fossa approach, minicraniotomy, subtotal petrosectomy

Meningoencephalic herniation is the herniation of meningeal and/or encephalic tissue in the middle ear or mastoid. It occurs in connection with infection, previous surgery, head trauma, or congenital tegmental defects. A patient with meningoencephalic herniation has a high risk of developing meningitis and epilepsy due to epileptogenic focus in the herniating tissues.

The patient may present with a pulsatile retrotympanic mass, cerebrospinal fluid (CSF) leakage, and aphasia. However, the most common manifestation is that of a conductive or mixed hearing loss with a draining ear or serous otitis media.

Herniation of meningeal and/or encephalic tissue into the middle ear is a form of pathology that—even if rarely found by the otologist—can be life-threatening for the patient due to possible infectious intracranial complications. Four different etiological types are possible: infectious, postsurgical, traumatic, and spontaneous. From a pathogenic point of view, all these types are characterized by a bony and dural defect located in the tegmen, through which meningeal and encephalic tissue can herniate. Therefore, once meningoencephalic herniation is suspected, surgical correction is required. The symptoms are often nonspecific, so that some cases are diagnosed during surgery.

When there is strong suspicion of herniation, neuroradiological assessment procedures have to be performed to establish a correct preoperative diagnosis. High-resolution computed tomography (CT) of the temporal bone, in particular, can demonstrate the exact limits and location of the bone defect, while magnetic resonance imaging (MRI) allows the nature of the tissue in the middle ear to be determined. The choice of surgical approach is directed by the etiology, the position and size of the bony defect, preoperative audiometry, the presence of chronic infection in the middle ear, and/or intraoperative active CSF leakage.

In our experience, 5% of revision canal wall down mastoidectomies are complicated by either meningoencephalic or dural herniations. A small herniation (< 1 cm²) can be pushed back intracranially and a piece of cartilage then inserted beneath the bone to ensure repositioning of the dura. The cartilage is covered with bone paste and fascia.

Middle-sized herniations (1–2 cm²) can be repaired by a combined approach. The brain tissue is treated with bipolar coagulation. Then, after pushing back the herniation intracranially, a sufficiently large piece of autologous or homologous cartilage is inserted extradurally through a small craniotomy to ensure repositioning. The bony defect is further repaired using bone paste and covered with temporalis fascia from the mastoid cavity.

In cases of large herniation (> 2 cm²), a middle cranial fossa approach is adopted. In this approach, the dura of the temporal lobe is carefully elevated until the neck of the hernia is identified and subjected to bipolar coagulation. The coagulated part is left in the middle ear or mastoid, where it acts as a barrier against infection. The defect is then reconstructed by placing a piece of temporalis fascia between the cerebral tissue and the dura; another piece of fascia is placed extradurally. Next, a piece of cartilage is placed between the bony defect and the dura for reinforcement.

The advantage of this approach is the opportunity to reach bony defects located anteriorly without any manipulation of the ossicular chain.

Subtotal petrosectomy with middle ear obliteration, in our opinion, represents the safest and most definitive treatment for meningoencephalic herniation. Performing a blind sac closure of the external auditory canal, obliterating the Eustachian tube, and filling the surgical cavity with fat completely isolate the middle ear and mastoid cavities from the external environment, minimizing the risks of recurrence and other complications such as CSF leakage. However, due to the resulting conductive hearing loss (generally around 60 dB), it should be reserved for cases with poor auditory reserve or extensive middle ear destruction with a limited possibility for reconstruction. Because of the closure of the external auditory canal, in subtotal petrosectomy postoperative radiologic follow-up is mandatory (CT scan, MRI scan with fat-suppression and diffusion-weighted images) to reveal presence of residual cholesteatoma.

Meningoencephalic herniation is depicted in the following figures (▶ Fig. 13.1, ▶ Fig. 13.2, ▶ Fig. 13.3, ▶ Fig. 13.4, ▶ Fig. 13.5, ▶ Fig. 13.6, ▶ Fig. 13.7, ▶ Fig. 13.8, ▶ Fig. 13.9, ▶ Fig. 13.10, ▶ Fig. 13.11, ▶ Fig. 13.12, ▶ Fig. 13.13, ▶ Fig. 13.14, ▶ Fig. 13.15, ▶ Fig. 13.16, ▶ Fig. 13.17, ▶ Fig. 13.18, ▶ Fig. 13.19, ▶ Fig. 13.20, ▶ Fig. 13.21, ▶ Fig. 13.22, ▶ Fig. 13.23, ▶ Fig. 13.24, ▶ Fig. 13.25, ▶ Fig. 13.26, ▶ Fig. 13.27, ▶ Fig. 13.28, ▶ Fig. 13.29).

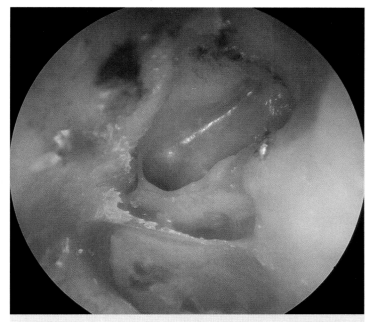

Fig. 13.1 Left meningoencephalic herniation in a patient who had previously undergone open tympanoplasty. The hernia protrudes into the attic through a small tegmental defect and appears otoscopically as a pulsatile retrotympanic mass.

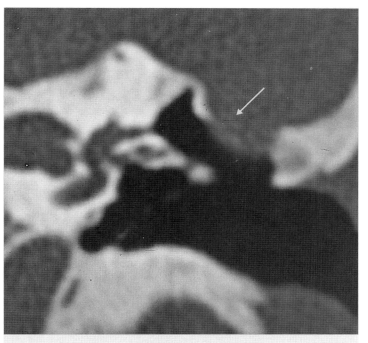

Fig. 13.2 CT scan of the case described in ▶ Fig. 13.1, coronal view. The osseous defect with the herniating tissue can be clearly visualized (*arrow*).

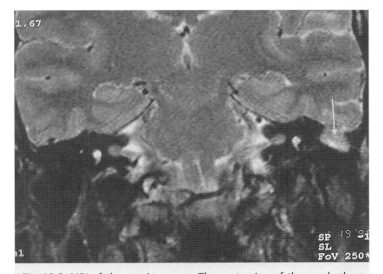

Fig. 13.3 MRI of the previous case. The protrusion of the cerebral tissue into the middle ear is visible (*arrow*).

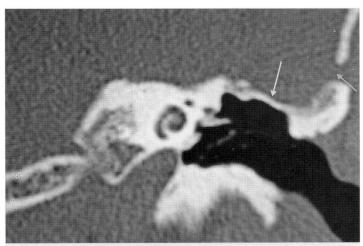

Fig. 13.4 Postoperative CT scan. The hernia was managed using a middle fossa approach. The bony defect was repaired using cartilage. The temporal craniotomy (*green arrow*) and the cartilage (*yellow arrow*) are clearly visible.

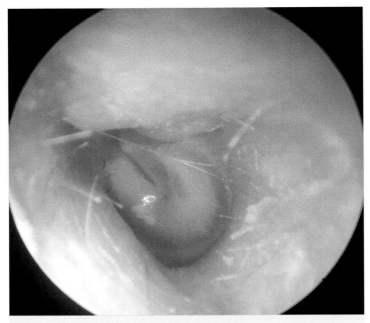

Fig. 13.5 Left meningoencephalic hernia. The superior wall of the external auditory canal is dehiscent. A soft, reducible, nonpulsating mass is observed. The patient had a history of head trauma with transverse fracture of the temporal bone that occurred 3 years before presentation. He complained of left hearing loss and the sensation of ear fullness.

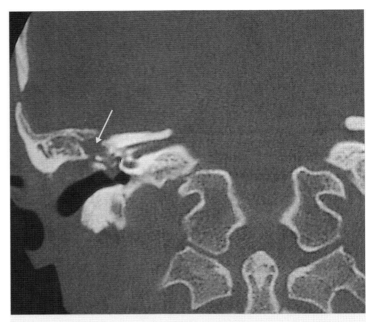

Fig. 13.6 Preoperative CT scan of the case in ▶ Fig. 13.5 demonstrating the herniation of cerebral tissue into the middle ear (*arrow*).

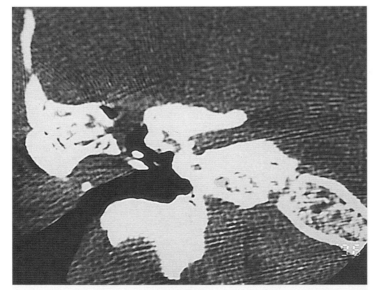

Fig. 13.7 CT scan of the previous case 1 year postoperatively. The hernia was managed using a middle fossa approach, placing a cartilaginous plate to reconstruct the bony defect after having sectioned the neck of the herniating tissue. The cerebral tissue, which is left in the ear during the operation, is resorbed with time as seen in the CT scan

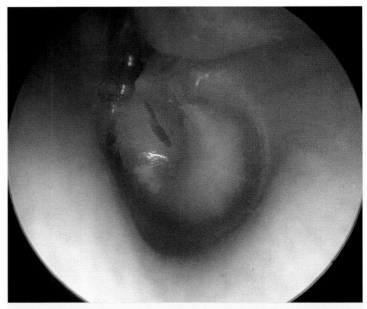

Fig. 13.8 Left ear. Otoscopy 6 months postoperatively in the same patient. The soft mass protruding from above into the external auditory canal has shrunk, indicating progressive atrophy of the herniated tissue left in the attic.

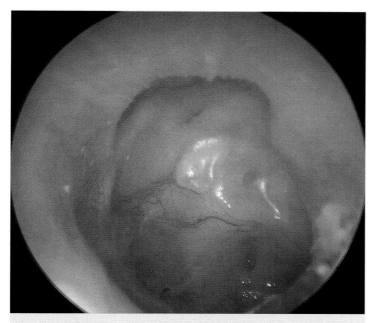

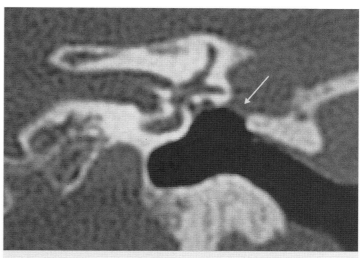

Fig. 13.10 CT scan of the case presented in ► Fig. 13.9.

Fig. 13.9 Left meningoencephalic herniation in a patient who had previously undergone multiple ear surgeries. The only manifestation was conductive hearing loss.

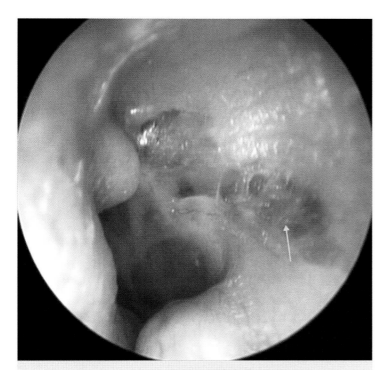

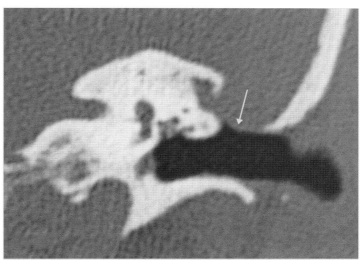

Fig. 13.12 CT scan of the same case. Meningoencephalic herniation is evident at the level of the tegmen antri (*arrow*).

Fig. 13.11 Posttraumatic meningoencephalic herniation in a patient with temporal bone fracture. The fracture line is evident with disruption of the posterior wall of the external auditory canal (*yellow arrow*). A pinkish pulsating retrotympanic mass could be visible in the whole attic (*green arrow*). Exostoses of the inferior and anterior walls of the external auditory canal are also visible. The patient underwent subtotal petrosectomy with obliteration of the middle ear.

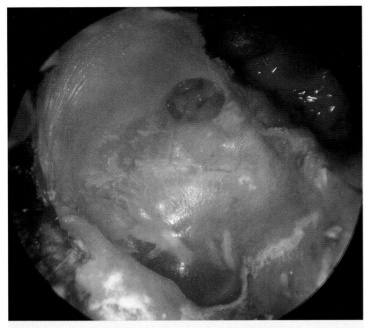

Fig. 13.13 A patient with a history of left open tympanoplasty presenting with conductive hearing loss. Otoscopy demonstrates a badly performed cavity with high facial ridge, secretions, granulations in the posterior wall of the cavity, and an attic defect through which a soft-tissue mass protrudes into the middle ear. A CT scan was performed that confirmed the presence of a meningoencephalic hernia (see subsequent figures).

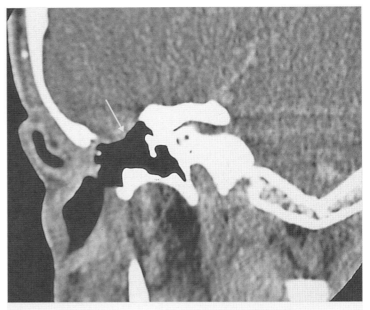

Fig. 13.14 CT scan, coronal view, soft-tissue window of the case presented in ▶ Fig. 13.13 demonstrating the herniating cerebral tissue into the cavity (*arrow*).

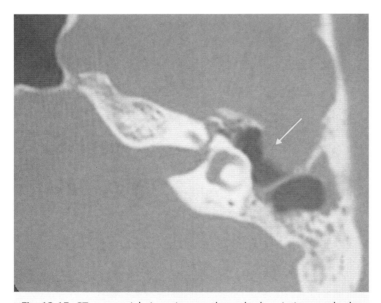

Fig. 13.15 CT scan, axial view. Arrows show the herniating cerebral tissue.

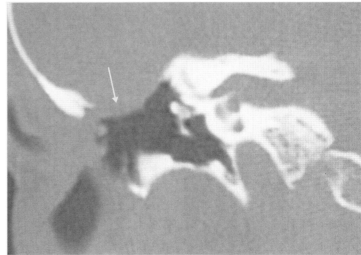

Fig. 13.16 CT scan, coronal view, bone window.

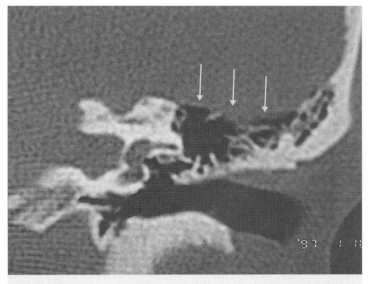

Fig. 13.17 CT scan of a patient with a congenital tegmental defect. This patient has a higher risk of meningitis following an episode of otitis.

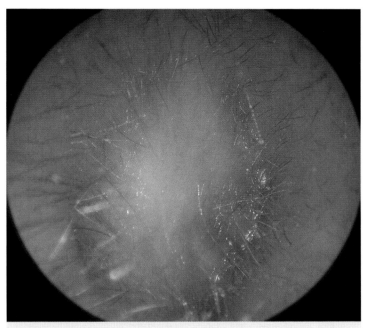

Fig. 13.18 Right ear. Meningoencephalic herniation in a plurioperated patient. The otoscopy shows a new tympanic membrane lateralized by a retrotympanic whitish mass. The patient complained of right ear anacusis and House–Brackmann grade III facial nerve palsy of 1-year duration.

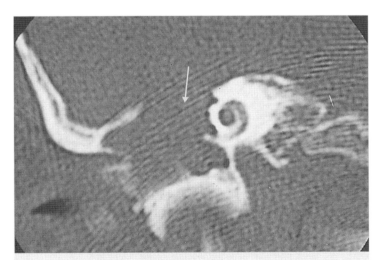

Fig. 13.19 CT scan revealed the presence of a mass occupying the surgical cavity with erosion of the cochlea and absence of the tegmen (*arrow*).

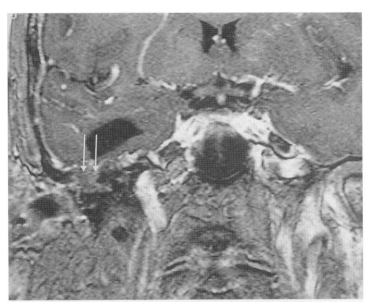

Fig. 13.20 MRI also demonstrated the presence of meningoencephalic herniation (*arrows*). During surgery, the cholesteatoma was confirmed together with a large encephalic herniation.

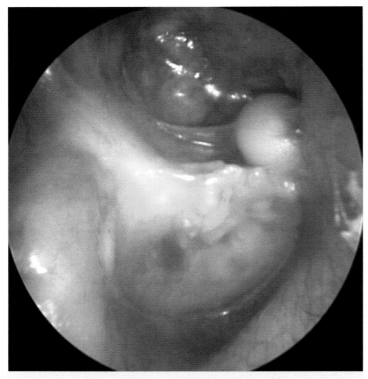

Fig. 13.21 Right ear. Open tympanoplasty. The tympanic membrane is normal. A residual cholesteatoma (pearl) is visible in the anterior attic. A posterosuperior bulging over the cholesteatoma is clearly seen. Iatrogenic meningoencephalic herniation was diagnosed.

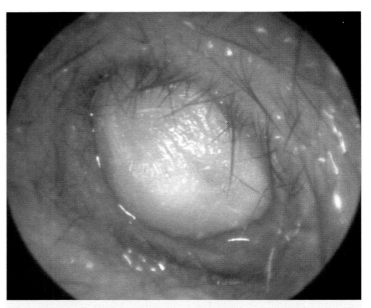

Fig. 13.22 Right ear. There is a pulsating polypoid mass protruding out of the external auditory canal. The patient underwent open tympanoplasty many years back. Cerebrospinal fluid leakage was present at the time of consultation and a meningoencephalic herniation was found on CT and MRI scans. A middle fossa approach was adopted to reduce the herniation.

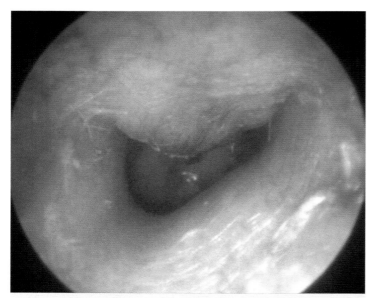

Fig. 13.23 Right posttraumatic meningoencephalic herniation. The superior wall of the external auditory canal is dehiscent. The CT scan showed a transverse fracture of the temporal bone. The patient also had sensorineural hearing loss.

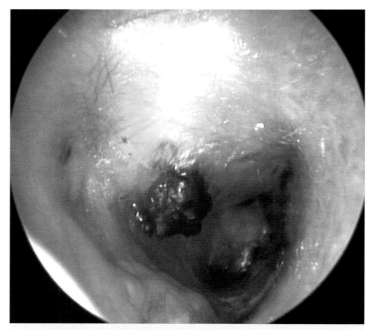

Fig. 13.24 Right ear. Patient with meningoencephalic herniation after a canal wall down tympanoplasty. The patient underwent subtotal petrosectomy with removal even of the residual cholesteatoma.

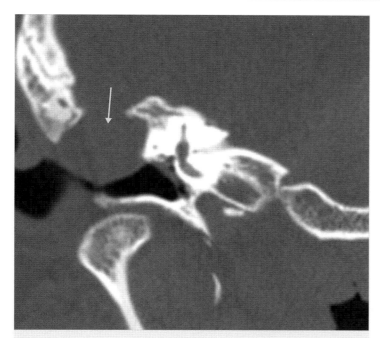

Fig. 13.25 CT scan, coronal view, of the previous case. A wide defect of the tegmen antri is visible, with a clear meningoencephalic herniation in the external auditory canal and in the mastoid cavity (*arrow*).

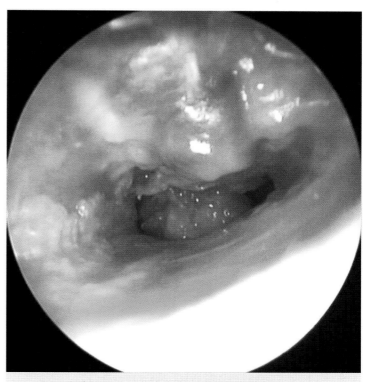

Fig. 13.26 Right ear. Residual cholesteatoma and meningoencephalic herniation. The patient underwent canal wall up tympanoplasty elsewhere 2 years before. Cholesteatoma filling the middle ear cleft is visible, as well as a bulging of the superior canal wall covered by granulation tissue. Even in this case a subtotal petrosectomy was further performed.

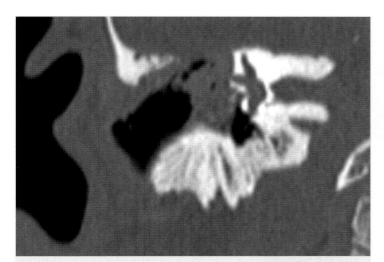

Fig. 13.27 CT scan, coronal view, of the same case. A large defect of the tegmen antri is present even in this case with meningoencephalic herniation and cholesteatoma filling the middle ear and mastoid.

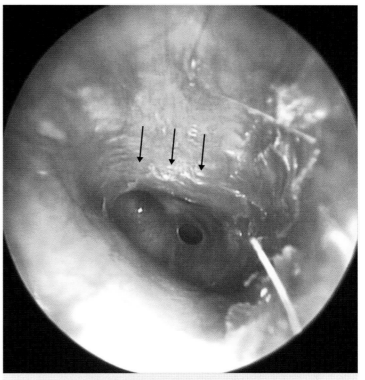

Fig. 13.28 Another case of meningoencephalic herniation in a previous closed tympanoplasty. There is a bulging of the attic corresponding to the herniation (*arrows*). A central perforation of the tympanic membrane is also present. The patient referred an episode of meningitis 6 months before our consultation. A subtotal petrosectomy was performed.

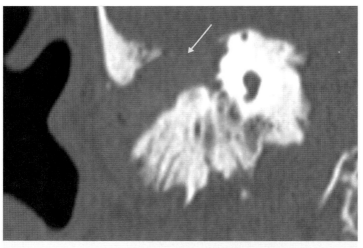

Fig. 13.29 CT scan of the same case, showing the bony defect of the tegmen (*arrow*), with meningoencephalic herniation and residual cholesteatoma.

13.1 Surgical Management

13.1.1 Transmastoid Approach

The surgical management of meningoencephalic herniation through transmastoid approach is shown in ▶ Fig. 13.30, ▶ Fig. 13.31, ▶ Fig. 13.32.

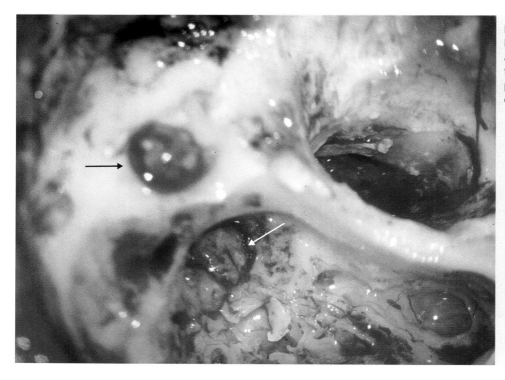

Fig. 13.30 A case of small meningoencephalic herniation repair. Mastoidectomy is performed and the antrum is opened. Scar and granulation tissue (*black arrow*) around the meningoencephalic herniation (*white arrow*) are carefully dissected.

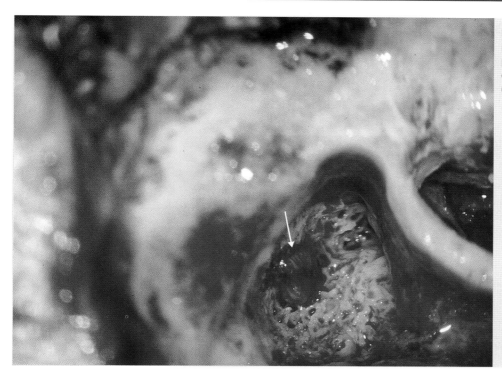

Fig. 13.31 With a bipolar coagulator, the tissue is coagulated and shrunk so that it can be pushed back into the cranium. A bony defect caused by the herniation is seen in the tegmen (*arrow*).

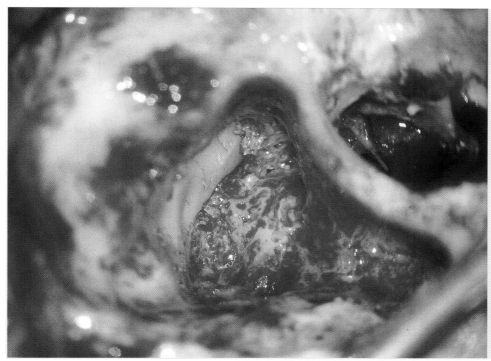

Fig. 13.32 The bony defect is repaired by inserting a thick cartilage between the tegmen and the middle fossa dura. The cartilage is further covered with the temporalis fascia.

13.1.2 Transmastoid Approach with Minicraniotomy

This surgical approach is shown in ▶ Fig. 13.33, ▶ Fig. 13.34, ▶ Fig. 13.35.

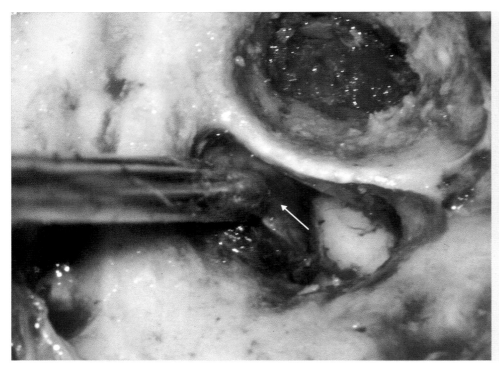

Fig. 13.33 A case of medium-size meningoencephalic herniation repair. Herniated tissue from the tegmen is seen in the antrum (*arrow*). Superiorly, the middle fossa dura just superior to the skull base is identified and the bone covering the dura is thinned, taking care not to damage the dura.

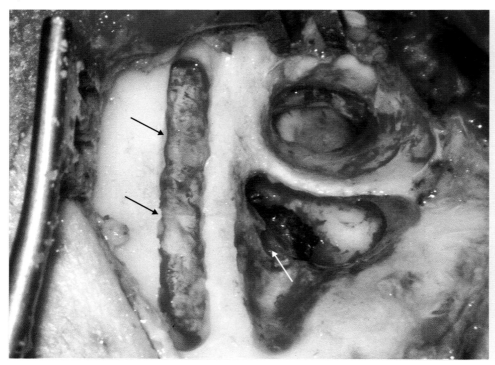

Fig. 13.34 The herniated brain tissue is coagulated and shrunk with a bipolar coagulator. A minicraniotomy in the middle fossa dura is accomplished by removing the cortical bone with a burr. The exposed middle fossa dura is seen (*arrows*).

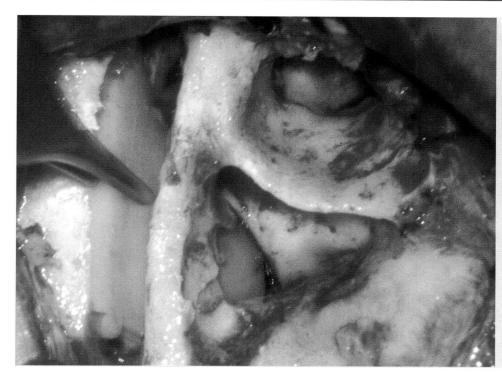

Fig. 13.35 From the minicraniotomy, a thick piece of cartilage that covers the bony defect with sufficient extension is inserted between the middle fossa plate and the dura. A large piece of temporalis fascia used to cover the bony defect is inserted between the cartilage and the middle fossa plate.

13.1.3 Subtotal Petrosectomy

This surgical approach is shown in ▶ Fig. 13.36, ▶ Fig. 13.37, ▶ Fig. 13.38, ▶ Fig. 13.39, ▶ Fig. 13.40, ▶ Fig. 13.41, ▶ Fig. 13.42, ▶ Fig. 13.43, ▶ Fig. 13.44, ▶ Fig. 13.45.

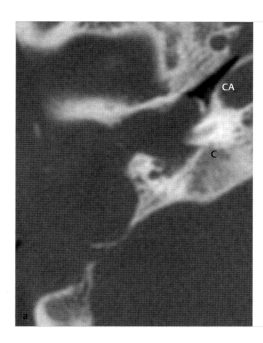
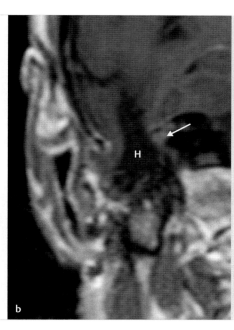

Fig. 13.36 The patient underwent middle ear surgery, which was followed by progressive hearing loss complicated by intractable otorrhea. Otoscopic examination showed a pinkish pulsating mass in the external auditory canal. Radiological examination revealed meningoencephalic herniation in the middle ear. In the axial CT **(a)**, a large amount of soft tissue with smooth border is seen. The coronal MRI **(b)** shows herniation of the brain tissue into the middle ear from the defect in the middle fossa plate (*arrow*). C, cochlea; CA, carotid artery; H, herniated tissue.

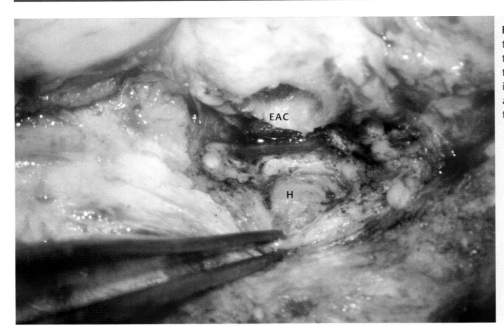

Fig. 13.37 A retroauricular incision is made and the musculoperiosteal layer covering the area of the mastoid is exposed. A circumferential cut at this level exposes meningoencephalic herniation in the external auditory canal. EAC, external auditory canal; H, meningoencephalic herniation.

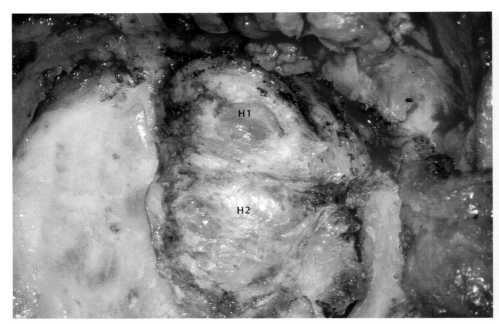

Fig. 13.38 Blind sac closure of the external auditory canal is conducted, and the musculoperiosteal layer is elevated to expose the large herniated tissue occupying the mastoid cavity. H1, herniation in the external auditory canal; H2, herniation in the mastoid.

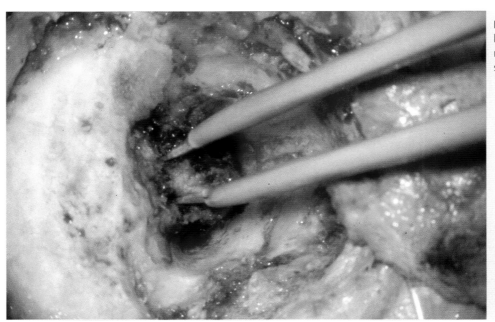

Fig. 13.39 The herniation is coagulated with the bipolar coagulator. The procedure shrinks herniated tissue and facilitates dissection from the surrounding structures.

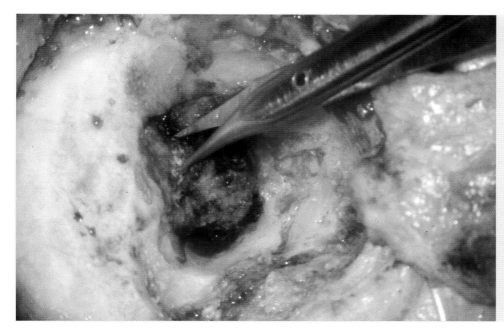

Fig. 13.40 The coagulated tissue is cut with scissors in piecemeal fashion.

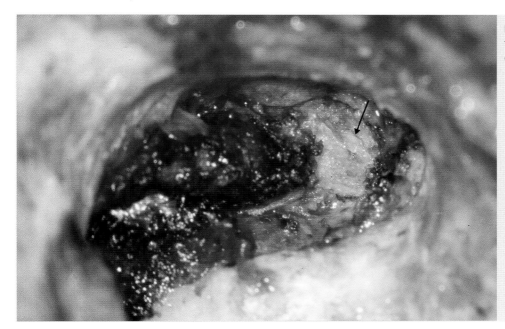

Fig. 13.41 Medially to the herniation in the tympanic cavity, entrapped skin has formed cholesteatoma (*arrow*).

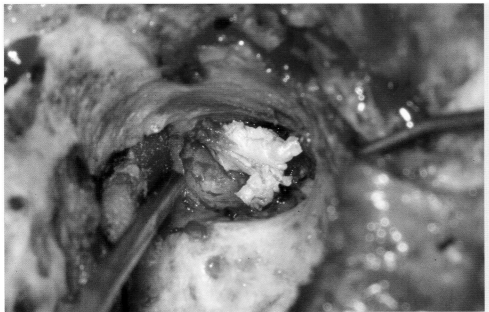

Fig. 13.42 The cholesteatoma is dissected from the tympanic cavity.

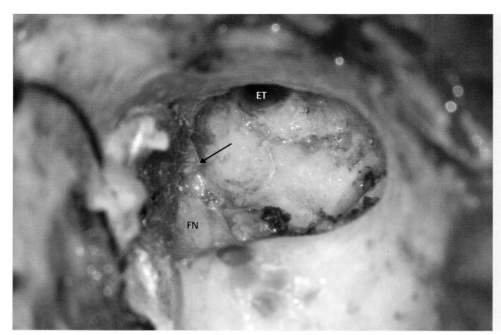

Fig. 13.43 All the skin and herniated tissue have been eradicated from the middle ear. The exposed facial nerve is seen running just superiorly to the cochleariform process (*arrow*). ET, Eustachian tube; FN, facial nerve.

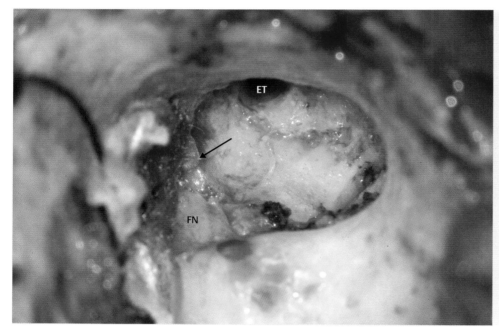

Fig. 13.44 The Eustachian tube is obliterated with pieces of periosteum. Fibrin glue is applied to ensure closure in this case.

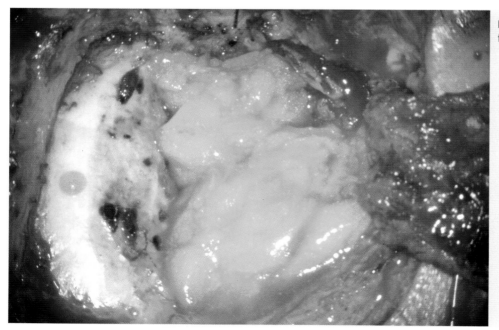

Fig. 13.45 The cavity is packed with abdominal fat.

Table 13.1 Gruppo Otologico published data on management of meningoencephalic herniation of the temporal bone (133 cases, 1984–2006)

Etiology/surgical approach	Etiology and surgical approach for meningoencephalic herniation			
	Transmastoid	Transmastoid with minicraniotomy	Middle cranial fossa	Subtotal petrosectomy
Spontaneous	3	1	21	8
Chronic otitis media with or without cholesteatoma	15	1	1	12
Iatrogenic	17	1	9	34
Traumatic	2	1	6	1
Total	37	4	37	55

Summary

Herniation of the meningeal and/or encephalic tissue into the middle ear space is a rare condition occurring most frequently postsurgically, spontaneously due to congenital defects, postinfection, and posttrauma. For herniation to occur, a bony defect should be present. Through this dehiscence, a meningocele, an encephalocele, or both can occur. The most appropriate term seems to be *meningoencephalic herniation*.

The condition can lead to serious sequelae such as CSF leak, meningitis, epilepsy, and aphasia. Therefore, once diagnosed, surgical correction should be performed. The herniated tissue is usually resected and the defect is reconstructed. The surgical approach is determined by the size of the defect. Small defects are managed using a transmastoid approach. In middle- and large-sized hernias and unserviceable hearing, a subtotal petrosectomy is the treatment of choice. The herniated part is left inside the middle ear or mastoid where it acts as a barrier against infection of the intracranial space. The external auditory canal is closed as a cul de sac, the Eustachian tube is sealed with periosteum and bone wax, and the surgical cavity is obliterated with abdominal fat. This avoids possible sources of infection from the external environment or from the nasal cavity.

A transmastoid approach combined with a craniotomy or a middle fossa approach can be also used for patients with normal hearing and medium- to large-sized defects.

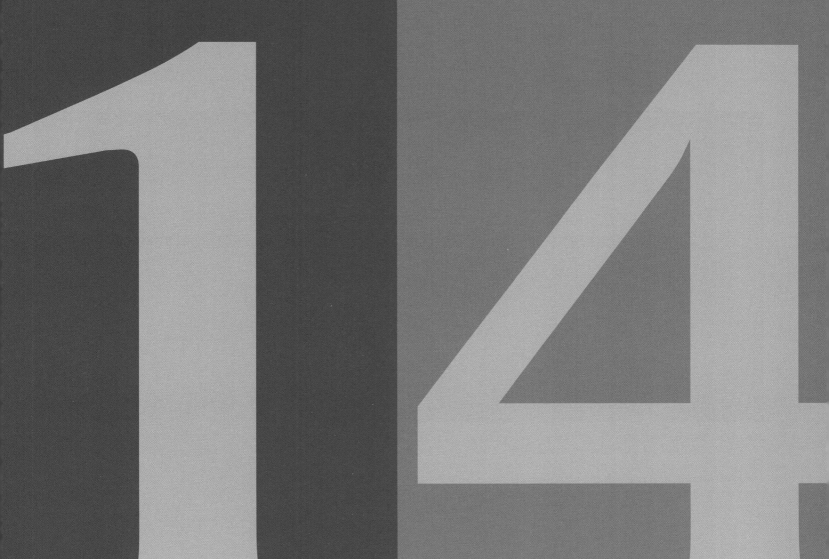

14 Postsurgical Conditions

Abstract

This chapter will show the most common postsurgical conditions, differentiating cases with normal postoperative healing and those with recurring pathology and/or immediate and late postoperative complications.

Keywords: myringotomy, ventilation tube, stapes surgery, myringoplasty, tympanoplasty, meatoplasty, blind-sac closure of the external auditory canal, hearing implants

As seen in the previous chapters, some otoscopic views may be difficult to interpret. This difficulty increases in cases involving previous surgery because of the distortion of the normal anatomy. The examiner should be competent and experienced enough to distinguish between cases with normal postoperative healing and those with recurring pathology and/or immediate and late postoperative complications. In this chapter, postoperative otoscopic views with and without complications and/or recurrence are presented.

14.1 Myringotomy and Insertion of Ventilation Tube

The indications of myringotomy and ventilation tube insertion have been discussed previously. Myringotomy is usually performed in the anteroinferior quadrant of the tympanic membrane in the region of the cone of light. The incision is made in a radial direction using a myringotomy knife. In cases with a hump of the anterior wall of the external auditory canal, myringotomy can be performed immediately inferior to the umbo in the posteroinferior quadrant. The incision should never be made in the posterosuperior quadrant to avoid injury to the ossicular chain. The operation is performed under general anesthesia in children. In adults, however, local anesthesia is sufficient.

After making a radial incision of the tympanic membrane, the middle ear effusion is aspirated and the ventilation tube is inserted. In the majority of cases, hearing improves immediately.

The patient is instructed to avoid water entering the ear by blocking it with cotton anointed with petrolatum when taking a shower or with rubber earplugs when swimming. Infection could occur if water were to enter the middle ear through the ventilation tube. Should this occur, ear lavage with a disinfectant solution consisting of 2% boric acid in 70% alcohol is indicated.

When the tube is obstructed by cerumen or crusts, the administration of hydrogen peroxide drops is usually sufficient to restore its patency. There are many types of commercially available ventilation tubes, but they can be generally grouped into short- and long-term tubes. Tubes with a larger inner flange usually remain in place longer. Once extruded, the myringotomy site closes spontaneously in approximately 98% of cases.

Refer to ▸ Fig. 14.1, ▸ Fig. 14.2, ▸ Fig. 14.3, ▸ Fig. 14.4, ▸ Fig. 14.5, ▸ Fig. 14.6, ▸ Fig. 14.7, ▸ Fig. 14.8, ▸ Fig. 14.9, ▸ Fig. 14.10, ▸ Fig. 14.11, ▸ Fig. 14.12, ▸ Fig. 14.13, ▸ Fig. 14.14, ▸ Fig. 14.15, ▸ Fig. 14.16.

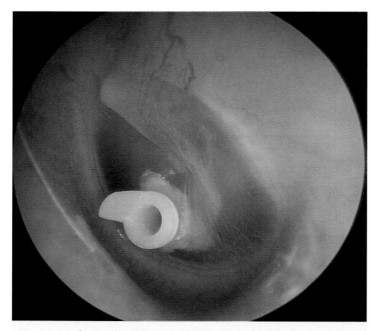

Fig. 14.1 Left ear. The Sultan ventilation tube. This type has two small wings: an outer one with which the tube can be held using the ear forceps and an inner one, viewed through the tympanic membrane, which facilitates tube insertion and prevents rapid extrusion. If properly inserted, the Sultan ventilation tube can remain for approximately 6 to 18 months before extrusion.

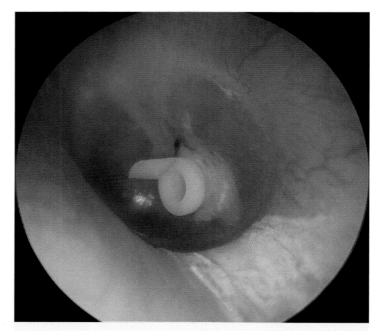

Fig. 14.2 Left ear. In this case, the tube has been placed inferior to the umbo due to the presence of an anterior hump in the anterior canal wall.

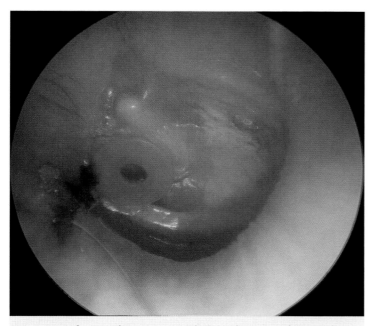

Fig. 14.3 Left ear. A long-term ventilation tube inserted 6 months after tympanoplasty because of an observed tendency for graft retraction. The graft is seen in an optimal condition with no evidence of retraction, indicating patency of the ventilation tube. This tube has been in situ for more than 10 years.

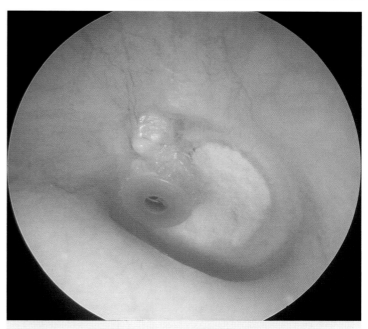

Fig. 14.4 Left ear. Long-term ventilation tube. A large tympanosclerotic plaque that formed 1 year after the tube insertion can be clearly seen. Such plaques result from hemorrhagic infiltrate between the epidermal and fibrous layers of the tympanic membrane secondary to the myringotomy and are asymptomatic.

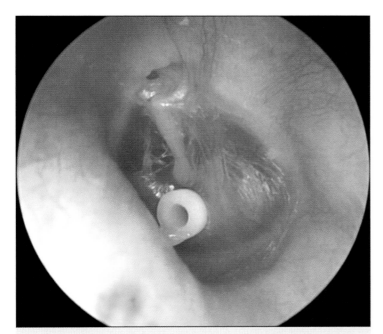

Fig. 14.5 Left ear. Sultan ventilation tube placed in the anteroinferior quadrant. Anterior hump of the external auditory canal is visible.

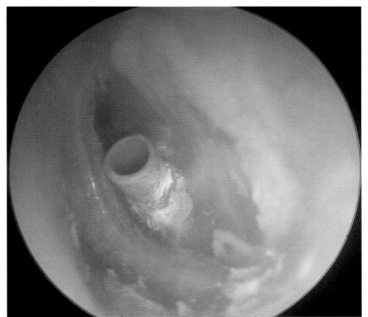

Fig. 14.6 Left ear. Example of a long-term "T" tube inserted in the anteroinferior quadrant of the tympanic membrane. After its insertion, the two wings of the tube open by virtue of their retained "memory," thereby preventing tube extrusion.

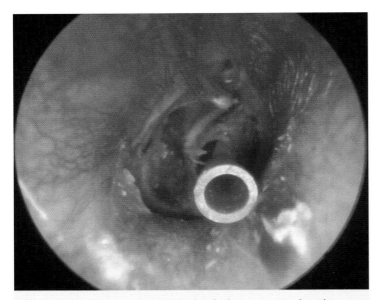

Fig. 14.7 Right ear. Another example of a long-term T tube. This type of tube unfortunately very often causes perforation of the tympanic membrane.

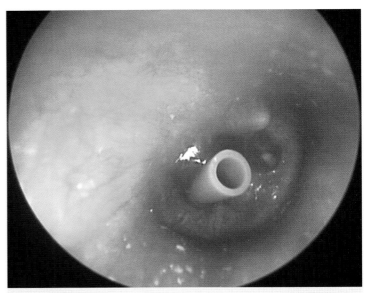

Fig. 14.8 Right ear. Long-term T tube placed in the posteroinferior quadrant.

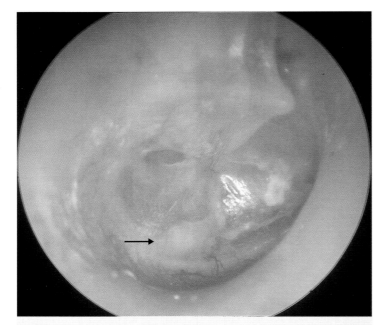

Fig. 14.9 Right ear. The consequences of a misplaced ventilation tube is shown. A healed myringotomy is seen in the posterosuperior quadrant (at 9 o'clock position). Two months later, the tube was extruded. During tube insertion, however, dislocation of the incus occurred. The dislocated incus fell to the hypotympanum where its body and short process can be clearly seen (*arrow*). In the anteroinferior quadrant, immediately under the umbo, another healed myringotomy site (this time correctly placed) is visible. In the latter, tube extrusion occurred 1 year late.

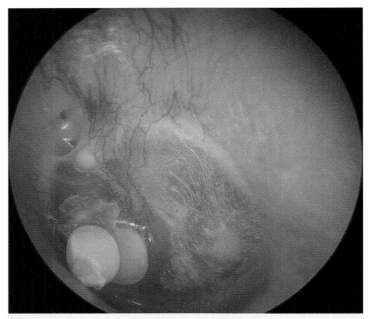

Fig. 14.10 Left ear. A ventilation tube in the process of extrusion. It is preferable not to take out the tube but rather wait for self-extrusion to occur. Closure of the myringotomy site occurs in approximately 98% of cases.

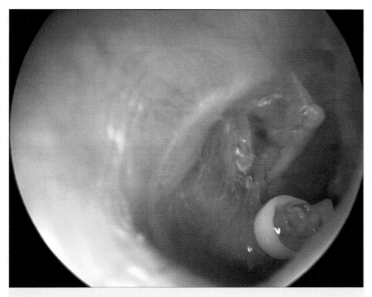

Fig. 14.11 Right ear. Sultan ventilation tube placed in the anteroinferior quadrant. The tube is blocked by cholesteatoma squamae. During myringotomy it is of utmost importance not to introduce skin inside the middle ear, thus avoiding the formation of an iatrogenic cholesteatoma.

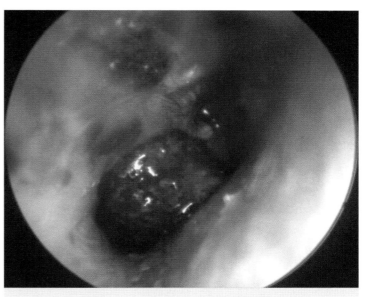

Fig. 14.12 Right ear. Granulation tissue after ventilation tube insertion. This complication is generally resolved with removal of the tube.

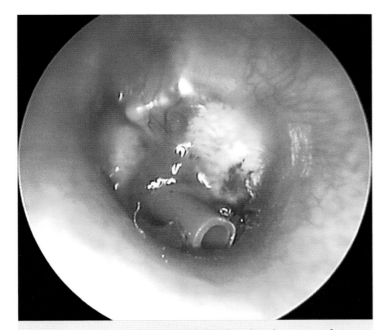

Fig. 14.13 Right ear. Long-term T tube placed in the anteroinferior quadrant. Infection with otorrhea and granulation tissue are present. Local antibiotics and steroids are sufficient for the healing.

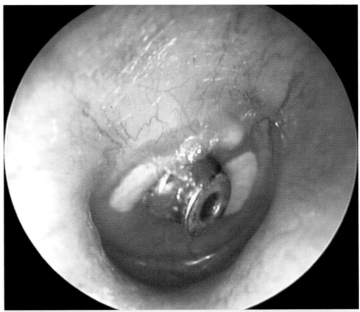

Fig. 14.14 Right ear. Partially extruded titanium tube. The ventilation tube has been placed in the area of the handle of the malleus. Ventilation tubes should be always placed away from the ossicles, thus avoiding injury of the ossicular chain and subsequent hearing loss.

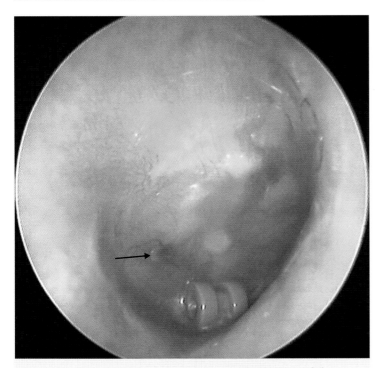

Fig. 14.15 Right ear. Extruded ventilation tube. The area of the previous myringotomy is visible as a scar in the posteroinferior quadrant (*arrow*).

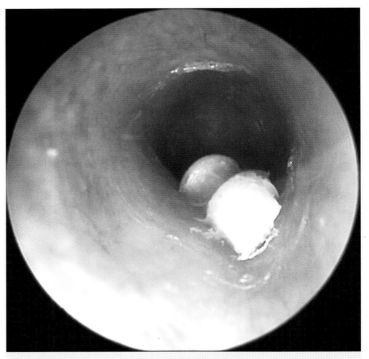

Fig. 14.16 Left ear. Extruded ventilation tube in the external auditory canal.

14.2 Stapes Surgery

Stapes surgery is performed when the footplate of the stapes is fixed in the oval window (i.e., in otosclerosis). This surgery is probably the finest otological procedure, requiring very delicate manipulation of instruments in a very narrow area with important structures all around.

It should be done only by experienced surgeons performing this procedure routinely. Occasional surgery should be avoided because miscarriage of the procedure may cost the hearing of the operated ear, and contralateral hearing is frequently abnormal.

Whenever possible, we perform stapedotomy as primary stapes surgery as it offers a calibrated hole in the footplate to stabilize both ends of the prosthesis. Compared with stapedectomy, the procedure also offers less trauma to the oval window and less possibility of damaging the inner ear. In addition, revision surgery, if required, is easier due to preserved anatomy.

Refer to ▶ Fig. 14.17, ▶ Fig. 14.18, ▶ Fig. 14.19, ▶ Fig. 14.20, ▶ Fig. 14.21, ▶ Fig. 14.22, ▶ Fig. 14.23, ▶ Fig. 14.24, ▶ Fig. 14.25, ▶ Fig. 14.26, ▶ Fig. 14.27.

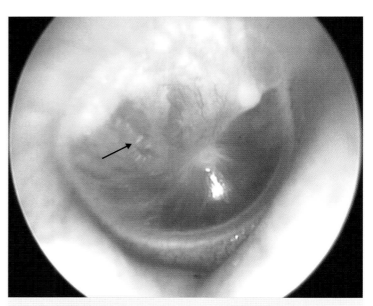

Fig. 14.17 Right ear. Schwartze's sign (*arrow*) is typical of otosclerosis, even if present in less than 10% of patients. This rosy glow visible through the tympanic membrane is due to vascular hyperemia of immature abnormal bone produced during the otosclerotic process.

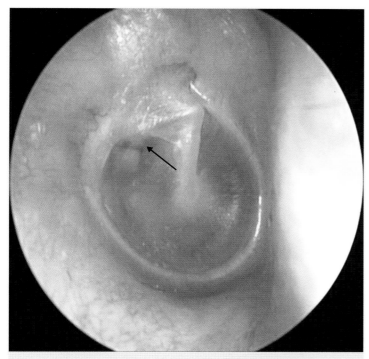

Fig. 14.18 Right ear. Otoscopy after stapedotomy. A small atticotomy is visible. The loop of the prosthesis has been correctly tightened all around the long process of the incus (*arrow*).

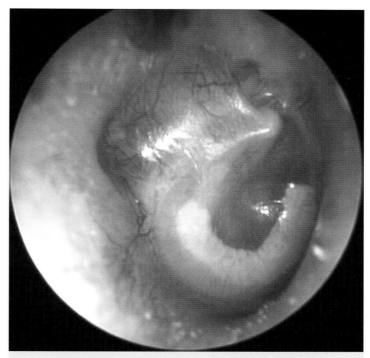

Fig. 14.19 Right ear. Otoscopy after stapedotomy. In this case, atticotomy is wider than that in ▶ Fig. 14.17, but no tympanic retraction occurred. The loop of the prosthesis is firmly fixed on the long process of the incus.

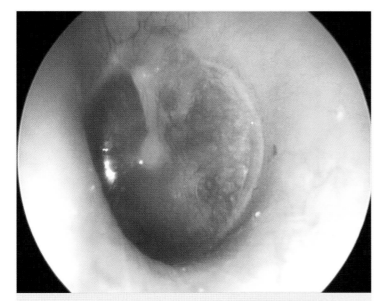

Fig. 14.20 Left ear. Another case of well-performed atticotomy for stapes surgery.

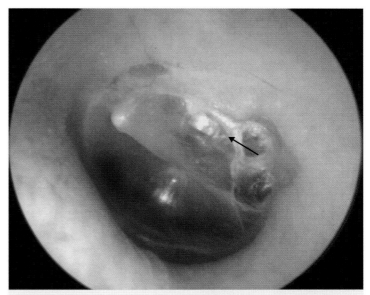

Fig. 14.21 Left ear. Otoscopy view after stapedotomy. The atticotomy is visible; the prosthesis, dislocated from the incus, has adhered to the tympanic membrane (*arrow*).

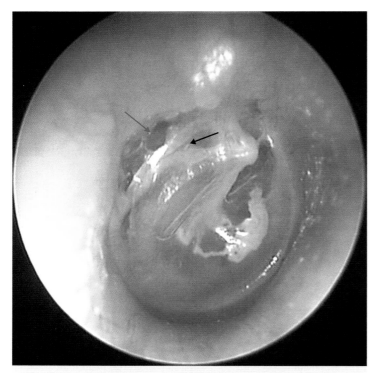

Fig. 14.22 Right ear. Otoscopy view after stapedotomy. A small retraction in the area of the atticotomy is visible (*red arrow*). Even in this case, the prosthesis, dislocated from the incus, has adhered to the tympanic membrane (*black arrow*).

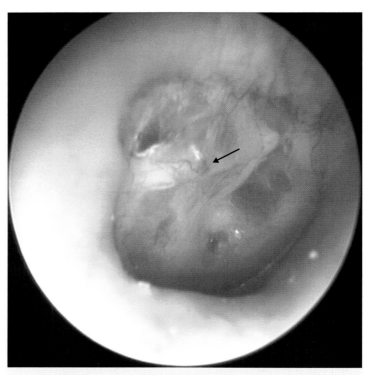

Fig. 14.23 Right ear. Otoscopy view after stapedotomy. The prosthesis is about to dislocate from the long process of the incus (*arrow*). The loop is loose, resulting in persistence of conductive hearing loss.

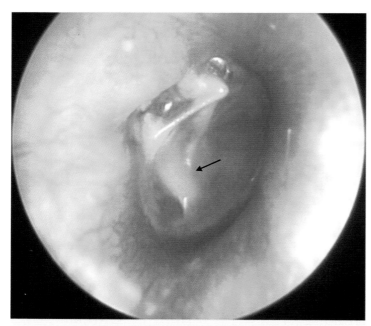

Fig. 14.24 Right ear. Dislocation of a Causse (Teflon) prosthesis (*arrow*) in a patient who underwent stapedotomy.

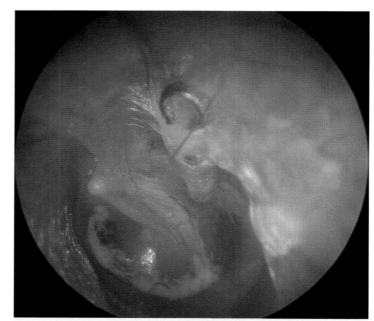

Fig. 14.25 Left ear. A rare case of extrusion of a stapes prosthesis. The metallic ring is seen extruding through a microperforation covered with epidermal squames. The Teflon shaft of the prosthesis can be visualized through the tympanic membrane.

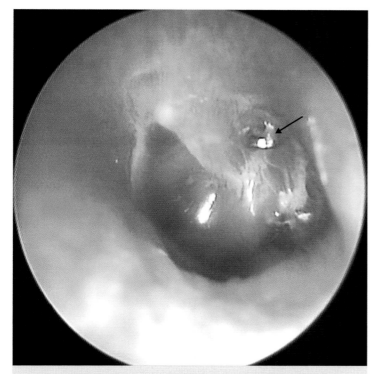

Fig. 14.26 Left ear. This 41-year-old woman underwent bilateral stapedotomy for otosclerosis elsewhere. After 2 years from the last surgery, she developed bilateral conductive hearing loss. On the left side, the prosthesis is clearly extruding for the middle ear (*arrow*).

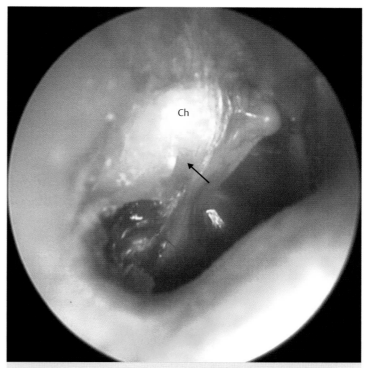

Fig. 14.27 Right ear. Same case. A clear iatrogenic cholesteatoma (Ch) is visible in the posterosuperior quadrant. The prosthesis (*black arrow*) is partially dislocated. A retraction pocket is present in the posteroinferior quadrant (*red arrow*). The patient underwent removal of the cholesteatoma through an endocanalar approach. A second-stage operation has been planned after 8 months.

14.3 Myringoplasty

The aim of reconstructing a tympanic membrane perforation is twofold: first, to allow the patient to have a normal social life with no restrictions, even regarding water entry into the ear, and second, to correct the hearing loss resulting from the perforation.

There are essentially two techniques for myringoplasty. The underlay technique is utilized in the presence of an anterior residue (at least the annulus) of the tympanic membrane, under which the graft can be placed. In the absence of any anterior residue of the membrane, the overlay technique is used. In such cases, the graft is positioned against the anterior wall of the external auditory canal.

Normally, the tympanic membrane forms an acute angle with the anterior wall of the external auditory canal. While performing myringoplasty, it is generally possible to respect this angulation when the annulus is present anteriorly.

The myringoplasty operation is considered a success when the reconstructed tympanic membrane is intact, is well epithelialized, and has normal angulation with the external auditory canal.

These characteristics allow the patient to have a normal social life (hearing improvement and possibility of water entry into the ear). Reperforation is a frequent complication of myringoplasty that occurs in approximately 5 to 10% of cases in the best series. Reperforation occurs more commonly in the underlay technique, particularly in the anterior quadrant where the graft is detached from the anterior residues of the tympanic membrane and falls into the middle ear. When an overlay technique is utilized, blunting of the anterior angle can occur with resultant conductive hearing loss. Lateralization, in which the graft is detached from the handle of the malleus, is another possible complication that leads to conductive hearing loss. It occurs mostly when the graft is placed lateral rather than medial to the handle of the malleus. Stenosis of the external auditory canal, either due to inflammatory reaction or as a result of bad repositioning of the meatal flaps, can also occur.

Refer to ▶ Fig. 14.28, ▶ Fig. 14.29, ▶ Fig. 14.30, ▶ Fig. 14.31, ▶ Fig. 14.32, ▶ Fig. 14.33, ▶ Fig. 14.34, ▶ Fig. 14.35, ▶ Fig. 14.36, ▶ Fig. 14.37, ▶ Fig. 14.38, ▶ Fig. 14.39, ▶ Fig. 14.40, ▶ Fig. 14.41.

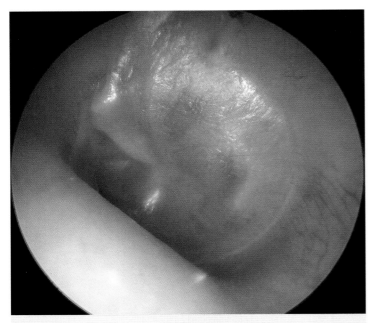

Fig. 14.28 Left ear. Normal aspect of the reconstructed tympanic membrane. The posterior quadrant is slightly elevated. In this case, a posterior perforation was grafted with temporalis fascia using an underlay technique.

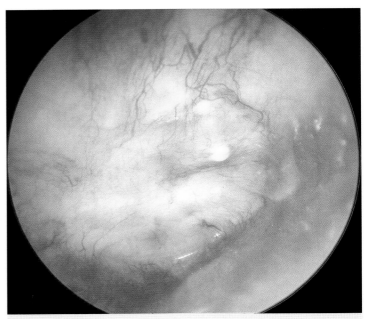

Fig. 14.29 Right ear. Myringoplasty with an underlay technique. The reconstructed tympanic membrane is thicker than normal. The anterior angle is maintained. The handle of the malleus is clearly visible except for the umbo, which is detached from the membrane. Tympanosclerotic plaques are also visible.

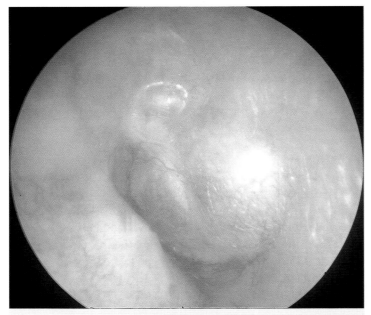

Fig. 14.30 Left ear. Another example of a tympanic membrane perforation that was repaired using an underlay technique with preservation of the anterior residue. The posterior quadrants are slightly lateralized, making it difficult to see the handle of the malleus.

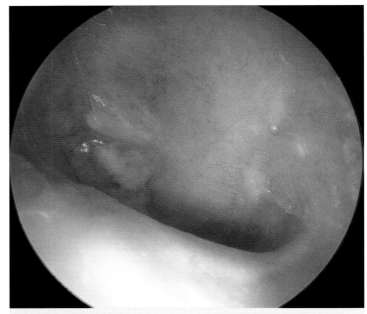

Fig. 14.31 Left ear. Similar case. The repaired tympanic membrane is well attached to the malleus except for the area of the umbo due to lateralization of the posteroinferior quadrant.

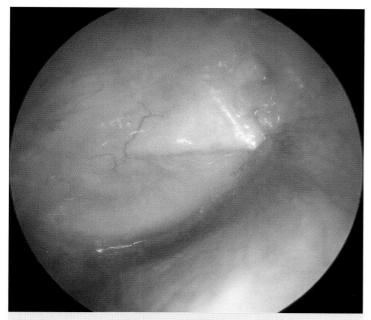

Fig. 14.32 Right ear. Underlay myringoplasty. The malleus is slightly medialized. The repaired tympanic membrane is whitish in its anterior quadrants and vascularized in the posterior ones. The anterior angle is normal.

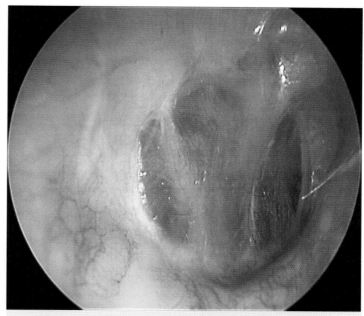

Fig. 14.33 Right ear. Underlay myringoplasty for a posterior perforation. The anterior angle is perfectly normal, as the thickness of the membrane.

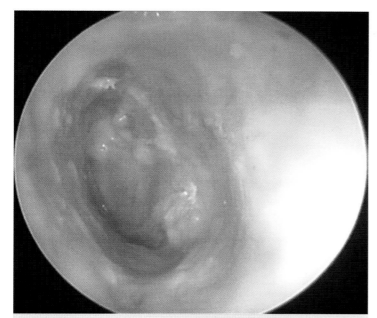

Fig. 14.34 Left ear. Another case of underlay myringoplasty for a posterior perforation. This image has been taken immediately after removal of the postoperative ear plugging (Gelfoam), approximately 30 days after surgery. The repaired tympanic membrane retains its normal position, with a perfect anterior angle.

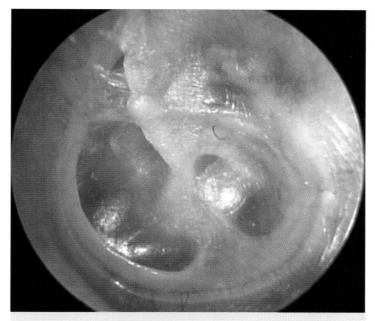

Fig. 14.35 Left ear. Underlay myringoplasty. The tympanic membrane is thicker on its posterior quadrants. A retraction of the anterior quadrants is also present. However, hearing function is normal.

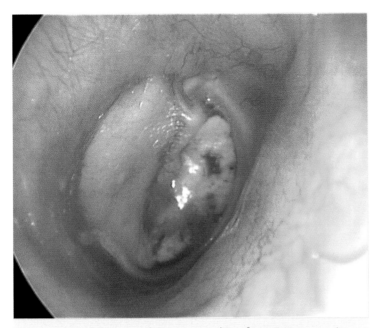

Fig. 14.36 Right ear. Cartilage myringoplasty for a mesotympanic retraction of the posterior quadrants with perforation (Grade V of Sadè classification). No epithelialization was found in the middle ear. Incus was not eroded. Cartilage could be useful in cases like this to reinforce the tympanic membrane, avoiding further retractions. Myringosclerosis of the anterior quadrants is also visible.

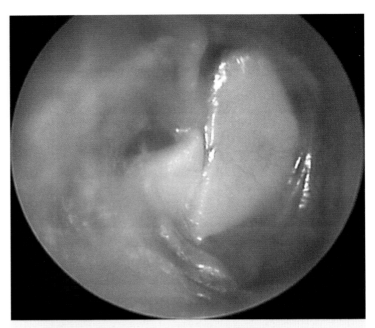

Fig. 14.37 Right ear. Revision myringoplasty with cartilage for subtotal perforation of the tympanic membrane. The use of cartilage avoids further reperforations in revision cases. Sometimes, sensation of fullness could be referred by the patient, even in case of complete closure of the air–bone gap.

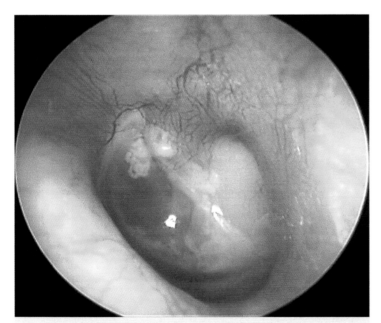

Fig. 14.38 Left ear. A case similar to that in ▶ Fig. 14.35.

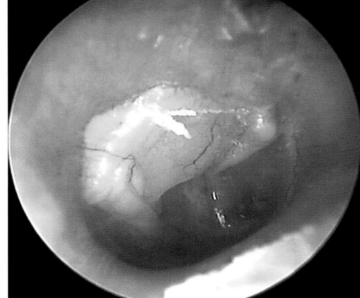

Fig. 14.39 Right ear. Myringoplasty for a posterosuperior retraction pocket without cholesteatoma. The long process of the incus was absent, resulting in conductive hearing loss. A thick piece of cartilage was put directly over the stapes, resulting in complete closure of the air–bone gap.

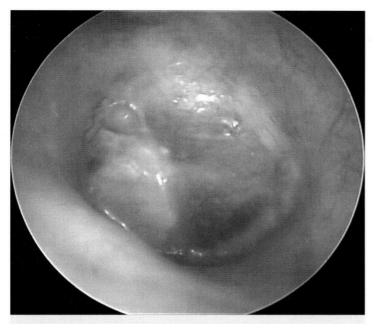

Fig. 14.40 Underlay myringoplasty for perforation of the anterior quadrants. A piece of cartilage was used to avoid anterior reperforation.

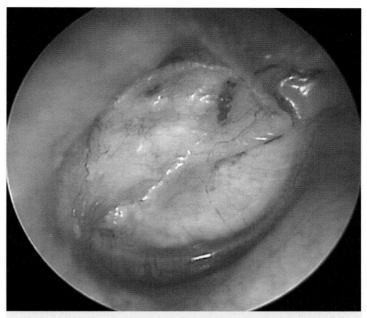

Fig. 14.41 Right ear. Myringoplasty with an underlay technique. The reconstructed membrane is thicker than normal, with a tympanosclerotic appearance. The anterior angle is maintained.

14.3.1 Failures and Complications

Refer to ▶ Fig. 14.42, ▶ Fig. 14.43, ▶ Fig. 14.44, ▶ Fig. 14.45, ▶ Fig. 14.46, ▶ Fig. 14.47, ▶ Fig. 14.48, ▶ Fig. 14.49, ▶ Fig. 14.50, ▶ Fig. 14.51, ▶ Fig. 14.52, ▶ Fig. 14.53, ▶ Fig. 14.54, ▶ Fig. 14.55, ▶ Fig. 14.56, ▶ Fig. 14.57.

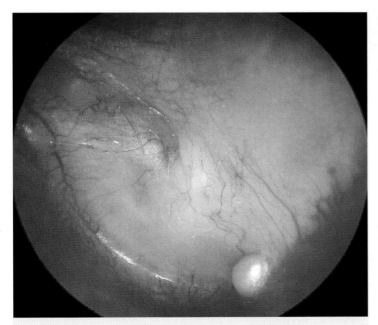

Fig. 14.42 Left ear. The repaired tympanic membrane retains a normal anterior angle and is well vascularized, though thicker than normal. A small cholesteatomatous pearl is observed. This pearl can be easily removed in the outpatient clinic under the microscope.

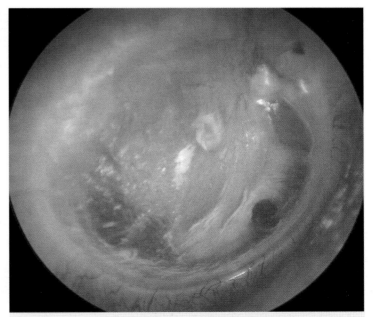

Fig. 14.43 Right ear. The repaired tympanic membrane has normal thickness. The short process of the malleus can be observed, although the handle is not visible due to lateralization.

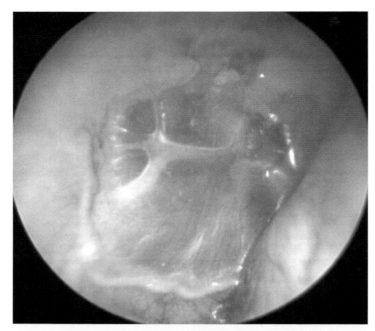

Fig. 14.44 Right ear. Even in this case the repaired tympanic membrane has normal thickness, but the graft is detached from the handle of the malleus.

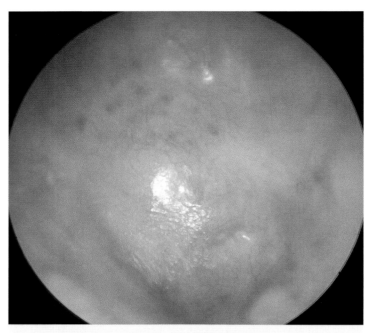

Fig. 14.45 The external auditory canal is wide but the repaired tympanic membrane is lateralized and shows blunting.

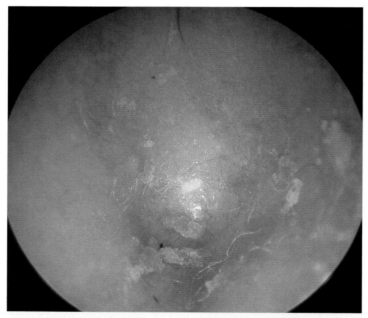

Fig. 14.46 Similar case. The reconstructed tympanic membrane is lateralized with marked blunting of the anterior angle.

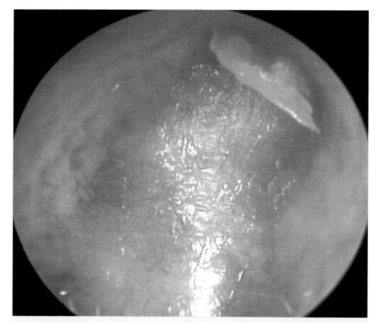

Fig. 14.47 Another case of lateralization of the reconstructed tympanic membrane with marked blunting of the anterior angle. Further revision has a high rate of failure.

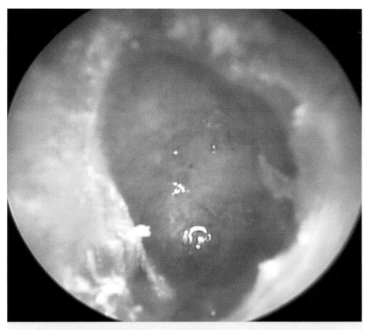

Fig. 14.48 Lateralization of the reconstructed tympanic membrane with initial stenosis of the external auditory canal.

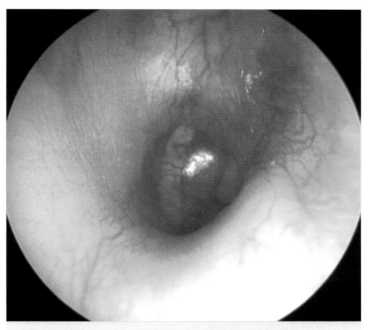

Fig. 14.49 Lateralization of the reconstructed tympanic membrane in an 8-year-old male patient. The posterior annulus is completely detached from the bony wall. The external auditory canal has not been calibrated during myringoplasty, so the anteroinferior quadrant is not completely under view. Middle ear effusion is also present (note the air bubble in the inferior quadrant).

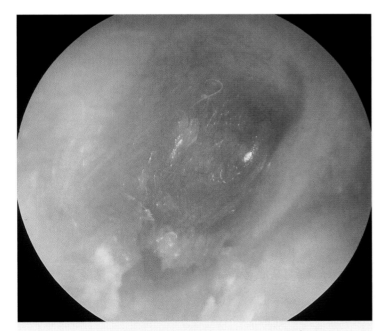

Fig. 14.50 Postoperative myringitis. The tympanic membrane is hyperemic, thickened, and lateralized following a tympanoplasty. The epidermal layer is substituted by granulation tissue. Myringitis is a rare complication that usually resolves with local steroid applications. In very rare cases, reoperation is necessary. The pathological tympanic membrane is removed followed by grafting.

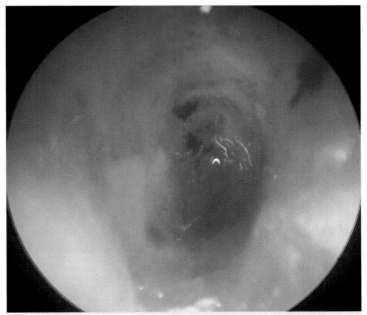

Fig. 14.51 A patient who has undergone quadruple myringoplasty. In these cases, myringitis and canal stenosis are frequent; therefore, it is necessary to remove the pathological tissues, perform canalplasty, and use free skin flaps.

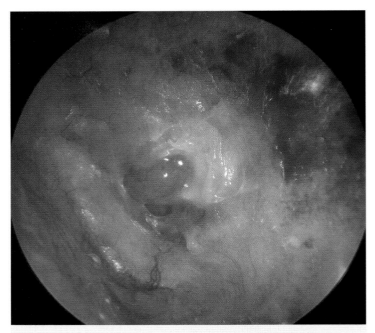

Fig. 14.52 Left ear. Reperforation of the tympanic membrane with granulations near the perforation. In such cases, curettage of the granulation and freshening of the edges under the microscope may lead to spontaneous closure of the perforation.

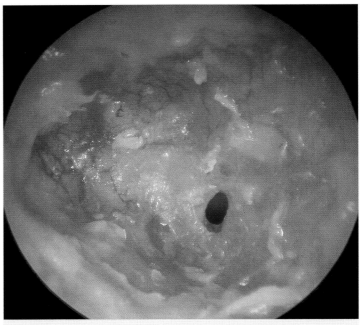

Fig. 14.53 Reperforation of the tympanic membrane. Myringitis with otorrhea can be appreciated. Lavage and freshening of the perforation edges as well as insertion of Gelfoam (in the middle ear) can favor spontaneous closure of the perforation.

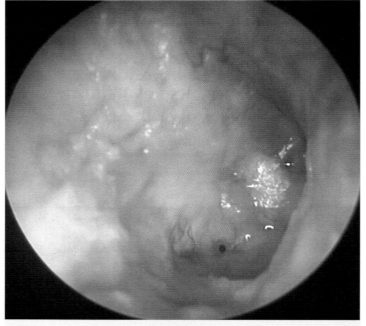

Fig. 14.54 Small reperforation of the tympanic membrane during an acute attack of otitis media. Otorrhea is also present. Local therapy (lavage and antibiotic drops) as well as nasal decongestants and oral antibiotics are helpful for the healing process. In this case, the perforation could close spontaneously.

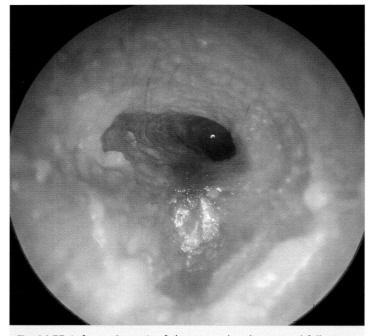

Fig. 14.55 Left ear. Stenosis of the external auditory canal following myringoplasty.

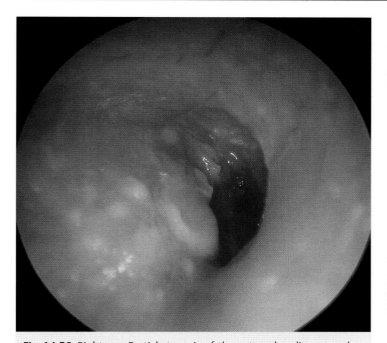

Fig. 14.56 Right ear. Partial stenosis of the external auditory canal following myringoplasty. For the management of this complication, it is usually sufficient to incise the skin of the canal and insert a plastic sheet for approximately 20 days, while using local medication of steroid lotion.

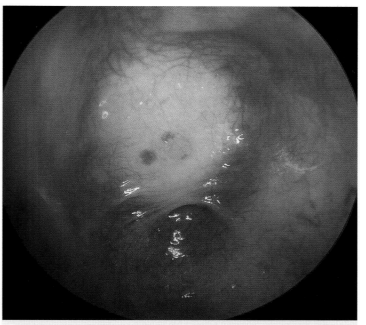

Fig. 14.57 Retrotympanic cholesteatoma following myringoplasty. This iatrogenic cholesteatoma can be explained by the entrapment of epidermal residues in the middle ear or malpositioning of the meatal flap at the level of the anterior angle. It can be managed by incision of the cholesteatoma sac, aspiration of its contents, and insertion of a plastic sheet in the external auditory canal for approximately 20 days to favor healing.

14.4 Tympanoplasty

Tympanoplasty operations can be classified into those without mastoidectomy, performed with chronic otitis media in which the tympanic membrane perforation is associated with necrosis of the ossicular chain, and those with mastoidectomy, performed in chronic suppurative otitis media with cholesteatoma. As mentioned previously, tympanoplasty with mastoidectomy can be either closed or open.

In closed tympanoplasty, the posterior wall of the external auditory canal is kept intact. This technique is employed in children and in patients with very pneumatized mastoids to avoid having a large cavity. Regular otoscopic follow-up is essential to identify the formation of a retraction pocket or a recurrent cholesteatoma. Should these occur, there should be no hesitation in switching to an open technique.

In open tympanoplasty, the posterior wall of the external auditory canal is removed. The indications of this technique in the treatment of cholesteatoma include: a wide erosion of the posterosuperior wall, cholesteatoma in the only hearing ear, bilateral cholesteatoma, cholesteatoma in patients with Down's syndrome, the presence of a contracted mastoid, a large labyrinthine fistula, and recurrent cholesteatoma following a closed tympanoplasty. Because the posterior canal wall is removed, the mastoid cavity is exteriorized and on otoscopy the external auditory canal and the mastoid appear as one communicating cavity. If properly performed, the cavity appears rounded in shape, dry, and well epithelialized. On the other hand, a badly performed cavity may appear wet, irregular, and be lined with granulation tissue in addition to accumulated debris. There may also be the possibility of a residual cholesteatoma. In cases of tympanoplasty, it is usually possible to see the reconstructed ossicular chain through the tympanic membrane. We generally prefer to utilize an autologous or homologous incus for reconstruction. In our experience (more than 7,000 tympanoplasties), we never encountered any case of extrusion when the incus was used. In contrast, variable rates of extrusion were noticed when biological materials (e.g., plastipore, ceramics, hydroxyapatite) were utilized.

Although the use of homologous ossicles has never been proven to transmit slow viruses (e.g., Creutzfeldt–Jakob disease), the theoretical risk makes it more prudent to use predominantly autologous tissue or biomaterial of better characteristics that might appear in the future.

Later on in this chapter, some otoscopic views of cases managed by the modified Bondy's technique are shown. This is an open technique indicated in epitympanic cholesteatoma with a good preoperative hearing in which the tympanic membrane and the ossicular chain are intact. Some cases of radical mastoidectomy are also shown. This technique is used mainly in elderly patients with sensorineural hearing loss in which the only goal of surgery is to have a dry and safe ear.

14.4.1 Canal Wall Up (Closed) Tympanoplasty

Closed tympanoplasty operations have been shown in ► Fig. 14.58, ► Fig. 14.59, ► Fig. 14.60, ► Fig. 14.61, ► Fig. 14.62, ► Fig. 14.63, ► Fig. 14.64, ► Fig. 14.65, ► Fig. 14.66, ► Fig. 14.67, ► Fig. 14.68, ► Fig. 14.69, ► Fig. 14.70, ► Fig. 14.71, ► Fig. 14.72, ► Fig. 14.73, ► Fig. 14.74, ► Fig. 14.75, ► Fig. 14.76, ► Fig. 14.77, ► Fig. 14.78, ► Fig. 14.79, ► Fig. 14.80, ► Fig. 14.81, ► Fig. 14.82, ► Fig. 14.83.

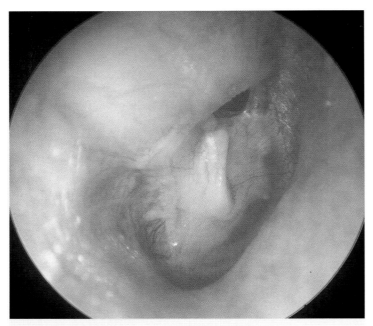

Fig. 14.58 Right ear. Staged closed tympanoplasty. The tympanic membrane has a normal angle and is well attached to the handle of the malleus. The cartilage used for reconstructing the attic is visible. In this region, a small self-cleaning retraction pocket can be seen.

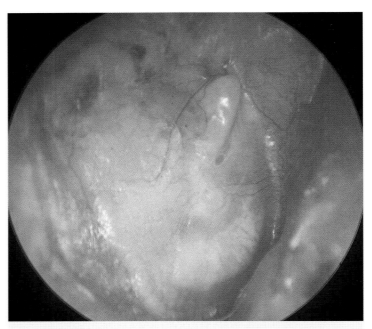

Fig. 14.59 Right ear. Staged closed tympanoplasty performed 10 years previously for the management of a cholesteatoma. The tympanic membrane is whitish, slightly thicker than normal, but retains a good anterior angle. The annulus is well seen anteriorly. The handle of the malleus is in a good position. There are no signs of resorption of the posterior canal wall.

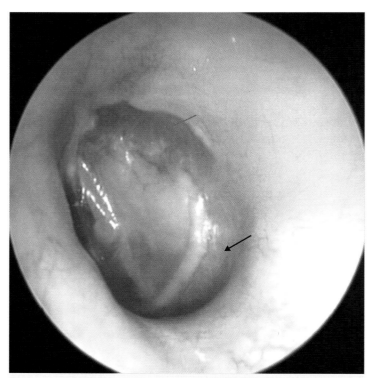

Fig. 14.60 Left ear. Staged closed tympanoplasty for a congenital cholesteatoma. An extended posterior tympanotomy was performed (*black arrow*). The cartilage used for ossiculoplasty is visible. There is a slight retraction of the attic (*red arrow*).

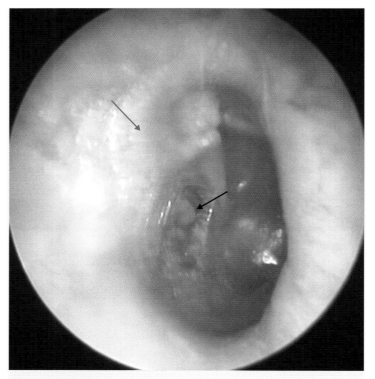

Fig. 14.61 Right ear. Closed tympanoplasty. The cartilage used for reconstructing the attic is visible (*red arrow*). The tendency to tympanic retraction is evident, mainly in the anteroinferior quadrant. A myringoincudopexy is also visible (*black arrow*).

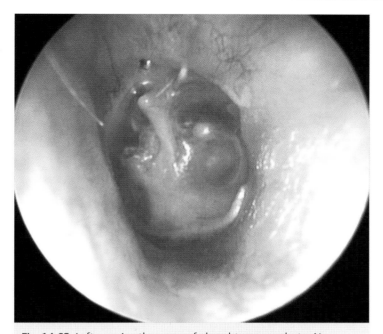

Fig. 14.62 Left ear. Another case of closed tympanoplasty. No cartilage was used for reconstruction and a small self-cleaning retraction pocket is visible in the attic. Hearing function was good due to a natural myringostapedopexy. In cases like this, a strict otoscopic follow-up should be adopted.

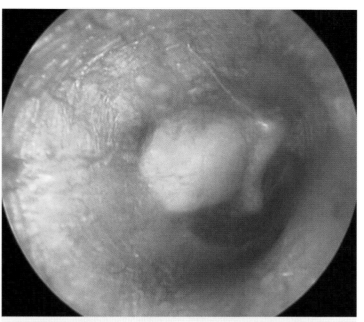

Fig. 14.63 Right ear. Another case of close tympanoplasty. A thick piece of cartilage was used both for reconstructing the attic and for ossiculoplasty. In this case, the long process of the incus was eroded, but was still in contact with the head of the stapes (see ▶ Fig. 14.64 for drawing).

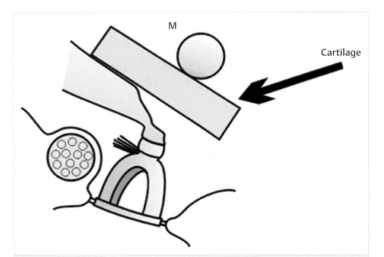

Fig. 14.64 In case of limited erosion of the incudostapedial joint, cartilage is placed medial to the handle of the malleus (M) and lateral to the long process of the incus.

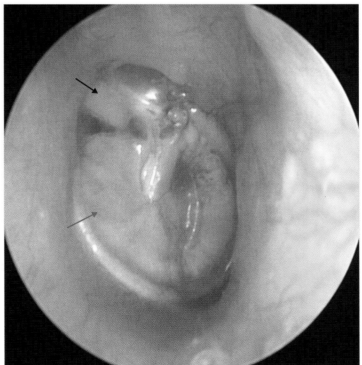

Fig. 14.65 Right ear. Staged closed tympanoplasty. Two pieces of cartilage were used for reconstructing the attic (black arrow) and the mesotympanic area (red arrow). The latter was used even for ossiculoplasty. Nevertheless, a tendency to attic retraction is visible.

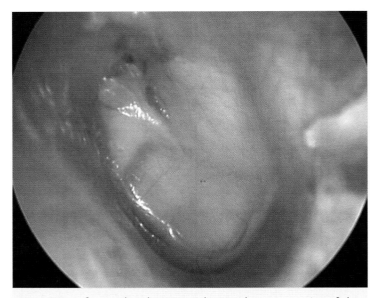

Fig. 14.66 Left ear. Closed tympanoplasty with reconstruction of the whole tympanic membrane with cartilage. The tympanic membrane and the handle of the malleus are excellently positioned.

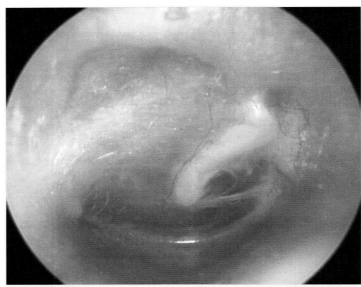

Fig. 14.67 Right ear. First-staged close tympanoplasty. The tympanic membrane is well positioned and the attic is not retracted. A second stage with ossiculoplasty has been further planned.

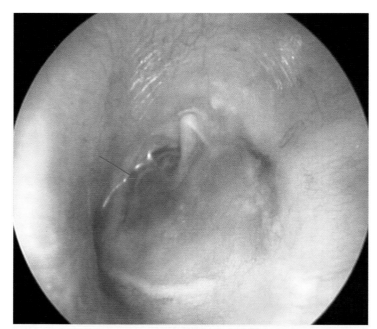

Fig. 14.68 Left ear. Another example of first-stage closed tympano-plasty without the use of cartilage. A thick piece of temporalis fascia was used for reconstructing the tympanic membrane. A second-stage procedure has been planned for ossiculoplasty. Middle ear effusion is evident in the anterosuperior quadrant (red arrow).

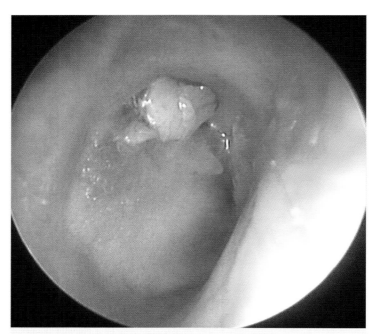

Fig. 14.69 Right ear. Staged closed tympanoplasty. The handle of the malleus was eroded by the cholesteatoma. Tympanic membrane was reconstructed with temporalis fascia. A piece of cartilage was used for reconstructing the attic. Slight medialization of the tympanic membrane is evident.

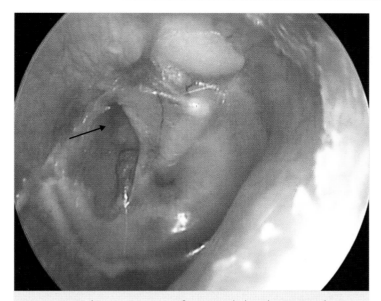

Fig. 14.70 Right ear. Otoscopy after staged closed tympanoplasty. Cartilage was used to reinforce the attic. Cholesteatoma eroded the incus and the stapes, resulting in absence of both the ossicles. A posterior retraction pocket is evident with myringoplatinopexy (*arrow*). In this case, a strict otoscopic follow-up should be adopted, even if a conversion to a canal wall down technique can be an option to avoid a recurrence of cholesteatoma.

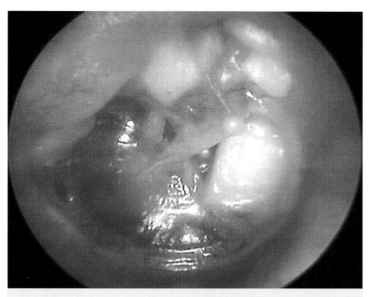

Fig. 14.71 Right ear. Closed tympanoplasty with cartilage reconstruction of the whole attic and anterior quadrant. The tympanic membrane is slightly retracted with myringoincudopexy. Regular otoscopic examinations are sufficient to follow up this case.

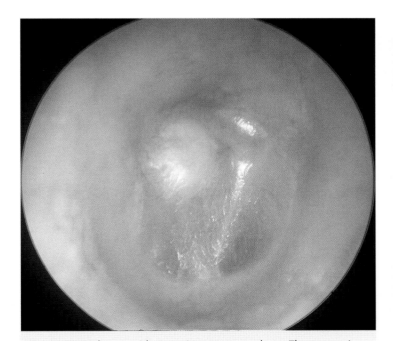

Fig. 14.72 Right ear with a previous tympanoplasty. The tympanic membrane is thin with mild blunting. The sculptured incus is visible.

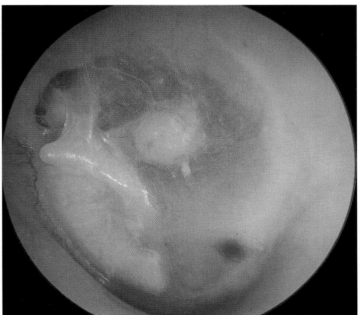

Fig. 14.73 Right ear with a previous tympanoplasty. The tympanic membrane is thin with mild blunting. The sculptured incus is visible.

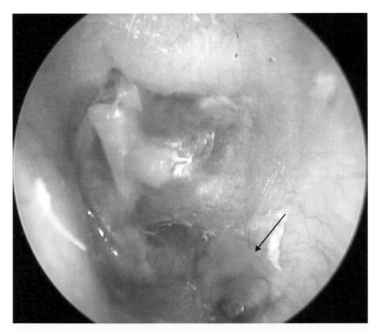

Fig. 14.74 Left ear. Closed tympanoplasty. The sculptured incus is visible. A thickening and bulging of the posteroinferior meatal skin is evident (*arrow*). A CT scan is indicated in this case to exclude the presence of a cholesteatoma.

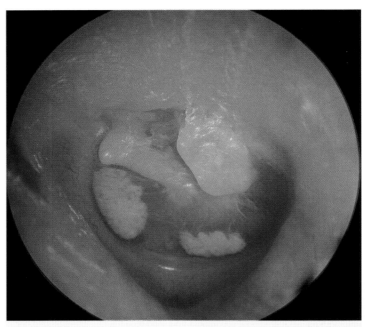

Fig. 14.75 Left ear. Ossiculoplasty. The tympanic membrane is retracted and the malleus is medialized. The sculptured incus is displaced posteriorly and is adherent to the posterior mesotympanum. Two tympanosclerotic plaques are noted anteriorly and interiorly.

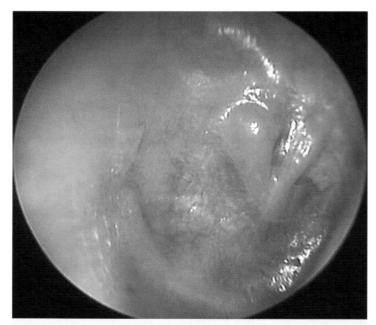

Fig. 14.76 Right ear. Closed tympanoplasty. The tympanic membrane is thick and in perfect position. The sculptured incus is in contact with both the malleus and the head of the stapes (see ▶ Fig. 14.77 for drawings).

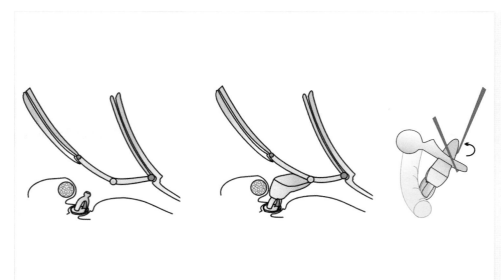

Fig. 14.77 Drawings of a reshaped incus graft for ossiculoplasty when the stapes is intact.

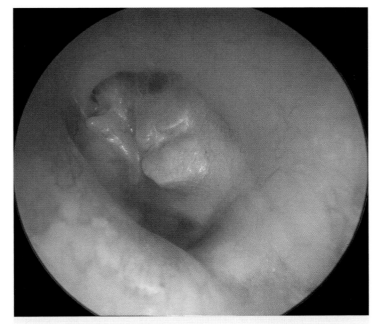

Fig. 14.78 Left ear. Posteriorly displaced incus that was used for ossiculoplasty. The trough created on the incus to fit the handle of the malleus is clearly seen. Revision surgery is necessary to reposition the displaced incus and improve the patient's hearing.

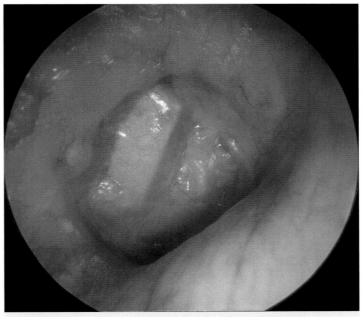

Fig. 14.79 Right ear. Slightly retracted reconstructed tympanic membrane. A T-shaped columella from homologous cartilage is visible. The columella has been placed between the tympanic membrane and the footplate of the stapes.

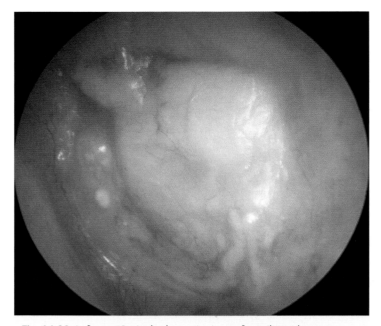

Fig. 14.80 Left ear. Ossiculoplasty. A piece of cartilage that was interposed between the reconstructed ossicular chain and the tympanic membrane can be visualized. It appears as a whitish thick mass that causes elevation of the posterior quadrants of the tympanic membrane.

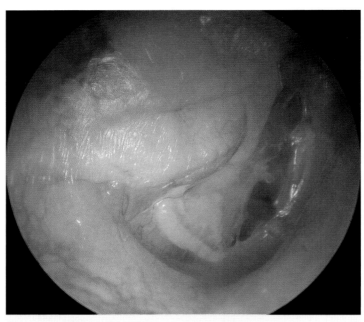

Fig. 14.81 Right ear. Closed tympanoplasty. Sculptured incus in a perfect position under the reconstructed tympanic membrane. The cartilage used to reconstruct the posterosuperior wall of the external auditory canal is also visible.

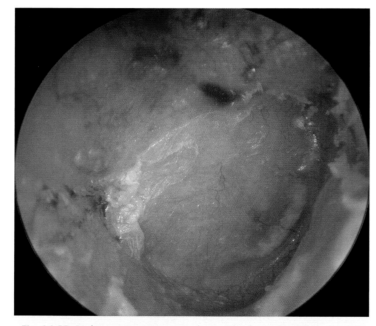

Fig. 14.82 Right ear. Posttympanoplasty. Good position of the tympanic membrane. In this case, it is difficult to identify the type of ossicular chain reconstruction due to the thickness of the tympanic membrane, particularly noted at its posterior quadrants.

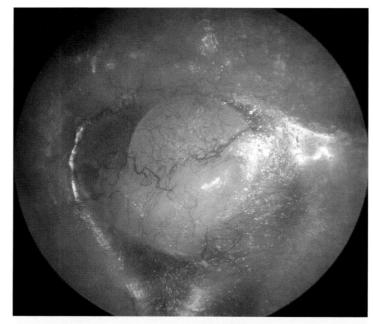

Fig. 14.83 Left ear. In the posterosuperior quadrant, a TORP (total ossicular replacement prosthesis) with its circular head is noted. The overlying cartilage is partially resorbed. There are no signs of extrusion.

Failures and Complications

Some failures and complications faced in closed tympanoplasty have been depicted in ► Fig. 14.84, ► Fig. 14.85, ► Fig. 14.86, ► Fig. 14.87, ► Fig. 14.88, ► Fig. 14.89, ► Fig. 14.90, ► Fig. 14.91, ► Fig. 14.92, ► Fig. 14.93, ► Fig. 14.94, ► Fig. 14.95, ► Fig. 14.96, ► Fig. 14.97, ► Fig. 14.98, ► Fig. 14.99, ► Fig. 14.100, ► Fig. 14.101, ► Fig. 14.102, ► Fig. 14.103, ► Fig. 14.104, ► Fig. 14.105, ► Fig. 14.106, ► Fig. 14.107, ► Fig. 14.108, ► Fig. 14.109, ► Fig. 14.110, ► Fig. 14.111, ► Fig. 14.112, ► Fig. 14.113.

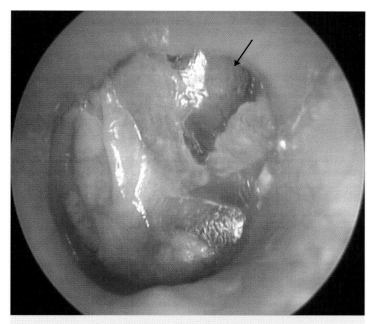

Fig. 14.84 Left ear. Closed tympanoplasty. There is a posterosuperior retraction with perforation and skin migration. A cholesteatoma seems to be observed in transparency (*arrow*).

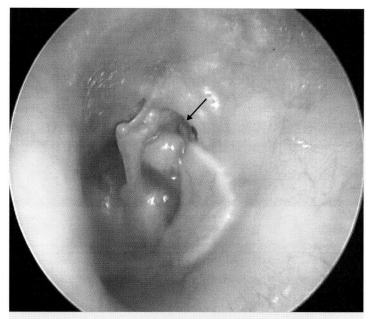

Fig. 14.85 Left ear. Closed tympanoplasty with sculptured incus and cartilage. A posterosuperior, not self-cleaning retraction pocket is evident (arrow) with a strong suspect of recurrent cholesteatoma. Conversion to an open tympanoplasty is the treatment of choice.

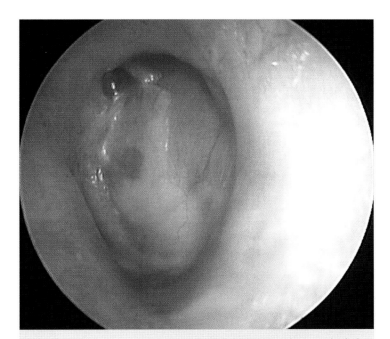

Fig. 14.86 Left ear. Another case of closed tympanoplasty with slight attic retraction. The patient complained of intermittent otorrhea, so a CT scan was performed with the presence of a recurrent cholesteatoma. An open tympanoplasty was further performed.

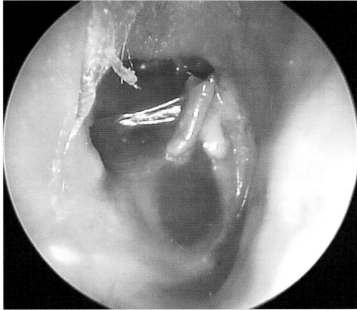

Fig. 14.87 A case similar to that of ▶ Fig. 14.86. There is a deep posterosuperior retraction with high suspect of recurrent cholesteatoma. The sculptured incus is misplaced. Revision tympanoplasty (open technique) was performed.

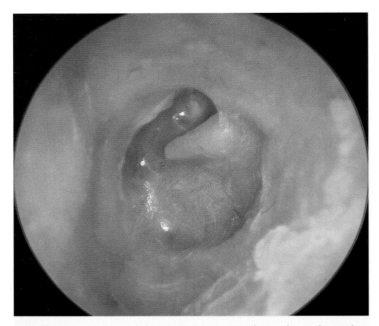

Fig. 14.88 Left ear. In the posterosuperior quadrant, the sculptured incus with the short process pointing anteriorly is seen through the retracted tympanic membrane. In cases with hearing loss, repeat surgery is indicated to reinforce the tympanic membrane and improve the hearing. Surgery entails dissection of the retraction pocket from the incus, and the placement of cartilage between the sculptured incus and the tympanic membrane. This cartilage prevents (or delays) the reformation of a retraction pocket and corrects the hearing deficit.

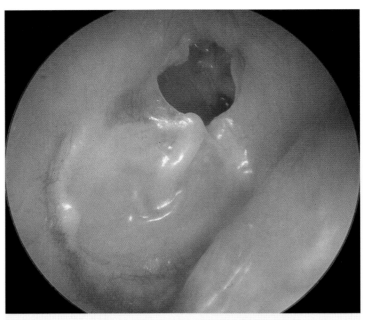

Fig. 14.89 Right ear. Recurrent epitympanic cholesteatoma following closed tympanoplasty. The reconstructed tympanic membrane (pars tensa) shows an optimal anterior angle and is perfectly attached to the handle of the malleus. In this case, transformation to an open technique is indicated while conserving the tympanic membrane and ossicular chain if there is no hearing loss.

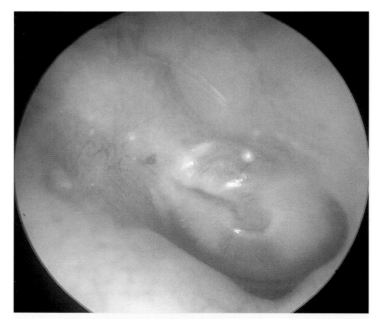

Fig. 14.90 Left ear. Another example of a closed tympanoplasty 2 years postoperatively. The attic was reconstructed using cartilage and bone pate and shows no signs of erosion. A small cholesteatomatous pearl is seen in the posterosuperior quadrant. It can be easily removed in the outpatient clinic under microscopic control.

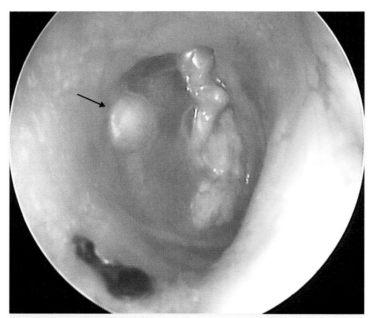

Fig. 14.91 Right ear. Residual cholesteatoma is visible as whitish bulging of the posterior tympanic membrane (arrow).

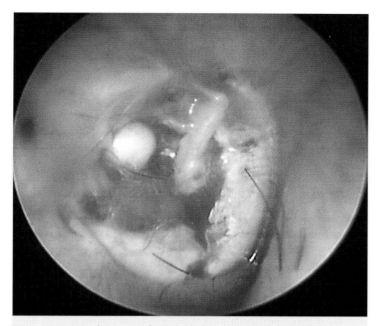

Fig. 14.92 Another case of residual cholesteatoma. Tympanosclerosis of anterior and inferior quadrants is visible. In case of a small pearl of cholesteatoma, a transcanal approach can be adopted.

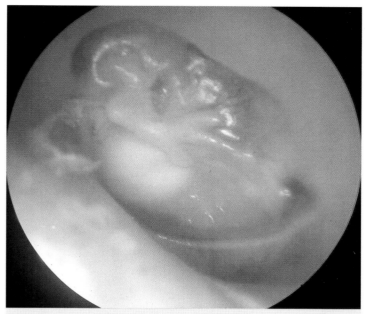

Fig. 14.93 Left ear. Good anterior angle of the reconstructed tympanic membrane. An anteromalleolar cholesteatomatous cyst is seen. An epitympanic retraction pocket that is adherent to the head of the malleus and body of the incus is also observed.

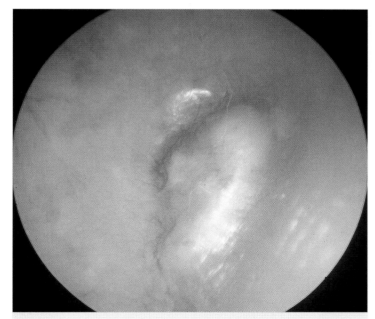

Fig. 14.94 Right ear. Posttympanoplasty. A white retrotympanic mass (cholesteatoma of the anterior angle) is noted causing bulging of the tympanic membrane. The cholesteatoma is probably the result of inadequate removal of the epithelium in an overlay technique. The entrapped skin led to the formation of the cholesteatoma.

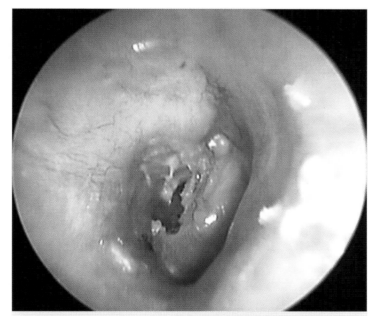

Fig. 14.95 Recurrent cholesteatoma after an exclusive endoscopic tympanoplasty. In this case, an open tympanoplasty was performed.

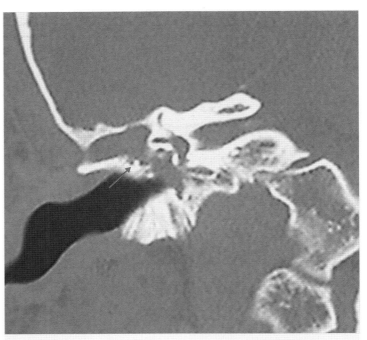

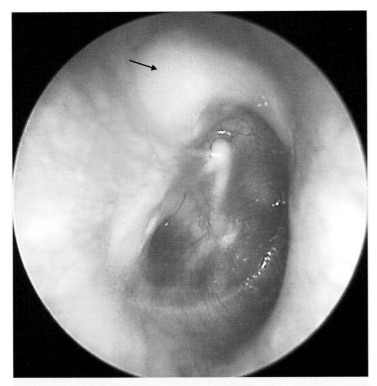

Fig. 14.96 Recurrent cholesteatoma in a closed tympanoplasty. Retraction of the attic with otorrhea is visible (*arrow*). A CT scan showed extension of the disease toward the attic, mesotympanum, and mastoid (see ▶ Fig. 14.97, ▶ Fig. 14.98). An open tympanoplasty was further performed.

Fig. 14.97 CT scan, coronal view. The cholesteatoma fills the attic and the middle ear cleft. The posterior wall of the external auditory canal is partially eroded (*arrow*).

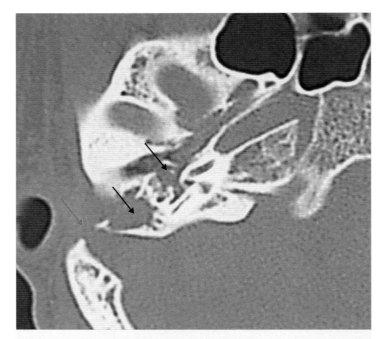

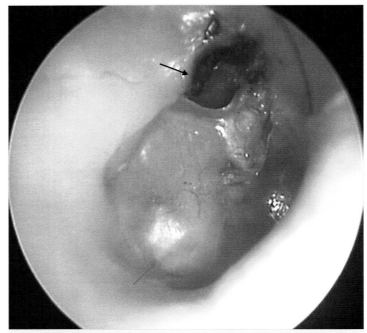

Fig. 14.98 CT scan of the same case, axial view. Recurrent cholesteatoma is visible (*black arrows*). The sigmoid sinus is uncovered from bone (*red arrow*). Care should be taken not to open it during the first surgical steps, in particular during creation of the muscoloperiosteal flap.

Fig. 14.99 Right closed tympanoplasty. A residual cholesteatoma close to the promontory (*red arrow*) and an epitympanic cholesteatoma (*black arrow*) are present. Even in this case a conversion to an open technique was performed.

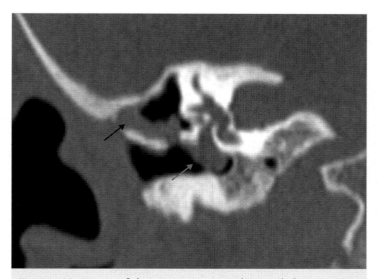

Fig. 14.100 CT scan of the same case, coronal view. Cholesteatoma in the area of the promontorium (*red arrow*) and attic (*black arrow*) is visible. Erosion of the posterior canal wall is also present.

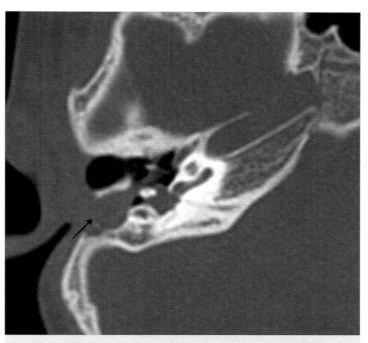

Fig. 14.101 CT scan of the same case, axial view. Residual cholesteatoma inside the closed cavity is shown (*arrow*).

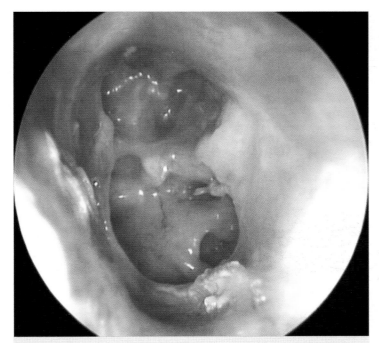

Fig. 14.102 Left ear. This patient was operated elsewhere for an epitympanic cholesteatoma with a transcanal atticotomy. The cavity is discharging and a deep posterosuperior retraction is evident, as well as a complete perforation of the reconstructed tympanic membrane. A canal wall down tympanoplasty was further performed with complete cholesteatoma removal.

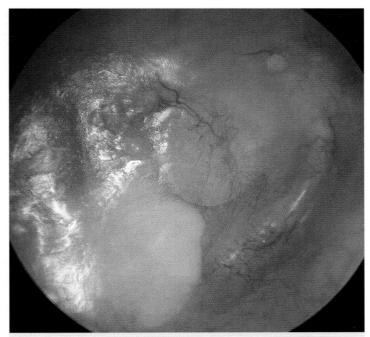

Fig. 14.103 Right ear. Example of a TORP that is visible through the tympanic membrane. The overlying cartilage, which is whitish in color, has been displaced into the posteroinferior quadrant. There are no signs of extrusion.

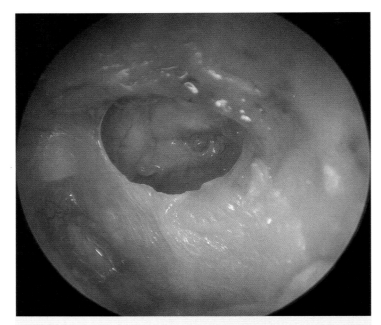

Fig. 14.104 Left ear. Posterosuperior perforation of the reconstructed tympanic membrane with extrusion of the TORP. The shaft of the prosthesis has caused an erosion of the footplate of the stapes (which appears through the perforation as a rounded dark area).

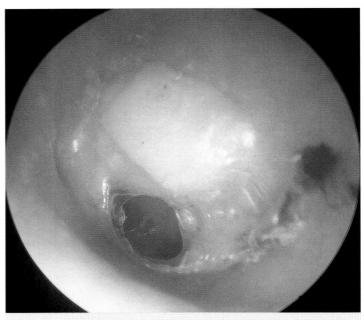

Fig. 14.105 Left ear. Anteroinferior reperforation due to an acute otitis media, occurring 3 years after a staged closed tympanoplasty. A rectangular cartilage used for ossiculoplasty is visible. The cartilage is well integrated in the tympanic membrane residue.

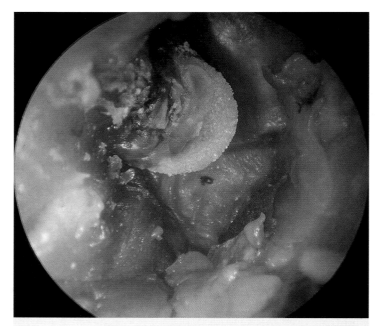

Fig. 14.106 Right ear. An example of TORP extrusion that occurred 1 year after a second-stage tympanoplasty. The head of the prosthesis can be seen despite the surrounding wax. The tympanic membrane residue is atelectatic.

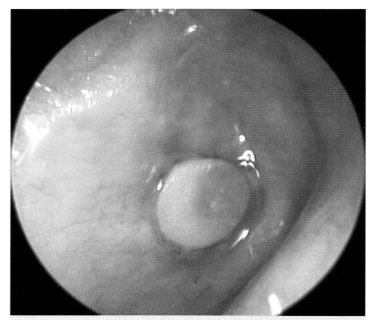

Fig. 14.107 Right ear. Another example of TORP extrusion with infection and otorrhea.

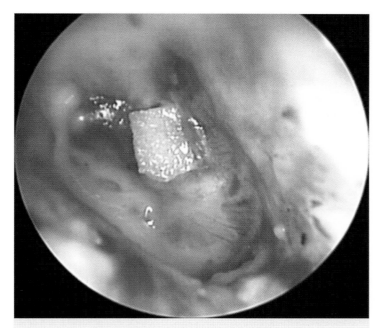

Fig. 14.108 Left ear. PORP extrusion with infection and otorrhea.

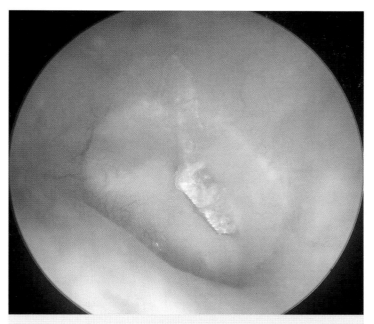

Fig. 14.109 Left ear. Gold prosthesis in the process of extrusion in a staged closed tympanoplasty.

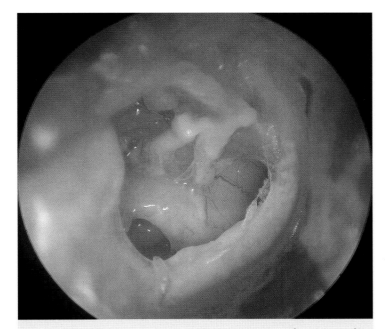

Fig. 14.110 Right ear. Posttympanoplasty. Large reperforation. In the posterosuperior quadrant, a Teflon prosthesis is interposed between the medialized malleus and the footplate of the stapes. The round window is visible in the posteroinferior quadrant. The anterior residue of the tympanic membrane is tympanosclerotic.

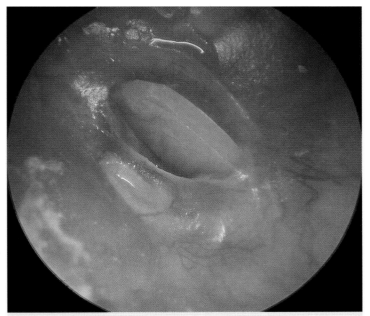

Fig. 14.111 Left ear. Silastic sheet in extrusion through a posterosuperior perforation. The handle of the malleus is clearly visible anteriorly. In general, Silastic is inserted in first stage tympanoplasty. This material is usually placed in the middle ear to favor the restoration of the normal mucosal lining of the middle ear and to avoid the formation of adhesions in the meantime. It is removed during the second-stage tympanoplasty, except in cases showing a tendency toward atelectasis.

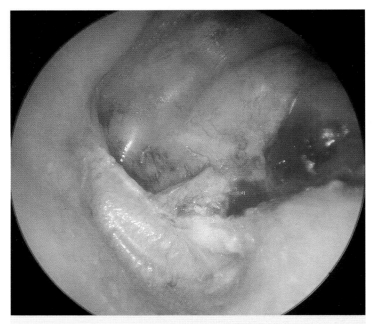

Fig. 14.112 Left ear. Total resorption of the posterior wall of the external auditory canal 3 years after a closed tympanoplasty. The otoscopic view is similar to that observed after an open tympanoplasty. Repeat surgery was necessary. The facial ridge was lowered and all bony irregularities were smoothed to avoid the retention of squamous debris with subsequent otorrhea. An adequate meatoplasty was also performed.

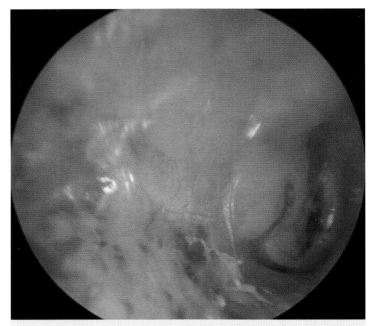

Fig. 14.113 Right ear. Partial resorption of the posterior wall of the external auditory canal approximately 7 to 8 mm from the annulus following a closed tympanoplasty. The atrophic area appears bluish due to lack of underlying bone. No cutaneous retraction is seen. However, due to the lack of bone, the skin can invaginate into the mastoid cavity giving rise to recurrent cholesteatoma. In such cases, regular long-term follow-up is indicated.

14.4.2 Canal Wall Down (Open) Tympanoplasty

Open tympanoplasty operations have been shown in ► Fig. 14.114, ► Fig. 14.115, ► Fig. 14.116, ► Fig. 14.117, ► Fig. 14.118, ► Fig. 14.119, ► Fig. 14.120, ► Fig. 14.121, ► Fig. 14.122, ► Fig. 14.123, ► Fig. 14.124, ► Fig. 14.125, ► Fig. 14.126.

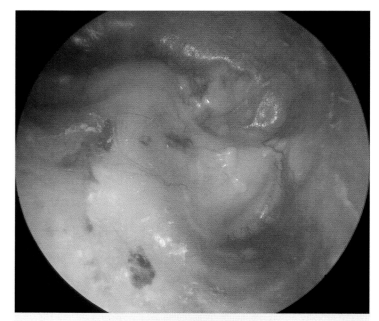

Fig. 14.114 Right ear. A well-performed open tympanoplasty. The cavity is epithelialized and the facial ridge is adequately lowered. In the attic region, the material used for obliteration can be noted.

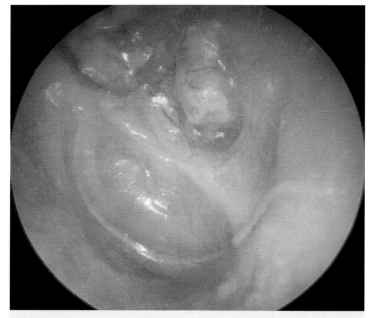

Fig. 14.115 Left ear. Open tympanoplasty. Attic obliteration with autologous bone.

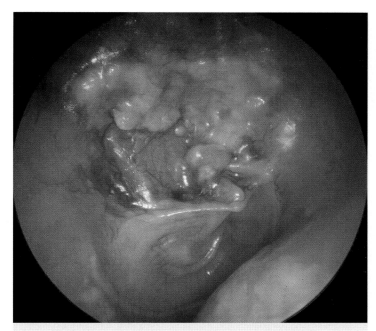

Fig. 14.116 Right ear. Open tympanoplasty. Partial obliteration of the attic with bone pate.

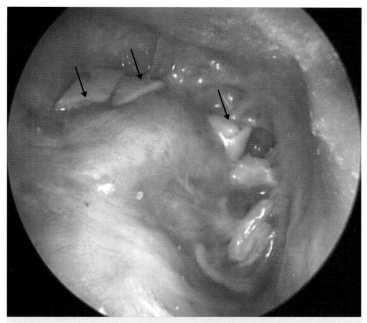

Fig. 14.117 Right ear. Open tympanoplasty. The cavity is perfectly epithelialized and regular. The facial ridge is adequately lowered. Pieces of cartilage were used for partial obliteration (*arrows*).

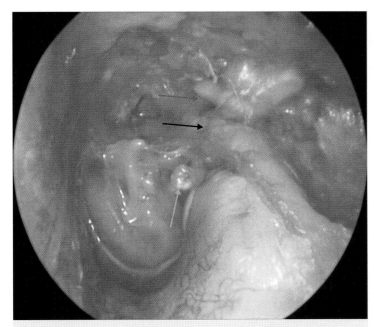

Fig. 14.118 Left ear. Another case of open tympanoplasty. The second portion of the facial nerve is uncovered (*black arrow*). Pieces of cartilage were used for obliteration of the posterior attic and the lateral semicircular canal is visible (*red arrow*). A myringostapedopexy is also present (*green arrow*).

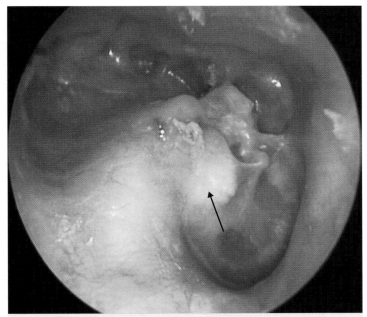

Fig. 14.119 Right ear. Another case of stable open cavity. A piece of cartilage was placed over the stapes for ossiculoplasty (*arrow*).

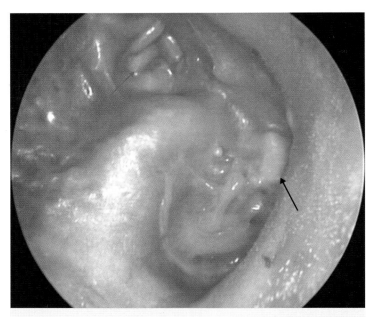

Fig. 14.120 Right ear, open tympanoplasty. Cartilage was placed in the supratubal recess (*black arrow*) and in the attic (*red arrow*). The cavity is perfectly epithelialized.

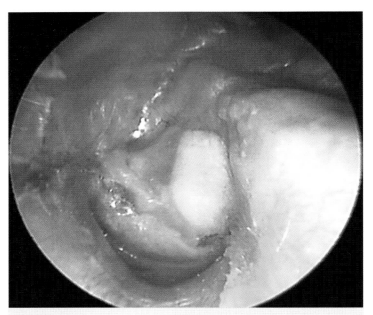

Fig. 14.121 Left ear. Case similar to that in ▶ Fig. 14.120. This 25-year-old male patient was scheduled for a staged canal wall down tympanoplasty for an extended cholesteatoma. At the first stage, the eroded incus was removed and a piece of cartilage placed over the stapes. After 8 months, the patient performed a CT scan which showed no residual cholesteatoma and a perfect contiguity between the cartilage and the stapes. Hearing function was near-normal. So, a second-stage was not further performed.

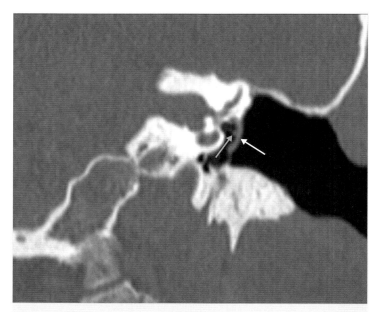

Fig. 14.122 CT scan of the same patient, coronal view. Note the cartilage (*white arrow*) perfectly in contact with the head of the stapes (*green arrow*).

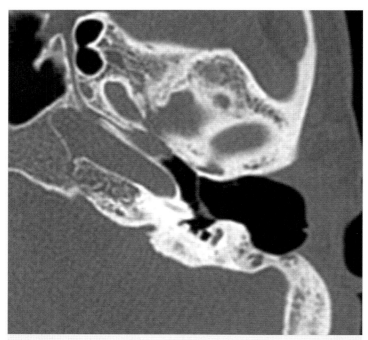

Fig. 14.123 CT scan, axial view, of the same case.

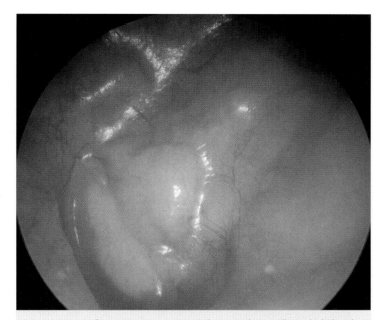

Fig. 14.124 Left ear. Open tympanoplasty with a well-epithelialized cavity. The tympanic membrane shows a tympanosclerotic plaque anteriorly; posteriorly, the ossicular chain reconstruction is observed.

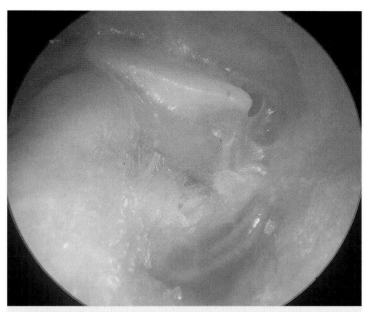

Fig. 14.125 Right ear. Open tympanoplasty. The cartilage used for obliteration of the attic is seen in the superior part.

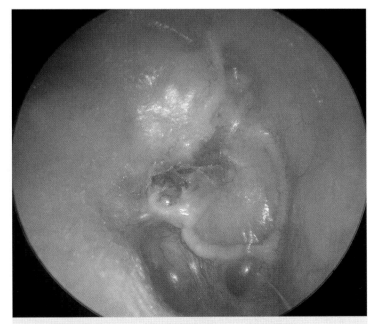

Fig. 14.126 Right ear. Open tympanoplasty. The tympanic bone was drilled in this case because it was involved with the cholesteatoma. The inferior annulus is visible. Superiorly, the chorda tympani is observed close to the incus used for reconstruction of the ossicular chain.

Radical Mastoidectomy

This technique is shown in ► Fig. 14.127, ► Fig. 14.128, ► Fig. 14.129, ► Fig. 14.130, ► Fig. 14.131.

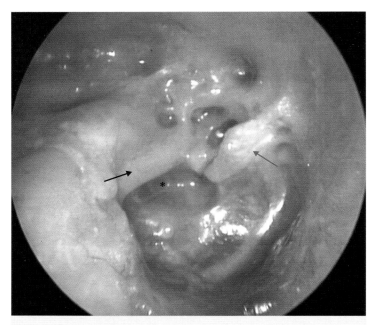

Fig. 14.127 Radical mastoidectomy in a 70-year-old patient with cholesteatoma of the mastoid and tympanic membrane atelectasis. In this case, the posterior tympanic retraction was not treated due to a pexy with the oval window (*asterisk*). The second portion of the facial nerve is uncovered (*black arrow*). Only a small remnant of the malleus is visible (*red arrow*).

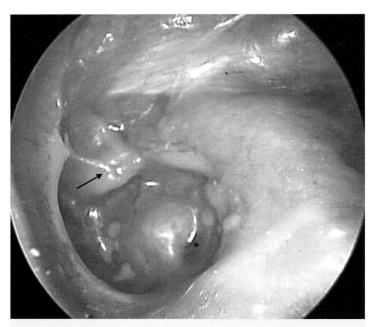

Fig. 14.128 Left ear. Another case of radical mastoidectomy. Even in this case the second portion of the facial nerve is uncovered. The atelectatic tympanic membrane is in direct contact with the oval window. The round window (*asterisk*) is visible, as well as the cochleariform process and the tensor tympani (*arrow*). There are no remnants of the ossicular chain.

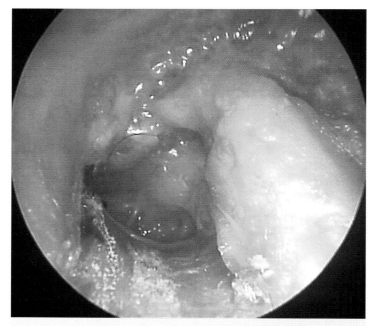

Fig. 14.129 Left ear. Another case of radical mastoidectomy. Complete atelectasis of the tympanic membrane is present.

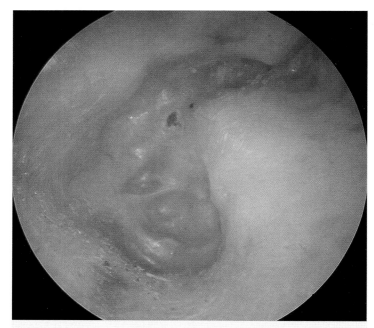

Fig. 14.130 The cavity is dry, smooth, and well epithelialized, and the facial ridge is low.

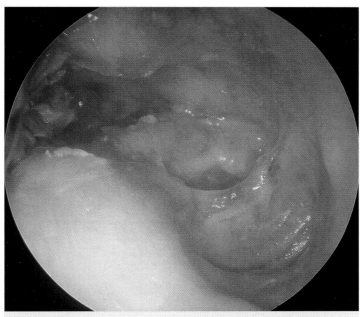

Fig. 14.131 Right ear. A patient with bilateral cholesteatoma. An open tympanoplasty with obliteration was performed. The material used for obliteration of the attic (cartilage and bone pate) has nearly totally resorbed. The cavity is humid, granulating, and wet. Hearing is poorer than that of the other side in which an open technique without obliteration was performed (see ► Fig. 14.132).

Modified Bondy's Technique Tympanoplasty

This technique is shown in ► Fig. 14.132, ► Fig. 14.133, ► Fig. 14.134, ► Fig. 14.135, ► Fig. 14.136, ► Fig. 14.137, ► Fig. 14.138, ► Fig. 14.139, ► Fig. 14.140, ► Fig. 14.141.

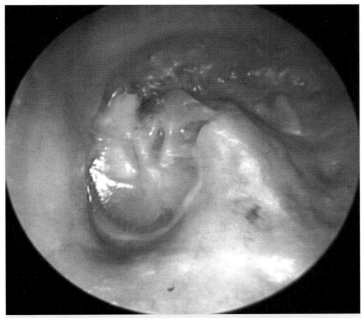

Fig. 14.132 Left ear. Example of a modified Bondy's technique. In this case, the preoperative pure tone average was 20 dB. The patient conserved his preoperative hearing. The modified Bondy's technique is indicated in epitympanic cholesteatoma with an intact tympanic membrane and ossicular chain. It is an open technique in which the attic and the mastoid are exteriorized and the facial ridge is lowered until the level of the annulus. The ossicular chain and the tympanic membrane are left in situ. If necessary, the attic is obliterated with a piece of cartilage; this procedure helps to reduce the risk of retractions around the ossicles. Fascia is then inserted with two anterior tongues; one is positioned under the incus body, the other between the handle of the malleus and the long process of the incus. A meatoplasty according to the size of the cavity is performed at the end of the procedure.

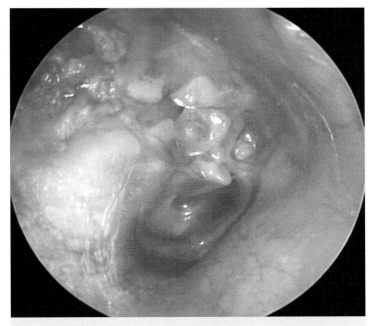

Fig. 14.133 Right ear. Modified Bondy's technique tympanoplasty. The attic is obliterated with cartilage.

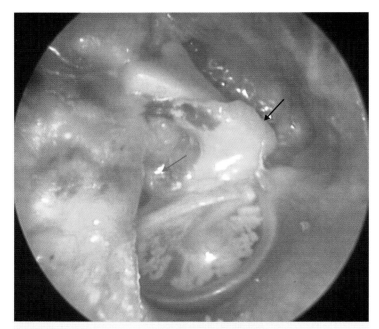

Fig. 14.134 Right ear. Modified Bondy's technique tympanoplasty. The incudomalleolar (*black arrow*) and the incudostapedial (*red arrow*) joints are visible. A piece of cartilage was placed behind the incus and in the posterior attic.

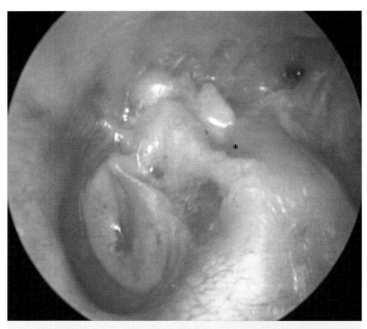

Fig. 14.135 Left ear. Another case of modified Bondy's technique tympanoplasty for epitympanic cholesteatoma. The second portion of the facial nerve is uncovered (*asterisk*).

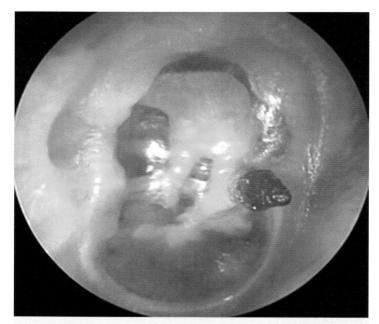

Fig. 14.136 Right ear. Spontaneous Bondy's cavity due to a self-cleaning retraction pocket. The whole attic is exposed and no erosion of the ossicular chain is present. The patient did not complained of otorrhea or hearing loss. Audiometry showed normal hearing. Even a CT scan excluded the presence of a cholesteatoma. The patient has been simply followed up with otoscopic examinations.

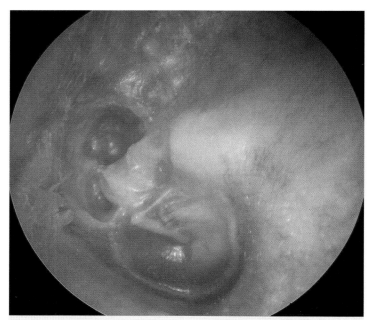

Fig. 14.137 Left ear. The modified Bondy's technique. Although an attic retraction is noted, recurrent cholesteatoma is uncommon with this technique. The tympanic membrane is retracted and middle ear effusion is noted. In this case, the insertion of a ventilation tube is indicated.

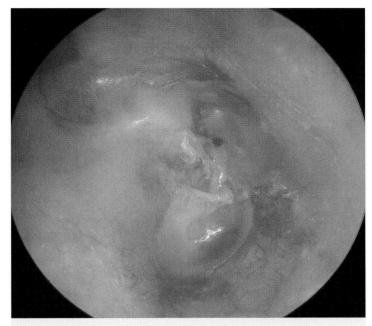

Fig. 14.138 Right ear. The modified Bondy's technique. The attic is obliterated with cartilage.

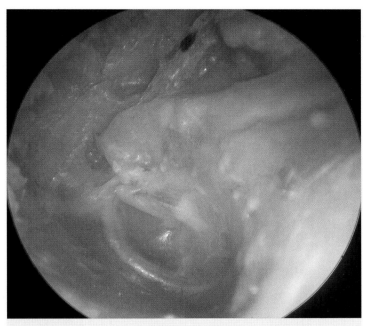

Fig. 14.139 Left ear. Another case of the modified Bondy's technique. As the incus was slightly eroded, a piece of cartilage was placed between it and the malleus. The attic was obliterated with cartilage.

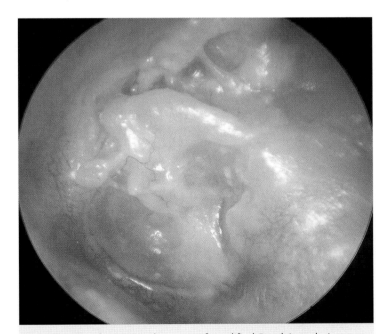

Fig. 14.140 Left ear. Another case of modified Bondy's technique tympanoplasty.

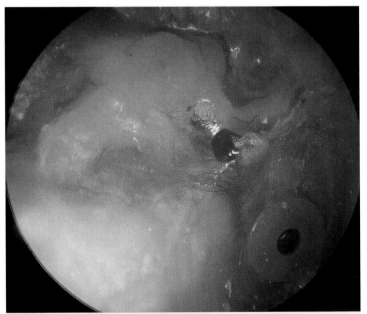

Fig. 14.141 Right ear. The modified Bondy's technique. A ventilation tube was inserted because of the presence of middle ear effusion that did not respond to medical treatment.

Failures and Complications

Some failures and complications faced in open tympanoplasty have been depicted in ► Fig. 14.142, ► Fig. 14.143, ► Fig. 14.144, ► Fig. 14.145, ► Fig. 14.146, ► Fig. 14.147, ► Fig. 14.148, ► Fig. 14.149, ► Fig. 14.150, ► Fig. 14.151, ► Fig. 14.152, ► Fig. 14.153, ► Fig. 14.154, ► Fig. 14.155.

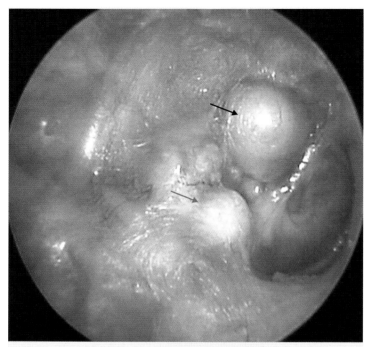

Fig. 14.142 Right ear. Residual cholesteatoma in a canal wall down tympanoplasty performed elsewhere. Two big cholesteatoma pearls are visible, respectively, in the attic (*black arrow*) and close to the facial ridge (*red arrow*), which has not been sufficiently lowered. A revision tympanoplasty was performed.

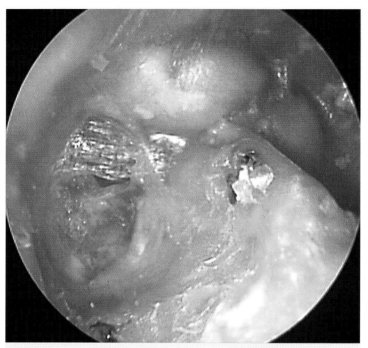

Fig. 14.143 Left ear. Another residual cholesteatoma in a canal wall down cavity. The attic shows a whitish bulging. The presence of a meningoencephalic herniation was excluded with the CT scan. Even in this case, the facial ridge is too high. A revision tympanoplasty was further performed.

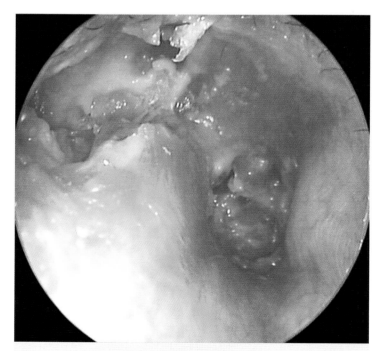

Fig. 14.144 Right ear. Recurrent cholesteatoma in a canal wall down tympanoplasty. The cavity is irregular (note the anterior hump of the external auditory canal and the insufficient exteriorization of the mastoid) and the facial ridge is too high. A subtotal perforation of the tympanic cavity is visible with fetid otorrhea. A revision tympanoplasty was performed.

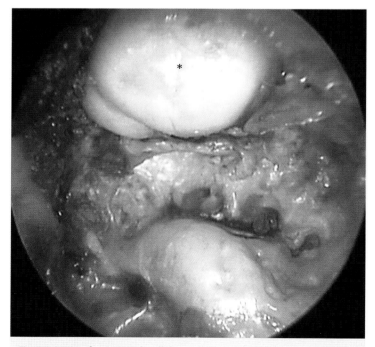

Fig. 14.145 Left ear. Canal wall down tympanoplasty with skin debris and wax accumulation. A whitish stiff bulging in the attic can be noted (*asterisk*). The CT scan (see ► Fig. 14.146) showed a bony mass, suggestive of neo-osteogenesis and trapped skin. A revision tympanoplasty, with removal of the bony mass and recurrent cholesteatoma, was further performed.

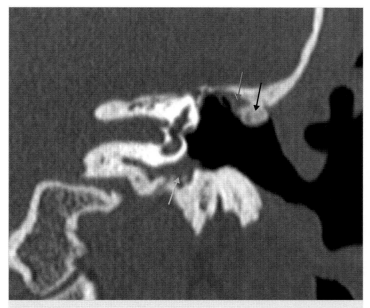

Fig. 14.146 CT scan, coronal view, of the previous case. The bony mass (*black arrow*) is visible in the attic. Trapped skin is present behind the neoformation (*red arrow*). Recurrent cholesteatoma can be noted in the hypotympanum (*green arrow*).

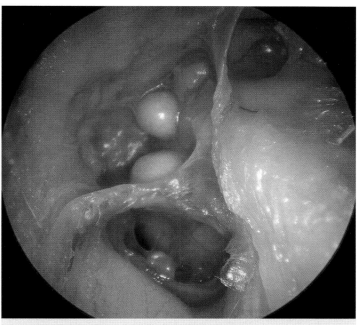

Fig. 14.147 Left ear. Open tympanoplasty. A large perforation of the reconstructed tympanic membrane is seen. Cholesteatomatous pearls are observed in the attic.

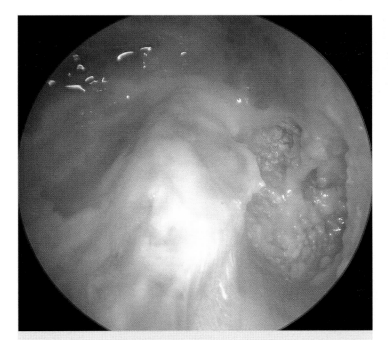

Fig. 14.148 Right ear. Another example of a badly performed open tympanoplasty. Purulent secretions and a high facial ridge are observed.

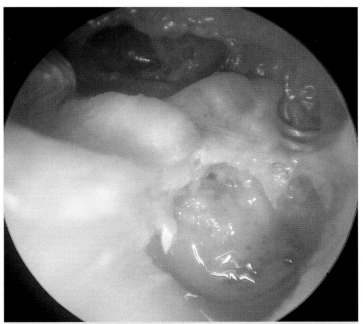

Fig. 14.149 Right ear. A badly performed open tympanoplasty. The cavity is irregular, with undermined borders and a very high facial ridge. Purulent secretion is present in the middle ear and the rest of the cavity.

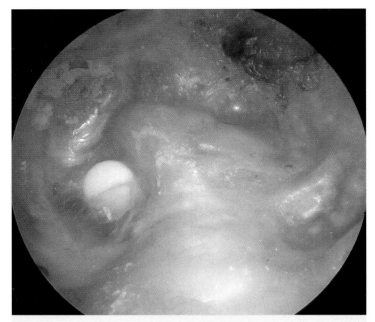

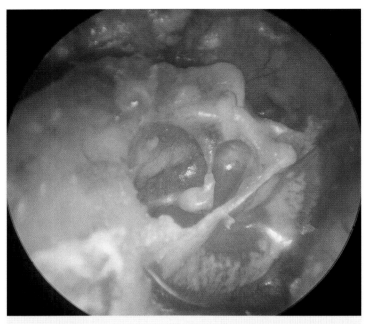

Fig. 14.150 Left ear. TORP in extrusion following a second- stage open tympanoplasty. In the first stage, a cholesteatoma involving the attic and mesotympanum and causing erosion of the ossicular chain was removed. In the second stage, a TORP was used for reconstruction. It was placed between the footplate of the stapes and the tympanic membrane. One year postoperatively, early extrusion of the prosthesis is observed. To avoid this complication, a tragal cartilage has to be placed between the prosthesis and the tympanic membrane.

Fig. 14.151 Right ear. In this case of a modified Bondy's technique, incus erosion occurred 3 years postoperatively due to the presence of a significant retraction pocket. The middle ear shows a catarrhal effusion.

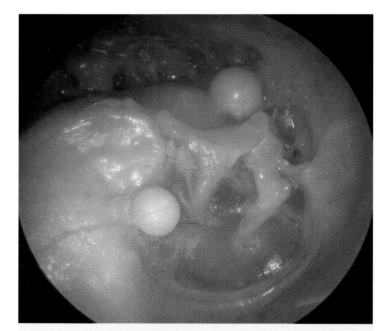

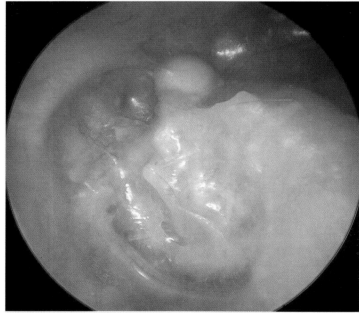

Fig. 14.152 Right ear. A modified Bondy's technique. Two cholesteatomatous pearls are present in the cavity. They are easily removed in the outpatient clinic. The attic, antrum, and mastoid were exteriorized. The ossicular chain was left in situ.

Fig. 14.153 Left ear. A cholesteatomatous pearl seen in the attic following a modified Bondy's technique.

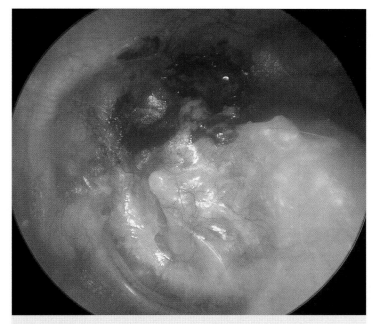

Fig. 14.154 Same patient after removal of the pearl in the outpatient clinic.

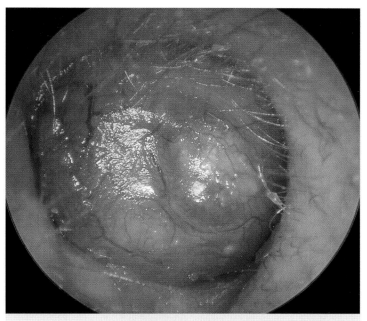

Fig. 14.155 Radical mastoidectomy. A mucosal cyst causes complete obstruction of the external auditory canal.

14.4.3 Meatoplasty, Blind-Sac Closure of the External Auditory Canal

Examples of meatoplasty have been shown in ▶ Fig. 14.156, ▶ Fig. 14.157, ▶ Fig. 14.158, ▶ Fig. 14.159, ▶ Fig. 14.160. See external auditory canal closure in ▶ Fig. 14.161, ▶ Fig. 14.162, ▶ Fig. 14.163.

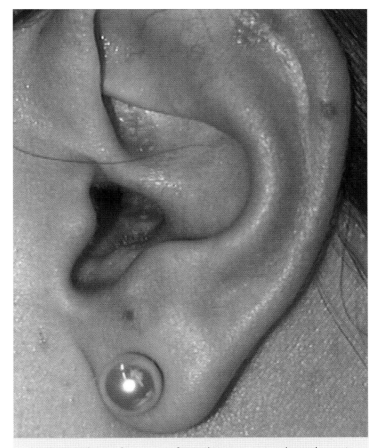

Fig. 14.156 The performance of an adequate meatoplasty that suits the dimension of the cavity is fundamental to assure proper aeration and prevent accumulation of epithelial debris and cerumen in the cavity.

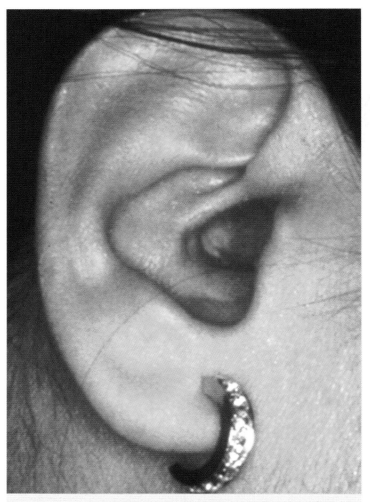

Fig. 14.157 Another example of meatoplasty performed in an open tympanoplasty.

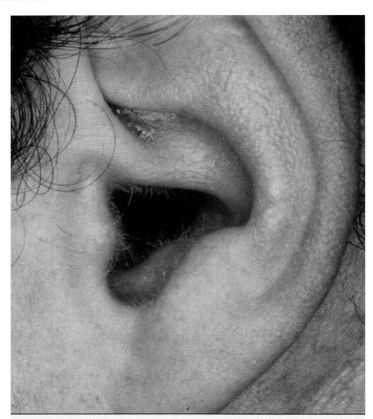

Fig. 14.158 A well-performed large meatoplasty in an open tympanoplasty, providing perfect aeration of the cavity.

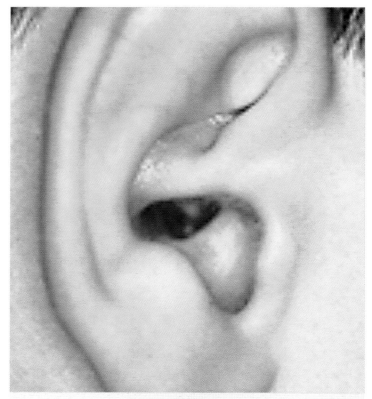

Fig. 14.159 Another example of a meatoplasty performed in a 10-year-old boy who underwent surgery for bilateral epitympanic cholesteatoma using a modified Bondy's technique.

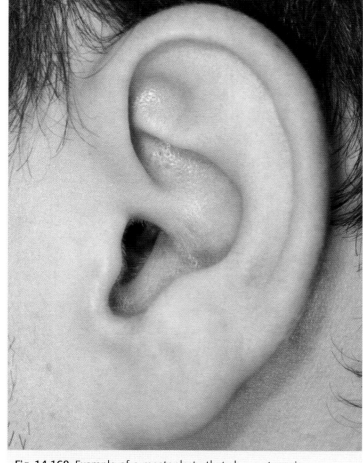

Fig. 14.160 Example of a meatoplasty that shows stenosis.

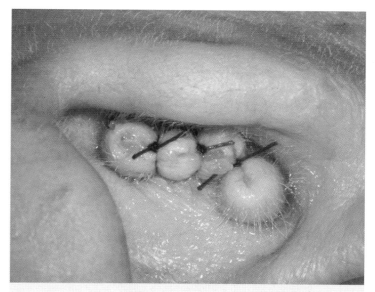

Fig. 14.161 Surgical picture of a blind-sac closure of the external auditory canal. The skin is everted and sutured with absorbable stitches. After some months, the closed wound tends to retract inside the external auditory canal with no aesthetic issues (see ► Fig. 14.162).

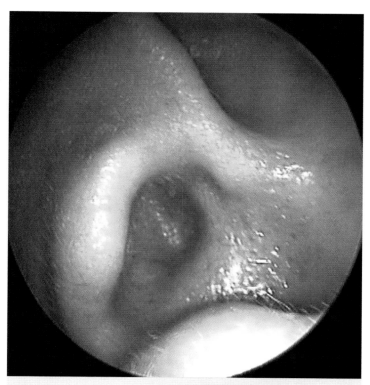

Fig. 14.162 Image of the same patient 2 months after surgery. The wound is completely closed and the skin infolded inside the external auditory canal.

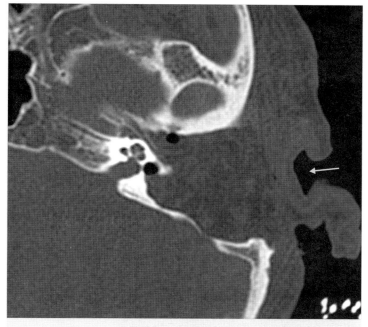

Fig. 14.163 CT scan, axial view, of the surgical cavity (obliterated with abdominal fat). The external auditory canal is blind-sac closed (*arrow*).

14.5 Hearing Implants

Hearing implantology is a set of surgical techniques aided by devices aimed at the functional rehabilitation of a patient affected by total or partial deafness. Hearing implants are not a replacement for an ear, but they can help many people who were effectively declared deaf. By stimulating the auditory nerve, signals are transmitted to the brain, which turns into "hearing."

Implants are key for many children or infants born with severe hearing loss who receive the devices so that they can grow up with auditory skills and have stronger language skills.

A cochlear implant (CI) is a surgically implanted electronic device that provides a sense of sound to a person who is profoundly deaf or severely hard of hearing. CI may help provide hearing in patients who are deaf because of damage to sensory hair cells in their cochleas. In those patients, the implants often can enable sufficient hearing for better understanding of speech. Newer devices and processing strategies allow recipients to hear better in noise, enjoy music, and even use their implant processors while swimming.

An auditory brainstem implant (ABI) is a surgically implanted electronic device that provides a sense of sound to a person who is profoundly deaf due to sensorineural hearing impairment (due to illness or injury damaging the cochlea or auditory nerve, and so precluding the use of a CI). The ABI uses similar technology as the CI, but instead of electrical stimulation being used to stimulate the cochlea, it is used to stimulate the brainstem of the recipient.

Active middle ear implants (Esteem Implantable Hearing System, Vibrant Soundbridge Middle Ear Implant System, Carina Implantable Hearing System) are surgically implanted hearing aids, which are placed within the middle ear, and are suggested as a therapy for certain patients with conductive, sensorineural, or mixed hearing loss for whom alternative treatments (e.g., conventional hearing aids, bone anchored hearing aids) are unsuitable. Active middle ear implants can be fully implantable or semi-implantable and work via electromagnetic or piezoelectric transducers.

A bone-anchored hearing implant (BAHI) is a type of hearing aid based on bone conduction. It is primarily suited to people who have conductive hearing losses, unilateral hearing loss, and mixed hearing losses who cannot otherwise wear "in the ear" or "behind the ear" hearing aids. A patient without external/middle ear function is one example where a BAHI could be useful where a conventional hearing aid with a mold in the ear canal opening is not possible to use. As the inner ear is normal, sound conducted via the skull bone could give normal/near-normal hearing.

Examples of hearing implantology have been shown in ► Fig. 14.164, ► Fig. 14.165, ► Fig. 14.166, ► Fig. 14.167.

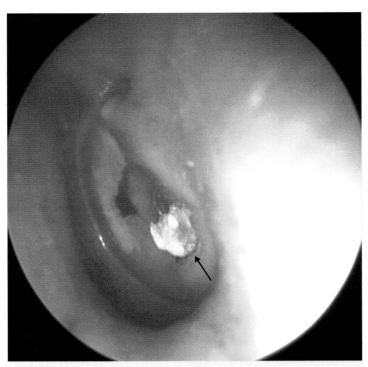

Fig. 14.164 Left ear. Extrusion of a Vibrant Soundbridge. Part of the Floating Mass Transducer (FMT) is outside the tympanic membrane (*arrow*).

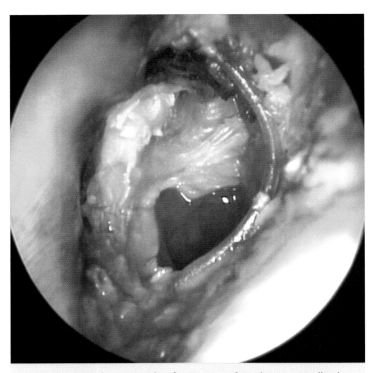

Fig. 14.165 Another example of extrusion of a Vibrant Soundbridge, placed at the same stage of a radical mastoidectomy for a recurrent cholesteatoma. The cavity is discharging and the conductor link with the FMT is extruded. Hearing rehabilitation with implantable devices has been introduced since more than 50 years with cochlear implants. In case of discharging cavities or cholesteatoma, we prefer to stage the procedures and perform a subtotal petrosectomy, to be radical in disease clearance and avoid extrusion of the implant.

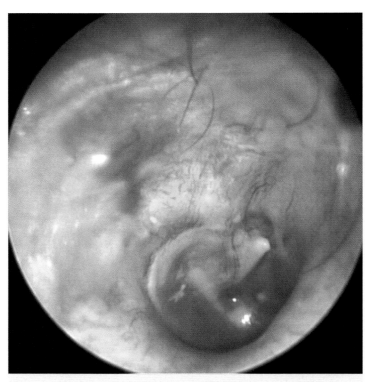

Fig. 14.166 Right ear. Otoscopy after cochlear implantation. The electrode of the implant is inserted in the round window through a posterior tympanotomy, after having performed a closed mastoidectomy.

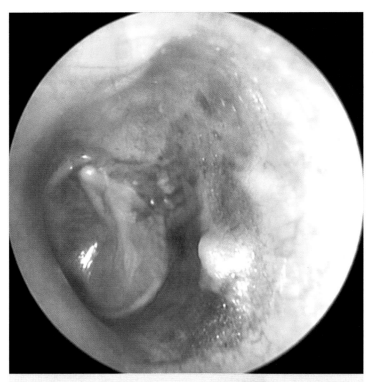

Fig. 14.167 Left ear. Extrusion of a cochlear implant. The receiver-stimulator is in contact with the skin of the posterior canal wall.

References

References

Amendola S, Falcioni M, Caylan R, Sanna M. Recurrent cholesteatoma in open vs closed technique tympanoplasties and its surgical management. Proceedings of the Fifth International Conference on Cholesteatoma and Mastoid Surgery; Alghero-Sardinia, Italy; September 1–6, 1996. Rome: CIC Edizioni Internazionali

Arìstegui M, Cokkeser Y, Saleh E, et al. Surgical anatomy of the extended middle cranial fossa approach. Skull Base Surg. 1994; 4(4):181–188

Arìstegui M, Falcioni M, Saleh E, et al. Meningoencephalic herniation into the middle ear: a report of 27 cases. Laryngoscope. 1995; 105(5, Pt 1):512–518

Austin DF. The significance of the retraction pockets in the treatment of cholesteatoma. In: McCabe BF, Sadè J, Abramson M, eds. Cholesteatoma: First International Conference. Birmingham, AL: Aesculapius; 1977:379–383

Bacciu A, Clemente IA, Piccirillo E, Ferrari S, Sanna M. Guidelines for treating temporal bone carcinoma based on long-term outcomes. Otol Neurotol. 2013; 34 (5):898–907

Bacciu A, Nusier A, Lauda L, Falcioni M, Russo A, Sanna M. Are the current treatment strategies for facial nerve schwannoma appropriate also for complex cases? Audiol Neurootol. 2013; 18(3):184–191

Bacciu A, Ait Mimoune H, D'Orazio F, Vitullo F, Russo A, Sanna M. Management of facial nerve in surgical treatment of previously untreated fisch class C tympanojugular paragangliomas: long-term results. J Neurol Surg B Skull Base. 2014; 75 (1):1–7

Bacciu A, Medina M, Ait Mimoune H, et al. Lower cranial nerves function after surgical treatment of Fisch Class C and D tympanojugular paragangliomas. Eur Arch Otorhinolaryngol. 2015; 272(2):311–319

Balyan FR, Celikkanat S, Aslan A, Taibah A, Russo A, Sanna M. Mastoidectomy in noncholesteatomatous chronic suppurative otitis media: is it necessary? Otolaryngol Head Neck Surg. 1997; 117(6):592–595

Bhatia S, Karmarkar S, DeDonato G, et al. Canal wall down mastoidectomy: causes of failure, pitfalls and their management. J Laryngol Otol. 1995; 109(7):583–589

Brackmann DE, Shelton C, Arriaga MA. 1994

Cama A, Verginelli F, Lotti LV, et al. Integrative genetic, epigenetic and pathological analysis of paraganglioma reveals complex dysregulation of NOTCH signaling. Acta Neuropathol. 2013; 126(4):575–594

Caparosa R. An Atlas of Surgical Anatomy and Techniques of the Temporal Bone. Springfield, IL: Thomas; 1972

Caylan R, Titiz A, De Donato G, et al. Meatoplasty technique in canal wall down procedures. Proceedings of the Fifth International Conference on Cholesteatoma and Mastoid Surgery; Alghero-Sardinia, Italy; September 1–6, 1996. Rome: CIC Edizioni Internazionali

Celikkanat SM, Saleh E, Khashaba A, et al. Cerebrospinal fluid leak after translabyrinthine acoustic neuroma surgery. Otolaryngol Head Neck Surg. 1995; 112 (6):654–658

Charachon R. La tympanoplastie. Grenoble: Presses Universitaires; 1990

Charachon R, Roulleau P, Bremond G, et al. 1987

Chole RA. Petrous apicitis: surgical anatomy. Ann Otol Rhinol Laryngol. 1985; 94 (3):251–257

Cody DTR, Taylor W. Mastoidectomy for acquired cholesteatoma: long-term results. In: McCabe BF, Sadè J, Abramson M, eds. Cholesteatoma: First International Conference. Birmingham, AL: Aesculapius; 1977:337–351

Cohen D. Locations of primary cholesteatoma. Am J Otol. 1987; 8(1):61–65

Coker NJ, Jenkins HA, Fisch U. Obliteration of the middle ear and mastoid cleft in subtotal petrosectomy: indications, technique, and results. Ann Otol Rhinol Laryngol. 1986; 95(1, Pt 1):5–11

Cokkeser Y, Naguib M, Aristegui M, et al. Revision stapes surgery: a critical evaluation. Otolaryngol Head Neck Surg. 1994; 111(4):473–477

Cokkeser Y, Aristegui M, Naguib M, Saleh E, Sanna M. Surgical anatomy of the vertebral artery at the craniovertebral junction. In: Mazzoni A, Sanna M, eds. Skull Base Surgery Update. Vol. 1. Amsterdam: Kugler; 1995;43–48

De Donato G, Caylan R, Falcioni M, et al. Facial nerve management and results in petrous bone cholesteatoma surgery. Proceedings of the Fifth International Conference on Cholesteatoma and Mastoid Surgery; Alghero-Sardinia, Italy; September 1–6, 1996. Rome: CIC Edizioni Internazionali

Deguine C. Longterm results in cholesteatoma surgery. Clin Otolaryngol Allied Sci. 1978; 3(3):301–310

De la Cruz A. The transcochlear approach to meningiomas and cholesteatoma of the cerebellopontine angle. In: Brackmann DE, ed. Neurological Surgery of the Ear and Skull Base. New York, NY: Raven Press; 1982:353–360

Derlacki EL, Clemis JD. Congenital cholesteatoma of the middle ear and mastoid. Ann Otol Rhinol Laryngol. 1965; 74(3):706–727

Dichiro G, Fisher RL, Nelson KB. The jugular foramen. J Neurosurg. 1964; 21:447–460

Donaldson A, Duckert LG, Lambert PM, Rubel EW. Anson and Donaldson Surgical Anatomy of the Temporal Bone. New York, NY: Raven Press; 1992

Dort JC, Fisch U. Facial nerve schwannomas. Skull Base Surg. 1991; 1(1):51–56

Falcioni M, De Donato G, Landolfi M, et al. The modified Bondy technique in the treatment of epitympanic cholesteatoma. Proceedings of the Fifth International Conference on Cholesteatoma and Mastoid Surgery; Alghero-Sardinia, Italy; September 1–6, 1996. Rome: CIC Edizioni Internazionali

Falcioni M, Sanna M. Usefulness of preoperative imaging in chronic ear surgery. Proceedings of the Sixth International Conference on Cholesteatoma and Ear Surgery; Cannes, France, June 29–July 2, 2000. Label Production

Falcioni M, Frisina A, Taibah A, Piccirillo E, De Donato G, Mancini F. Surgical treatment of labyrinthine fistula in chronic ear surgery. Proceedings of the Sixth International Conference on Cholesteatoma and Ear Surgery; Cannes, France, June 29–July 2, 2000. Label Production

Falcioni M, Caruso A, Avanzini P, Piccioni L, Russo A. Facial nerve iatrogenic palsy in chronic ear surgery. Proceedings of the Sixth International Conference on Cholesteatoma and Ear Surgery; Cannes, France, June 29–July 2, 2000. Label Production

Falcioni M, Russo A, Taibah A, Sanna M. Facial nerve tumors. Otol Neurotol. 2003; 24 (6):942–947

Farrior JB. Anterior facial nerve decompression. Otolaryngol Head Neck Surg. 1985; 93(6):765–768

Farrior JB. The canal wall in tympanoplasty and mastoidectomy. Arch Otolaryngol. 1969; 90(6):706–714

Farrior JB. Systematized approach to surgery for cholesteatoma. Arch Otolaryngol. 1973; 97(2):188–190

Fisch U. Infratemporal fossa approach to tumours of the temporal bone and base of the skull. J Laryngol Otol. 1978; 92(11):949–967

Fisch U. Infratemporal fossa approach for glomus tumors of the temporal bone. Ann Otol Rhinol Laryngol. 1982; 91(5, Pt 1):474–479

Fisch U. The infratemporal fossa approach for nasopharyngeal tumors. Laryngoscope. 1983; 93(1):36–44

Fisch U. Tympanoplasty, Mastoidectomy, and Stapes Surgery. Stuttgart: Thieme; 1994

Fisch U, Esslen E. Total intratemporal exposure of the facial nerve. Pathologic findings in Bell's palsy. Arch Otolaryngol. 1972; 95(4):335–341

Fisch U, Mattox D. Microsurgery of the Skull Base. New York, NY: Thieme; 1988

Fisch U, Fagan P, Valavanis A. The infratemporal fossa approach for the lateral skull base. Otolaryngol Clin North Am. 1984; 17(3):513–552

Flood LM, Kemink JL. Surgery in lesions of the petrous apex. Otolaryngol Clin North Am. 1984; 17(3):565–575

Friedberg J. Congenital cholesteatoma. Laryngoscope. 1994; 104(3, Pt 2) Suppl:1–24

Gamoletti R, Bellomi A, Sanna M, Zini C, Scandellari R. Histology of extruded Plasti-Pore ossicular prostheses. Otolaryngol Head Neck Surg. 1984; 92(3):342–345

Gacek RR. Surgical landmark for the facial nerve in the epitympanum. Ann Otol Rhinol Laryngol. 1980; 89(3, Pt 1):249–250

Gantz BJ, Fisch U. Modified transotic approach to the cerebellopontile angle. Arch Otolaryngol. 1983; 109(4):252–256

Glasscock ME, III. Surgical technique for open mastoid procedures. Laryngoscope. 1982; 92(12):1440–1442

Glasscock ME, III, Harris PF, Newsome G. Glomus tumors: diagnosis and treatment. Laryngoscope. 1974; 84(11):2006–2032

Glasscock ME, Miller GW. Intact canal wall tympanoplasty in the management of cholesteatoma. Laryngoscope. 1976; 86(11):1639–1657

Glasscock ME, Shambaugh GE. Surgery of the Ear. 4th ed. Philadelphia, PA: Saunders; 1990

Goodhill V. Tragal perichondrium and cartilage in tympanoplasty. Arch Otolaryngol. 1967; 85(5):480–491

Guild SR. A hitherto unrecognized structure, the glomus jugularis in man. Anat Rec. 1941; 79((Suppl 2)):28

Guild SR. The glomus jugulare, a nonchromaffin paraganglion, in man. Ann Otol Rhinol Laryngol. 1953; 62(4):1045–1071

Hakuba A, Nishimura S, Jang BJ. A combined retroauricular and preauricular trans-petrosal-transtentorial approach to clivus meningiomas. Surg Neurol. 1988; 30 (2):108–116

Hoffman RA. Cerebrospinal fluid leak following acoustic neuroma removal. Laryngoscope. 1994; 104(1, Pt 1):40–58

House WF. Surgical exposure of the internal auditory canal and its contents through the middle, cranial fossa. Laryngoscope. 1961; 71:1363–1385

House WF. Middle cranial fossa approach to the petrous pyramid: report of 50 cases. Arch Otolaryngol. 1963; 78:460–469

House WF, Hitselberger WE. Transtemporal bone microsurgical removal of acoustic neuromas: total versus subtotal removal of acoustic tumors. Arch Otolaryngol. 1964;80:751–752

House WF, Sheehy JL. Functional restoration in tympanoplasty. Arch Otolaryngol. 1963; 78:304–309

House WF, Glasscock ME, III. Glomus tympanicum tumors. Arch Otolaryngol. 1968; 87(5):550–554

House WF, Hitselberger WE. The transcochlear approach to the skull base. Arch Otolaryngol. 1976; 102(6):334–342

House JL, Hitselberger WE, House WF. Wound closure and cerebrospinal fluid leak after translabyrinthine surgery. Am J Otol. 1982; 4(2):126–128

House JW, Brackmann DE. Facial nerve grading system. Otolaryngol Head Neck Surg. 1985; 93(2):146–147

Jackler RK. Overview of surgical neuro-otology. In: Jackler RK, Brackmann DE, eds. Neuro-otology. Baltimore, MD: Mosby; 1993;651–684

Jackson CG. Surgery of Skull Base Tumors. New York, NY: Churchill Livingstone; 1991

Jackson CG, Glasscock ME, III, McKennan KX, et al. The surgical treatment of skull-base tumors with intracranial extension. Otolaryngol Head Neck Surg. 1987; 96 (2):175–185

Jackson CG, Cueva RA, Thedinger BA, Glasscock ME, III. Conservation surgery for glomus jugulare tumors: the value of early diagnosis. Laryngoscope. 1990; 100(10, Pt 1):1031–1036

Jansen C. The combined approach for tympanoplasty (report on 10 years' experience). J Laryngol Otol. 1968; 82(9):779–793

Jansen C. Posterior tympanotomy: experiences and surgical details. Otolaryngol Clin North Am. 1972; 5(1):79–96

Jansen C. Intact canal wall tympanoplasty. In: Shambaugh G, Shea J, eds. Fifth International Workshop on Middle Ear Microsurgery. Huntsville, AL: Strode; 1977:370–375

Jenkins HA, Fisch U. Glomus tumors of the temporal region. Technique of surgical resection. Arch Otolaryngol. 1981; 107(4):209–214

Karmarkar S, Bhatia S, Saleh E, et al. Cholesteatoma surgery: the individualized technique. Ann Otol Rhinol Laryngol. 1995; 104(8):591–595

Karmarkar S, Bhatia S, Khashaba A, Saleh E, Russo A, Sanna M. Congenital cholesteatomas of the middle ear: a different experience. Am J Otol. 1996; 17(2):288–292

Krmpotic-Nemanic J, Draf W, Helms J. Surgical Anatomy of the Head and Neck. Berlin: Springer; 1985

Kveton JF, Cooper MH. Microsurgical anatomy of the jugular foramen region. Am J Otol. 1988; 9(2):109–112

Landolfi M, Taibah A, Russo A, Szymanski M, Shaan M, Sanna M. Revalidation of the Bondy technique. In: Nakano Y, ed. Cholesteatoma and Mastoid Surgery. Amsterdam: Kugler; 1993:719–721

Lang J. Topographical anatomy of the skull base and adjacent tissues. In: Scheunemann H, Schurmann K, Helms J, eds. Tumors of the Skull Base. Berlin: de Gruyter; 1986:3–28

Lau T, Tos M. Treatment of sinus cholesteatoma. Long-term results and recurrence rate. Arch Otolaryngol Head Neck Surg. 1988a; 114(12):1428–1434

Lau T, Tos M. Sinus cholesteatomas: Recurrencies and observation time. Acta Otolaryngol. 1988b; 105 suppl 449:191–193

Lau T, Tos M. Tensa retraction cholesteatoma: treatment and long-term results. J Laryngol Otol. 1989; 103(2):149–157

Levenson MJ, Michaels L, Parisier SC. Congenital cholesteatomas of the middle ear in children: origin and management. Otolaryngol Clin North Am. 1989; 22(5):941–954

Liden-Jerger. Tympanoplasty-procedures, interpretation and variables. In: Feldman AS, Wilber LA, eds. Acoustic Impedance and Admittance—The Measurement of Middle Ear Function. Baltimore, MD: Williams and Wilkins; 1976:103–155

Lope Ahmad RA, Sivalingam S, Konishi M, De Donato G, Sanna M. Oncologic outcome in surgical management of jugular paraganglioma and factors influencing outcomes. Head Neck. 2013; 35(4):527–534

Magnan J, Brémond G. Les conditions de guérison de l'otite chronique cholestéatomateuse. Ann Otolaryngol Chir Cervicofac. 1985; 102(8):565–573

Magnan J, Chays A, Gignac D, Bremond G. Reconstruction of posterior canal wall: long-term results. In: Charachon R, Garcia- Ibanez E, eds. Long-Term Results and Indications in Otology and Otoneurosurgery. Amsterdam: Kugler; 1991:57–61

Magnan J, Sanna M. Endoscopy in Neuro-otology. Stuttgart: Thieme; 1999

Mancini F, Taibah AK, Falcioni M. Complications and their management in tympanomastoid surgery. Otolaryngol Clin North Am. 1999; 32(3):567–583

Marquet J. Eradication of cholesteatoma. In: Tos M, Thomsen J, Peitersen E, eds. Cholesteatoma and Mastoid Surgery. Amsterdam: Kugler; 1989: 811–816

Martin C, Prades JM. Removal of selected infralabyrinthine lesions without facial nerve mobilization. Skull Base Surg. 1992; 2(4):220–226

May M. Total facial nerve exploration: transmastoid, extralabyrinthine, and subtemporal indications and results. Laryngoscope. 1979; 89(6, Pt 1):906–917

Mazzoni A. Internal auditory canal arterial relations at the porus acusticus. Ann Otol Rhinol Laryngol. 1969; 78(4):797–814

Mazzoni A. Internal auditory artery supply to the petrous bone. Ann Otol Rhinol Laryngol. 1972; 81(1):13–21

Mazzoni A. Jugulo-petrosectomy. Arch Ital Otyol Rhinol Laring. 1974; 2:20–35

Mazzoni A, Sanna M. The petro-occipital trans-sigmoid approach to the posterolateral skull base: results and indications. Paper presented at the Third Annual Meeting of the North American Skull Base Society; Acapulco, Mexico; February 15–20, 1992

Medina M, Prasad SC, Patnaik U, et al. The effects of tympanomastoid paragangliomas on hearing and the audiological outcomes after surgery over a long-term follow-up. Audiol Neurootol. 2014; 19(5):342–350

Michaels L. An epidermoid formation in the developing middle ear: possible source of cholesteatoma. J Otolaryngol. 1986; 15(3):169–174

Morimitsu T, Nagai T, Nagai M, et al. Pathogenesis of cholesteatoma based on clinical results of anterior tympanotomy. Auris Nasus Larynx. 1989; 16 Suppl 1:S9–S14

Nadol JB, Jr. Causes of failure of mastoidectomy for chronic otitis media. Laryngoscope. 1985; 95(4):410–413

Nager GT. Pathology of the Ear and Temporal Bone. Baltimore, MD: Williams and Wilkins; 1993

Naguib MB, Aristegui M, Saleh E, et al. Surgical anatomy of the petrous apex as it relates to the enlarged middle cranial fossa approaches. Otolaryngol Head Neck Surg. 1994; 111(4):488–493

Naguib MB, Aristegui M, Saleh E, Cokkeser Y, Russo A, Sanna M. Surgical management of epitympanic cholesteatoma with intact ossicular chain: the modified Bondy technique. Otolaryngol Head Neck Surg. 1994; 111(5):545–549

Nakano Y. Cholesteatoma surgery and mastoid obliteration. In: Nakano Y, ed. Cholesteatoma and Mastoid Surgery. Amsterdam: Kugler; 1993:769–773

Neely JG, Alford BR. Facial nerve neuromas. Arch Otolaryngol. 1974; 100(4):298–301

Omran A, De Denato G, Piccirillo E, Leone O, Sanna M. Petrous bone cholesteatoma: management and outcomes. Laryngoscope. 2006; 116(4):619–626

Palva T. Reconstruction of ear canal and middle ear in chronic otitis. Acta Otolaryngol Suppl. 1964; 188 suppl:188–, 228

Palva T, Mäkinen J. The meatally based musculoperiosteal flap in cavity obliteration. Arch Otolaryngol. 1979; 105(7):377–380

Palva T, Palva A, Kärjä J. Cavity obliteration and ear canal size. Arch Otolaryngol. 1970; 92(4):366–371

Pandya Y, Piccirillo E, Mancini F, Sanna M. Management of complex cases of petrous bone cholesteatoma. Ann Otol Rhinol Laryngol. 2010; 119(8):514–525

Paparella MM, Jung TTK. Intact bridge tympanomastoidectomy (I.B.M.)-combining essential features of open vs. closed procedures. J Laryngol Otol. 1983; 97 (7):579–585

Paparella MM, Jung TTK. Intact-bridge tympanomastoidectomy. Otolaryngol Head Neck Surg. 1984; 92(3):334–338

Paparella MM, Shumrick DA. Otolaryngology. 3 Vols. Philadelphia, PA: Saunders; 1988

Pellet W, Cannoni M, Pech A. The widened transcochlear approach to jugular foramen tumors. J Neurosurg. 1988; 69(6):887–894

Piazza P, Di Lella F, Bacciu A, Di Trapani G, Ait Mimoune H, Sanna M. Preoperative protective stenting of the internal carotid artery in the management of complex head and neck paragangliomas: long-term results. Audiol Neurootol. 2013; 18 (6):345–352

Piccioni L, Piccirillo E, Falcioni M, De Donato G, Russo A, Taibah AK. Middle ear cholesteatoma in children. Proceedings of the Sixth International Conference on

Cholesteatoma and Ear Surgery; Cannes, France; June 29–July 2, 2000. Label Production

Plester D. Tympanic membrane homografts in ear surgery. Acta Otorhinolaryngol Belg. 1970; 24(1):34–37

Portmann M. The Ear and Temporal Bone. New York, NY: Masson; 1979

Prasad SC, Shin SH, Russo A, Di Trapani G, Sanna M. Current trends in the management of the complications of chronic otitis media with cholesteatoma. Curr Opin Otolaryngol Head Neck Surg. 2013; 21(5):446–454

Prasad SC, D'Orazio F, Medina M, Bacciu A, Sanna M. State of the art in temporal bone malignancies. Curr Opin Otolaryngol Head Neck Surg. 2014; 22(2):154–165

Prasad SC, Mimoune HA, D'Orazio F, et al. The role of wait-and-scan and the efficacy of radiotherapy in the treatment of temporal bone paragangliomas. Otol Neurotol. 2014; 35(5):922–931

Prasad SC, Mimoune HA, Khardaly M, Piazza P, Russo A, Sanna M. Strategies and long-term outcomes in the surgical management of tympanojugular paragangliomas. Head Neck. 2016; 38(6):871–885

Prasad SC, Giannuzzi A, Nahleh EA, Donato G, Russo A, Sanna M. Is endoscopic ear surgery an alternative to the modified Bondy technique for limited epitympanic cholesteatoma? Eur Arch Otorhinolaryngol. 2016; 273(9):2533–2540

Proctor B. Surgical anatomy of the posterior tympanum. Ann Otol Rhinol Laryngol. 1969; 78(5):1026–1040

Proctor B. Surgical Anatomy of the Ear and Temporal Bone. Stuttgart: Thieme; 1989

Rambo JHT. A new operation to restore hearing in conductive deafness of chronic suppurative origin. AMA Arch Otolaryngol. 1957; 66(5):525–532

Rambo JHT. Musculoplasty for restoration of hearing in chronic suppurative ears. Arch Otolaryngol. 1969; 89(1):184–190

Rhoton AL, Jr, Buza R. Microsurgical anatomy of the jugular foramen. J Neurosurg. 1975; 42(5):541–550

Rhoton AL, Jr, Pulec JL, Hall GM, Boyd AS, Jr. Absence of bone over the geniculate ganglion. J Neurosurg. 1968; 28(1):48–53

Russo A, Taibah A, Landolfi M, et al. Congenital cholesteatoma. Proceedings of the Fourth International Conference on Cholesteatoma and Mastoid Surgery; Niigata, Japan; September 8–12, 1992. Amsterdam: Kugler Publications

Russo A, Taibah AK, De Donato G, Falcioni M, Sanna M. Congenital cholesteatomas: A different experience. Proceedings of the Fifth International Conference on Cholesteatoma and Mastoid Surgery; Alghero-Sardinia, Italy; September 1–6, 1996. Rome: CIC Edizioni Internazionali

Sadè J. Postoperative cholesteatoma recurrence. In: McCabe BF, Sadè J, Abramson M, eds. Cholesteatoma: First International Conference. Birmingham, AL: Aesculapius; 1977:284–289

Sadè J. Secretory Otitis Media and Its Sequelae. New York, NY: Churchill Livingstone; 1979

Saleh EA, Aristegui M, Taibah AK, Mazzoni A, Sanna M. Management of the high jugular bulb in the translabyrinthine approach. Otolaryngol Head Neck Surg. 1994a; 110(4):397–399

Saleh EA, Taibah AK, Achilli V, Aristegui M, Mazzoni A, Sanna M. Posterior fossa meningioma: surgical strategy. Skull Base Surg. 1994b; 4(4):202–212

Saleh E, Achilli V, Naguib M, et al. Facial nerve neuromas: diagnosis and management. Am J Otol. 1995a; 16(4):521–526

Saleh E, Naguib M, Aristegui M, Cokkeser Y, Sanna M. Lower skull base: anatomic study with surgical implications. Ann Otol Rhinol Laryngol. 1995b; 104(1):57–61

Saleh E, Naguib M, Aristegui M, Cokkeser Y, Russo A, Sanna M. Surgical anatomy of the jugular foramen area. In: Mazzoni A, Sanna M, eds. Skull Base Surgery Update. Vol. 1. Amsterdam: Kugler; 1995c:3–8

Samii M, Draf W. Surgery of the Skull Base. Berlin: Springer; 1989

Sanna M. Anatomy of the posterior mesotympanum. In: Zini C, Sheehy JL, Sanna M, eds. Microsurgery of Cholesteatoma of the Middle Ear. Milan: Ghedini; 1980:69–73

Sanna M. Ossicular chain reconstruction in closed tympanoplasties. In: Zini C, Sheehy JL, Sanna M, eds. Microsurgery of Cholesteatoma of the Middle Ear. Milan: Ghedini; 1980:91–96

Sanna M. Congenital cholesteatoma of the middle ear. In: Zini C, Sheehy JL, Sanna M, eds. Microsurgery of Cholesteatoma of the Middle Ear. Milan: Ghedini; 1980:149–156

Sanna M. Cholesteatoma in children (Experience of 2nd ENT clinic of Parma). In: Zini C, Sheehy JL, Sanna M, eds. Microsurgery of Cholesteatoma of the Middle Ear. Milan: Ghedini; 1980:157–160

Sanna M. Proceedings of the Fifth International Conference on Cholesteatoma and Mastoid Surgery; Alghero-Sardinia, Italy; September 1–6, 1996. Rome: CIC Edizioni Internazionali

Sanna M, Magnani M, Gamoletti R. Ossicular chain reconstruction with plastipore prostheses. Am J Otol. 1981; 2(3):225–229

Sanna M, Mazzoni A. The modified transcochlear approach to the tumors of the petroclival area and prepontine cistern. Paper presented at the Third Annual Meeting of the North American Skull Base Society; Acapulco, Mexico; February 15–20, 1992

Sanna M, Zini C, Scandellari R, Jemmi G. Residual and recurrent cholesteatoma in closed tympanoplasty. Am J Otol. 1984; 5(4):277–282

Sanna M, Zini C. "Congenital cholesteatoma" of the middle ear. A report of 11 cases. Am J Otol. 1984; 5(5):368–373

Sanna M, Gamoletti R, Magnani M, Bacciu S, Zini C. Failures with Plasti-Pore ossicular replacement prostheses. Otolaryngol Head Neck Surg. 1984; 92(3):339–341

Sanna M. Management of labyrinthine fistulae. In: Marquet J, ed. Surgery and Pathology of the Middle Ear. Boston, MA: Martinus Niihoff; 1985

Sanna M, Gamoletti R, Scandellari R, Delogu P, Magnani M, Zini C. Autologous fitted incus versus Plastipore PORP in ossicular chain reconstruction. J Laryngol Otol. 1985; 99(2):137–141

Sanna M, Gamoletti R, Bortesi G, Jemmi G, Zini C. Posterior canal wall atrophy after intact canal wall tympanoplasty. Am J Otol. 1986; 7(1):74–75

Sanna M, Zini C, Gamoletti R, et al. Prevention of recurrent cholesteatoma in closed tympanoplasty. Ann Otol Rhinol Laryngol. 1987a; 96(3, Pt 1):273–275

Sanna M, Zini C, Gamoletti R, et al. The surgical management of childhood cholesteatoma. J Laryngol Otol. 1987b; 101(12):1221–1226

Sanna M, Zini C, Gamoletti R, et al. Surgical treatment of cholesteatoma in children. Adv Otorhinolaryngol. 1987c; 37:110–116

Sanna M, Zini C, Bacciu S, et al. Surgery for cholesteatoma in children. Proceedings of the Third International Conference on Cholesteatoma and Mastoid Surgery; Copenhagen, Denmark; June 5–9, 1988. Amsterdam: Kugler & Ghedini Publications

Sanna M, Zini C, Gamoletti R, Taibah AK, Russo A, Scandellari R. Closed versus open technique in the management of labyrinthine fistulae. Am J Otol. 1988; 9(6):470–475

Sanna M, Zini C, Gamoletti R, Pasanisi E. Primary intratemporal tumours of the facial nerve: diagnosis and treatment. J Laryngol Otol. 1990; 104(10):765–771

Sanna M, Shea CM, Gamoletti R, Russo A. Surgery of the 'only hearing ear' with chronic ear disease. J Laryngol Otol. 1992; 106(9):793–798

Sanna M, Zini C, Bacciu S, et al. Management of labyrinthine fistula. Proceedings of the Fourth International Conference on Cholesteatoma and Mastoid Surgery; Niigata, Japan; September 8–12, 1993. Amsterdam: Kugler Publications

Sanna M, Zini C, Gamoletti R, et al. Petrous bone cholesteatoma. Skull Base Surg. 1993; 3(4):201–213

Sanna M, Mazzoni A, Saleh EA, Taibah AK, Russo A. Lateral approaches to the median skull base through the petrous bone: the system of the modified transcochlear approach. J Laryngol Otol. 1994; 108(12):1036–1044

Sanna M, Mazzoni A, Taibah A, Saleh E, Russo A, Khashaba A. The modified transcochlear approaches to the skull base: results and indications. In: Mazzoni A, Sanna M, eds. Skull Base Surgery Update. Vol. 1. Amsterdam: Kugler; 1995a:315–323

Sanna M, Saleh E, Russo A, et al. Atlas of Temporal Bone and Lateral Skull Base Surgery. Stuttgart: Thieme; 1995b

Sanna M Atlas of Acoustic Neurinoma Microsurgery. Stuttgart: Thieme; 1998

Sanna M, Russo A, De Donato G, et al. Color Atlas of Otoscopy. Stuttgart: Thieme; 1999

Sanna M, Agarwal M, Khrais T, Di Trapani G. Modified Bondy's technique for epitympanic cholesteatoma. Laryngoscope. 2003; 113(12):2218–2221

Sanna M, Piazza P, Ditrapani G, Agarwal M. Management of the internal carotid artery in tumors of the lateral skull base: preoperative permanent balloon occlusion without reconstruction. Otol Neurotol. 2004; 25(6):998–1005

Sanna M, Russo A, Khrais T, Jain Y, Augurio AM. Canalplasty for severe external auditory meatus exostoses. J Laryngol Otol. 2004; 118(8):607–611

Sanna M, De Donato G, Piazza P, Falcioni M. Revision glomus tumor surgery. Otolaryngol Clin North Am. 2006; 39(4):763–782, vii

Sanna M, Khrais T, Mancini F, Russo A, Taibah A. The Facial Nerve in Temporal Bone and Lateral Skull Base Surgery. Stuttgart: Thieme; 2006

Sanna M, Bacciu A, Falcioni M, Taibah AK. Surgical management of jugular foramen schwannomas with hearing and facial nerve function preservation: a series of 23 cases and review of the literature. Laryngoscope. 2006; 116(12):2191–2204

Sanna M, Saleh E, Khrais T et al. Atlas of Microsurgery of the Lateral Skull Base. 2nd ed. Stuttgart: Thieme; 2007

Sanna M, Bacciu A, Falcioni M, Taibah A, Piazza P. Surgical management of jugular foramen meningiomas: a series of 13 cases and review of the literature. Laryngoscope. 2007; 117(10):1710–1719

Sanna M, Bacciu A, Pasanisi E, Taibah A, Piazza P. Posterior petrous face meningiomas: an algorithm for surgical management. Otol Neurotol. 2007; 28(7):942–950

Sanna M, Bacciu A, Pasanisi E, Piazza P, Fois P, Falcioni M. Chondrosarcomas of the jugular foramen. Laryngoscope. 2008; 118(10):1719–1728

Sanna M, Dispenza F, Flanagan S, De Stefano A, Falcioni M. Management of chronic otitis by middle ear obliteration with blind sac closure of the external auditory canal. Otol Neurotol. 2008; 29(1):19–22

Sanna M, Fois P, Russo A, Falcioni M. Management of meningoencephalic herniation of the temporal bone: Personal experience and literature review. Laryngoscope. 2009; 119(8):1579–1585

Sanna M, Dispenza F, Mathur N, De Stefano A, De Donato G. Otoneurological management of petrous apex cholesterol granuloma. Am J Otolaryngol. 2009; 30 (6):407–414

Sanna M, Facharzt AA, Russo A, Lauda L, Pasanisi E, Bacciu A. Modified Bondy's technique: refinements of the surgical technique and long-term results. Otol Neurotol. 2009; 30(1):64–69

Sanna M, Piazza P, De Donato G, Menozzi R, Falcioni M. Combined endovascular-surgical management of the internal carotid artery in complex tympanojugular paragangliomas. Skull Base. 2009; 19(1):26–42

Sanna M, De Donato G, Di Lella F, Falcioni M, Aggrawal N, Romano G. Nonvascular lesions of the jugular foramen: the gruppo otologico experience. Skull Base. 2009; 19(1):57–74

Sanna M, Fois P, Pasanisi E, Russo A, Bacciu A. Middle ear and mastoid glomus tumors (glomus tympanicum): an algorithm for the surgical management. Auris Nasus Larynx. 2010; 37(6):661–668

Sanna M, Pandya Y, Mancini F, Sequino G, Piccirillo E. Petrous bone cholesteatoma: classification, management and review of the literature. Audiol Neurootol. 2011; 16(2):124–136

Sanna M, Shin SH, De Donato G, et al. Management of complex tympanojugular paragangliomas including endovascular intervention. Laryngoscope. 2011; 121 (7):1372–1382

Sanna M, Sunose H, Mancini F, Russo A, Taibah A. Middle Ear and Mastoid Microsurgery. 2nd ed. Stuttgart: Thieme; 2012

Sanna M, Piazza P, Shin S, Flanagan S, Mancini F. Microsurgery of Skull Base Paragangliomas. Stuttgart: Thieme; 2013

Sanna M, Shin SH, Piazza P, et al. Infratemporal fossa approach type a with transcondylar-transtubercular extension for Fisch type C2 to C4 tympanojugular paragangliomas. Head Neck. 2014; 36(11):1581–1588

Saunders WH, Paparella MM. Atlas of Ear Surgery. St. Louis, MO: Mosby; 1971

Sbaihat A, Bacciu A, Pasanisi E, Sanna M. Skull base chondrosarcomas: surgical treatment and results. Ann Otol Rhinol Laryngol. 2013; 122(12):763–770

Schuknecht HF. Pathology of the Ear. 2nd ed. Malvern: Lea & Febiger; 1993

Schuknecht HF, Gylya JA. Anatomy of the Temporal Bone with Surgical Implications. Philadelphia, PA: Lea and Febiger; 1986

Shambaugh GE, Glasscock ME III. Surgery of the Ear. 3rd ed. Philadelphia, PA: Saunders; 1980

Shaan M, Landolfi M, Taibah A, Russo A, Szymanski M, Sanna M. Modified Bondy technique. Am J Otol. 1995; 16(5):695–697

Shea JJ, Homsy CA. The use of Proplast TM in otologic surgery. Laryngoscope. 1974; 84(10):1835–1845

Shea MC, Jr, Gardner G, Jr. Mastoid obliteration using homograft bone. Preliminary report. Arch Otolaryngol. 1970; 92(4):358–365

Sheehy JL. Surgery of chronic otitis media. In: Coates BM, Schenk HD, Miller MV, eds. Otolaryngology. Hagerstown: Prior; 1965

Sheehy JL. The intact canal wall technique in management of aural cholesteatoma. J Laryngol Otol. 1970a; 84(1):1–31

Sheehy JL. Tympanoplasty with mastoidectomy–a re-evaluation. Laryngoscope. 1970b; 80(8):1212–1230

Sheehy JL. Surgery of chronic otitis media: In: English GM, ed. Otolaryngology. Vol. 2. Hagerstown: Harper and Row; 1972: l–86

Sheehy JL. Cholesteatoma surgery: canal wall down procedures. Ann Otol Rhinol Laryngol. 1988; 97(1):30–35

Sheehy JL. Surgery for chronic otitis media. In: English GM, ed. Otolaryngology. 2nd ed. Vol. I. Philadelphia, PA: Lippincott; 1990: l–86

Sheehy JL, Patterson ME. Intact canal wall tympanoplasty with mastoidectomy. A review of eight years' experience. Laryngoscope. 1967; 77(8):1502–1542

Sheehy JL, Brackmann DE, Graham MD. Cholesteatoma surgery: residual and recurrent disease. A review of 1,024 cases. Ann Otol Rhinol Laryngol. 1977; 86(4, Pt 1):451–462

Shin SH, Sivalingam S, De Donato G, Falcioni M, Piazza P, Sanna M. Vertebral artery involvement by tympanojugular paragangliomas: management and outcomes with a proposed addition to the fisch classification. Audiol Neurootol. 2012; 17 (2):92–104

Shin SH, Piazza P, De Donato G, et al. Management of vagal paragangliomas including application of internal carotid artery stenting. Audiol Neurootol. 2012; 17 (1):39–53

Sivalingam S, Konishi M, Shin SH, Lope Ahmed RA, Piazza P, Sanna M. Surgical management of tympanojugular paragangliomas with intradural extension, with a proposed revision of the Fisch classification. Audiol Neurootol. 2012; 17(4):243–255

Smyth GDL. A preliminary report of a technique in tympanoplasty designed to eliminate the cavity problem. J Laryngol Otol. 1962; 76:460–463

Smyth G. Combined approach tympanoplasty. Arch Otolaryngol. 1969; 89(2):250–251

Smyth GD, Dowe AC. Cartilage canalplasty. Laryngoscope. 1971; 81(5):786–792

Taibah A, Russo A, Landolfi M, Shaan M, Sanna M. Open technique in cholesteatoma. Proceedings of the Fourth International Conference on Cholesteatoma and Mastoid Surgery; Niigata, Japan; September 8–12, 1993. Amsterdam: Kugler Publications

Taibah A, Russo A, Caylan R, Landolfi M, Mancini F, Sanna M. Canal wall down procedures: Causes of failure and pitfalls. Proceedings of the Fifth International Conference on Cholesteatoma and Mastoid Surgery; Alghero-Sardinia, Italy; September 1–6, 1996. Rome: CIC Edizioni Internazionali

Takahashi S, Nakano Y. Tympanoplasty with mastoid obliteration using hydroxyapatite granules. In: Yanagihara N, Suzucki Y, eds. Transplants and Implants in Otology. Amsterdam: Kugler; 1992;159–163

Tos M. Obliteration of the cavity in mastoidectomy. Acta Otolaryngol. 1969; 67 (5):516–520

Tos M. Pathogenesis and pathology of chronic secretory otitis media. Ann Otol Rhinol Laryngol Suppl. 1980; 89(3, Pt 2):91–97

Tos M. Modification of combined-approach tympanoplasty in attic cholesteatoma. Arch Otolaryngol. 1982; 108(12):772–778

Tos M. Manual of Middle Ear Surgery. Vol. 1: Approaches. Myringoplasty. Ossiculoplasty. Tympanoplasty. Stuttgart: Thieme; 1993

Tos M. Manual of Middle Ear Surgery. Vol. 2: Mastoid Surgery and Reconstructive Procedures. Stuttgart: Thieme; 1995

Tos M. Manual of Middle Ear Surgery. Vol. 3: Surgery of the External Auditory Canal. Stuttgart: Thieme; 1997

Tos M, Lau T. Attic cholesteatoma. Recurrence rate related to observation time. Am J Otol. 1988; 9(6):456–464

Tos M, Stangerup SE. The causes of asymmetry of the mastoid air cell system. Acta Otolaryngol. 1985; 99(5–6):564–570

Tos M, Stangerup SE, Andreassen UK. Size of the mastoid air cells and otitis media. Ann Otol Rhinol Laryngol. 1985; 94(4, Pt 1):386–392

Wigand ME, Trillsch K. Surgical anatomy of the sinus epitympani. Ann Otol Rhinol Laryngol. 1973; 82(3):378–383

Wullstein H. The restoration of the function of the middle ear, in chronic otitis media. Ann Otol Rhinol Laryngol. 1956; 65(4):1021–1041

Wullstein HL, Wullstein SR. Tympanoplasty: Osteoplastic Epitympanotomy. Stuttgart: Thieme; 1990

Wullstein SR. Osteoplastic epitympanotomy. Ann Otol Rhinol Laryngol. 1974; 83 (5):663–669

Yanagihara N, Gyo K, Sasaki Y, Hinohira Y. Prevention of recurrence of cholesteatoma in intact canal wall tympanoplasty. Am J Otol. 1993; 14(6):590–594

Zini C. Homotransplantation de dent en tympanoplastie. Rev Laryngol. 1970; 91:258–261

Zini C, Sanna M, Jemmi G, Gandolfi A. Transmastoid extralabyrinthine approach in traumatic facial palsy. Am J Otol. 1985; 6(3):216–221

Zini C, Sanna M, Bacciu S, Delogu P, Gamoletti R, Scandellari R. Molded tympanic heterograft. An eight-year experience. Am J Otol. 1985; 6(3):253–256

Zini C, Sheehy JL, Sanna M. Microsurgery of Cholesteatoma of the Middle Ear. Milan: Ghedini; 1993

Zöllner C, Büsing CM. How useful is tricalcium phosphate ceramic in middle ear surgery? Am J Otol. 1986; 7(4):289–293

Zöllner F. Tympanoplasty. In: Coates G, Schenck HP, Miller MV, eds. Otolaryngology. Vol. 1. Hagerstown: Prior; 1959

Index